Blockchain and IoT Approaches for Secure Electronic Health Records (EHR)

Kavita Saini
Galgotias University, India

J.N. Singh
Galgotias University, India

A volume in the Advances in Healthcare Information Systems and Administration (AHISA) Book Series

IGI Global
PUBLISHER of TIMELY KNOWLEDGE

Published in the United States of America by
IGI Global
Medical Information Science Reference (an imprint of IGI Global)
701 E. Chocolate Avenue
Hershey PA, USA 17033
Tel: 717-533-8845
Fax: 717-533-8661
E-mail: cust@igi-global.com
Web site: http://www.igi-global.com

Library of Congress Cataloging-in-Publication Data

CIP DATA PROCESSING

2024 Medical Information Science Reference
ISBN 9798369316627 | ISBN(sc) 9798369345146 | eISBN 9798369316634

This book is published in the IGI Global book series Advances in Healthcare Information Systems and Administration (AHISA) (ISSN: 2328-1243; eISSN: 2328-126X)

British Cataloguing in Publication Data
A Cataloguing in Publication record for this book is available from the British Library.

Advances in Healthcare Information Systems and Administration (AHISA) Book Series

ISSN:2328-1243
EISSN:2328-126X

Editor-in-Chief: Anastasius Moumtzoglou, Hellenic Society for Quality & Safety in Healthcare and P. & A. Kyriakou Children's Hospital, Greece

MISSION

The **Advances in Healthcare Information Systems and Administration (AHISA) Book Series** aims to provide a channel for international researchers to progress the field of study on technology and its implications on healthcare and health information systems. With the growing focus on healthcare and the importance of enhancing this industry to tend to the expanding population, the book series seeks to accelerate the awareness of technological advancements of health information systems and expand awareness and implementation.

Driven by advancing technologies and their clinical applications, the emerging field of health information systems and informatics is still searching for coherent directing frameworks to advance health care and clinical practices and research. Conducting research in these areas is both promising and challenging due to a host of factors, including rapidly evolving technologies and their application complexity. At the same time, organizational issues, including technology adoption, diffusion and acceptance as well as cost benefits and cost effectiveness of advancing health information systems and informatics applications as innovative forms of investment in healthcare are gaining attention as well. **AHISA** addresses these concepts and critical issues.

COVERAGE

- Management of Emerging Health Care Technologies
- IS in Healthcare
- Medical Informatics
- Measurements and Impact of HISA on Public and Social Policy
- Clinical Decision Support Design, Development and Implementation
- IT security and privacy issues
- E-Health and M-Health
- Virtual health technologies
- Nursing Expert Systems
- Role of informatics specialists

IGI Global is currently accepting manuscripts for publication within this series. To submit a proposal for a volume in this series, please contact our Acquisition Editors at Acquisitions@igi-global.com or visit: http://www.igi-global.com/publish/.

The Advances in Healthcare Information Systems and Administration (AHISA) Book Series (ISSN 2328-1243) is published by IGI Global, 701 E. Chocolate Avenue, Hershey, PA 17033-1240, USA, www.igi-global.com. This series is composed of titles available for purchase individually; each title is edited to be contextually exclusive from any other title within the series. For pricing and ordering information please visit http://www.igi-global.com/book-series/advances-healthcare-information-systems-administration/37156. Postmaster: Send all address changes to above address.

Titles in this Series

For a list of additional titles in this series, please visit:
http://www.igi-global.com/book-series/advances-healthcare-information-systems-administration/37156

Lightweight Digital Trust Architectures in the Internet of Medical Things (IoMT)
Ahdi Hassan (Global Institute for Research Education and Scholarship, The Netherlands) Pronaya Bhattacharya (Amity University, Kolkata, India) Subrata Tikadar (Amity University, Kolkata, India) Pushan Kumar Dutta (Amity University, Kolkata, India) and Martin Sagayam (Karunya Institute of Technology and Sciences, India)
Medical Information Science Reference • copyright 2024 • 448pp • H/C (ISBN: 9798369321096) • US $380.00 (our price)

Federated Learning and Privacy-Preserving in Healthcare AI
Umesh Kumar Lilhore (School of Computing, Galgotias University, Greater Noida, India) Sarita Simaiya (School of Computing, Galgotias University, Greater Noida, India) Manoharan Poongodi (Hamad Bin Khalifa University, Qatar) and Vishal Dutt (Department of Computer Science and Engineering, Chandigarh University, India)
Medical Information Science Reference • copyright 2024 • 351pp • H/C (ISBN: 9798369318744) • US $380.00 (our price)

Converging Pharmacy Science and Engineering in Computational Drug Discovery
Rati Kailash Prasad Tripathi (Assam University, India) and Shrikant Tiwari (Galgotias University, India)
Medical Information Science Reference • copyright 2024 • 322pp • H/C (ISBN: 9798369328972) • US $425.00 (our price)

Inclusivity and Accessibility in Digital Health
Muhammad Anshari (Universiti Brunei Darussalam, Brunei) Mohammad Nabil Almunawar (Universiti Brunei Darussalam, Brunei) and Patricia Ordonez de Pablos (The University of Oviedo, Spain)
Medical Information Science Reference • copyright 2024 • 349pp • H/C (ISBN: 9798369314630) • US $380.00 (our price)

For an entire list of titles in this series, please visit:
http://www.igi-global.com/book-series/advances-healthcare-information-systems-administration/37156

IGI Global
PUBLISHER of TIMELY KNOWLEDGE

701 East Chocolate Avenue, Hershey, PA 17033, USA
Tel: 717-533-8845 x100 • Fax: 717-533-8661
E-Mail: cust@igi-global.com • www.igi-global.com

Table of Contents

Detailed Table of Contents

Preface

Welcome to *Blockchain and IoT Approaches for Secure Electronic Health Records (EHR)*, a comprehensive exploration of the transformative potential of blockchain technology in the healthcare industry. As editors of this volume, we are excited to present a collection of chapters that delve into the intersection of blockchain, Internet of Things (IoT), and healthcare, offering insights into how these technologies can revolutionize the management of electronic health records.

In recent years, blockchain technology has emerged as more than just the foundation for digital currencies. Its inherent characteristics, such as decentralization, transparency, and tamper-proof data storage, make it an ideal solution for securing sensitive information like electronic health records. This book aims to highlight the relevance and applications of blockchain in healthcare, showcasing how it can enhance data security, streamline processes, and improve patient outcomes.

The chapters in this book cover a wide range of topics, from the fundamentals of blockchain technology to its practical applications in securing patient data and facilitating secure payments. We begin by providing an overview of blockchain's role in healthcare, examining its scope, opportunities, and challenges. Subsequent chapters delve into specific applications, including securing electronic health records, combating drug counterfeiting, and enhancing healthcare data security using blockchain.

We also explore the integration of blockchain with other emerging technologies, such as IoT, to create secure healthcare digital systems. By leveraging the combined power of blockchain and IoT, healthcare providers can remotely monitor patients, deliver clinical services, and conduct research, particularly crucial during the COVID-19 pandemic.

This book is intended for a wide audience, including undergraduate and postgraduate students, software engineers, researchers, and industry professionals. It offers a comprehensive overview of blockchain technology in healthcare, providing valuable insights into its potential impact on the industry.

We extend our gratitude to the contributing authors for their expertise and dedication in shaping this volume. Their insights and research have enriched the content of this book, making it a valuable resource for anyone interested in exploring the transformative potential of blockchain in healthcare.

We hope that this book serves as a catalyst for further research and innovation in the field of blockchain and healthcare. As the healthcare industry continues to evolve, we believe that blockchain technology will play an increasingly vital role in ensuring the security, integrity, and accessibility of electronic health records.

Chapter 1: "Guardians of Health Data: Empowering Secure Electronic Health Records With IoMT and Blockchain," by Babu et al. from Hindustan Institute of Technology and Science, India, explores the symbiotic relationship between the Internet of Medical Things (IoMT) and Blockchain technology in securing electronic health records (EHRs). This chapter delves into the significance and applications of IoMT while addressing concerns over data security, with Blockchain emerging as a promising solution. Insights into the potential benefits, emerging trends, and ethical considerations in the IoMT and Blockchain healthcare landscape are provided, offering valuable perspectives for stakeholders in the healthcare industry.

Chapter 2: "Challenges in Designing and Implementing Blockchain-Enabled Frameworks for Healthcare Records," by Bindya C A from REVA, India, navigates the complexities of integrating blockchain technology into healthcare data management systems. The chapter addresses unique challenges such as privacy concerns and regulatory compliance, offering guidance for researchers, practitioners, and policymakers. By shedding light on these challenges, the research aims to inform the development of robust and effective blockchain-enabled frameworks for healthcare records, fostering a more interconnected and secure healthcare ecosystem.

Chapter 3: "Safeguarding the Future: Cutting-Edge Time-Stamping Services and Blockchain Technologies for Maintaining EHR Data Integrity," by Rita Komalasari from Yarsi University, Indonesia, emphasizes the criticality of data integrity in electronic health records (EHRs). The chapter discusses the role of time-stamping services and blockchain technologies in ensuring data security over time. With groundbreaking results and conclusions, this research sets new standards for long-term data security in EHR and related fields.

Chapter 4: "Securing Sensitive Patient Data in Healthcare Settings Using Blockchain Technology," by Thanga Selvi R from Vel Tech Rangarajan DR Sagunthala R&D Institute of Science and Technology, India, presents a blockchain-based solution for enhancing the security and privacy of patient data. By empowering users with control over their confidential information, the proposed system addresses concerns associated with traditional EHR systems, offering improved data security and accessibility.

Chapter 5: "A Systematic Review: Future Prospects and Challenges of IoT-Based EHRs in Healthcare Industry Using Blockchain Technology," by Manikandan N from SRM Institute of Science and Technology, India, conducts a comprehensive review of IoT-based EHRs in healthcare and explores the potential of blockchain technology in addressing security and privacy issues. This chapter provides valuable insights for academics, practitioners, and policymakers seeking to leverage blockchain to enhance healthcare data security.

Chapter 6: "Human-Centric AI Applications for Remote Patient Monitoring," by Sunil Kadyan from Manav Rachna University Faridabad, India, introduces a human-centric IoT gadget for remote patient monitoring, leveraging machine learning models to enhance healthcare operations. With real-time physiological data analysis and predictive modelling, this research offers innovative solutions for personalized patient care.

Chapter 7: "A Deep Learning Approach for Medicine Preparation Machines With SVM and CNN Integration," by Anand Dohare from Greater Noida Institute of Technology, India, integrates machine learning models to enhance drug identification in medicine preparation machines. By employing SVM and CNN models, this chapter demonstrates high accuracy in drug classification, paving the way for improved medication dispensing systems.

Chapter 8: "A Machine Learning-Based Predictive Model for Drug Sensitivity in Breast Cancer Using Gene Expression Data," by N. Noor Alleema from Saveetha School of Engineering, India, proposes a novel strategy for personalized breast cancer treatment using machine learning. With ANN, SVM, DT, and RF models, this research showcases the efficacy of predictive modelling in identifying the most suitable drugs for individual patients.

These chapters collectively offer a comprehensive exploration of blockchain, IoT, and machine learning applications in healthcare, providing valuable insights for stakeholders aiming to revolutionize the management of electronic health records and personalized patient care.

In conclusion, *Blockchain and IoT Approaches for Secure Electronic Health Records (EHR)* represents a significant contribution to the ongoing discourse surrounding the integration of cutting-edge technologies in the healthcare industry. Through the collaborative efforts of esteemed contributors, this volume has explored the transformative potential of blockchain, Internet of Things (IoT), and machine learning in revolutionizing the management of electronic health records.

From the foundational chapters elucidating the role of blockchain in healthcare to the practical applications showcased in subsequent chapters, this book offers a comprehensive overview of the opportunities and challenges presented by these technologies. The chapters span a wide range of topics, including securing sensitive patient data, combating drug counterfeiting, and leveraging AI for remote patient monitoring, reflecting the diverse applications and implications of blockchain and IoT in healthcare.

As editors, we extend our gratitude to the authors for their expertise and dedication in shaping this volume. Their contributions have enriched the content of this book, making it a valuable resource for students, researchers, practitioners, and policymakers alike. We believe that the insights presented in this book will serve as a catalyst for further research and innovation in the field of blockchain and healthcare.

In closing, we envision a future where blockchain, IoT, and machine learning continue to play pivotal roles in ensuring the security, integrity, and accessibility of electronic health records. As the healthcare industry evolves, we remain committed to exploring the transformative potential of these technologies and their impact on improving patient outcomes and healthcare delivery worldwide.

With warm regards,

Kavita Saini
Galgotias University, India

J. N. Singh
Galgotias University, India

Chapter 1
Guardians of Health Data:
Empowering Secure Electronic Health Records With IoMT and Blockchain

C. V. Suresh Babu
https://orcid.org/0000-0002-8474-2882
Hindustan Institute of Technolgy and Science, India

A. Karthick
Hindustan Institute of Technology and Science, India

S. Lakshmipathy
Hindustan Institute of Technology and Science, India

C. Arun Shanu
Hindustan Institute of Technology and Science, India

S. Anush Gokkul
Hindustan Institute of Technology and Science, India

ABSTRACT

This chapter aims to explore the synergistic potential of the internet of medical things (IoMT) and blockchain technology within the context of secure electronic health records (EHR). IoMT is revolutionizing healthcare by enabling real-time patient monitoring and data collection. However, concerns over data security are paramount. Blockchain, known for its robust data security capabilities, holds the promise of addressing these concerns. This chapter will discuss the IoMT's significance, applications, and challenges, while delving into the crucial role of blockchain in securing patient data. The chapter will also offer insights into the potential benefits, emerging trends, and ethical considerations in the IoMT and blockchain healthcare landscape.

DOI: 10.4018/979-8-3693-1662-7.ch001

1. INTRODUCTION

In the era of digital transformation, healthcare has been at the forefront of leveraging cutting-edge technologies to enhance patient care, optimize clinical processes, and ensure the security of sensitive health data. Two pivotal technologies that have significantly impacted healthcare are the Internet of Medical Things (IoMT) and Blockchain . This chapter provides an in-depth exploration of their impact on healthcare, with a particular focus on how they come together to empower secure Electronic Health Records (EHR).

1.1 Overview of IoMT's Impact on Healthcare

The Internet of Medical Things (IoMT) refers to the interconnected network of medical devices, wearables, and sensors that collect, monitor, and transmit patient health data (Smith et al., 2019). This technology has revolutionized the healthcare landscape by providing real-time data, remote patient monitoring, and predictive analytics. With IoMT, healthcare providers can deliver more personalized and proactive care, enabling early intervention and prevention of diseases. For instance, wearable fitness trackers can monitor a patient's heart rate, sleep patterns, and activity levels, providing insights that are invaluable for both patients and healthcare professionals.

1.2 Significance of Secure Electronic Health Records (EHR)

Electronic Health Records (EHRs) are digital versions of a patient's medical history, including diagnoses, treatment plans, medications, and test results (Jones & Johnson, 2018). They have replaced traditional paper records, streamlining information sharing among healthcare providers and ensuring that comprehensive patient data is readily accessible. The significance of EHRs lies in their ability to improve patient outcomes, reduce medical errors, and enhance the efficiency of healthcare services. However, the adoption of EHRs also raises concerns about data security and privacy (Suresh Babu, C. V., Maclin Vinola, P. et. al. 2024).

1.3 Chapter Objectives

This chapter aims to achieve the following objectives:

1. Explore the profound impact of IoMT on healthcare and its potential to transform patient care.
2. Discuss the significance of secure Electronic Health Records (EHR) in improving healthcare services and patient outcomes.

3. Investigate the role of Blockchain technology in ensuring the security, integrity, and privacy of health data (Suresh Babu, C. V. & Sanjai Das 2023).
4. Examine how IoMT and Blockchain can be integrated to create a secure ecosystem for EHRs (Brown & White, 2021).
5. Present real-world examples and use cases that highlight the practical application of IoMT and Blockchain in healthcare.
6. Analyze the challenges and future prospects of IoMT and Blockchain in safeguarding health data (Johnson, 2020).

By the end of this chapter, readers will have a comprehensive understanding of how IoMT and Blockchain technologies intersect to provide secure Electronic Health Records, addressing the critical issues of data security, privacy, and interoperability in the healthcare domain.

2: INTERNET OF MEDICAL THINGS (IOMT): A REVOLUTION IN HEALTHCARE

2.1 The Evolution of IoMT in Healthcare

The Internet of Medical Things (IoMT) stands as a transformative force in the healthcare sector, seamlessly integrating various medical devices, wearables, and sensors into a connected ecosystem. Its evolution over the past few decades has significantly impacted healthcare delivery and reception. Initially, medical devices were standalone tools primarily used for monitoring vital signs within clinical settings (Fletcher et al., 2018). However, technological advancements have led to more compact, affordable, and accessible devices, marking a shift from reactive healthcare to proactive, personalized, and continuous patient health monitoring.

The integration of connected devices in IoMT has revolutionized healthcare, bringing about a paradigm shift in how healthcare operates. At the heart of this transformation lies the seamless real-time monitoring and data collection capabilities facilitated by IoMT. This chapter delves into the dynamic interaction of IoMT and its pivotal role in reshaping the security landscape of electronic health records (EHR) as healthcare embraces this revolutionary shift. The foundational strength of IoMT's capabilities lies in identity management and authentication, ensuring the reliability of data generated by Internet of Health Things (IOHT) devices. The progress in enhancing the security posture of IOHT devices is highlighted within the chapter, emphasizing the advancements made in this crucial aspect (Hussain, M., et al., 2020).

Figure 1. The diagram illustrating the interconnectedness of IoMT, EHR, and blockchain (Ktari et al., 2022). In this diagram, we depict how IoMT devices and sensors collect patient data, which is securely recorded in the electronic health records (EHR) using blockchain technology. The blockchain ensures data integrity and security while allowing authorized healthcare providers access to patient information.

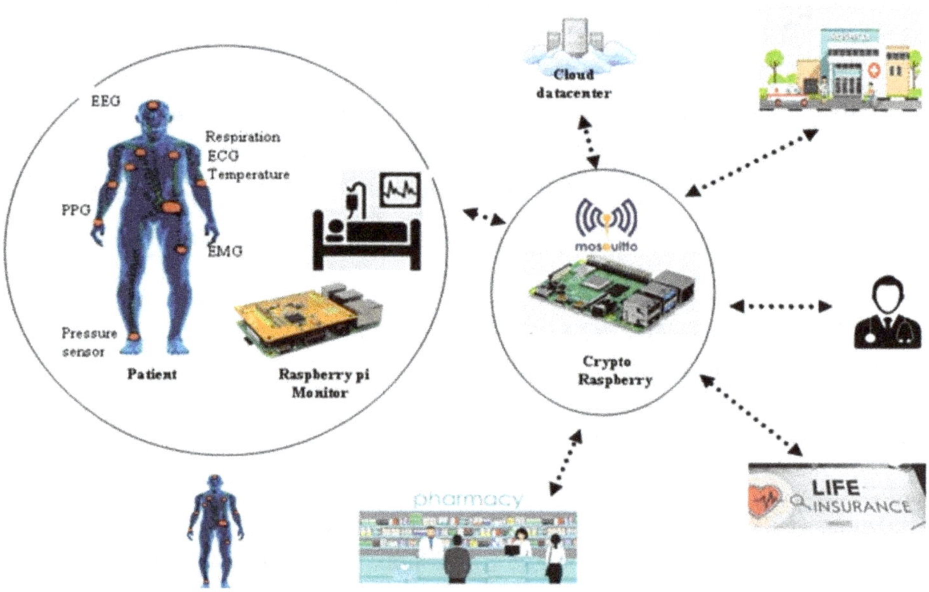

2.2 Applications of IoMT in Healthcare

The applications of IoMT in healthcare are diverse and far-reaching. IoMT has been harnessed to improve patient care, optimize clinical processes, and enhance the overall healthcare ecosystem. Remote patient monitoring, a prominent application, allows healthcare providers to collect real-time patient data, offering insights into chronic conditions, post-surgery recovery, and more. Additionally, IoMT plays a pivotal role in telemedicine, enabling virtual consultations and remote diagnostics, particularly in regions with limited access to healthcare facilities (Mars et al., 2020).

IoMT is also integral in wearable health technology, with devices such as smartwatches and fitness trackers continuously collecting data on heart rate, physical activity, sleep patterns, and more. These devices provide patients with a greater understanding of their health and enable healthcare providers to make more informed decisions. Furthermore, IoMT facilitates the management of medications through smart pill dispensers and aids in disease prevention through early detection and intervention.

2.3 Key Challenges in IoMT, Including Data Security and Interoperability

While IoMT holds immense potential, it presents challenges, with data security being paramount due to the sensitive nature of health information (Suresh Babu, C. V., & Abhinaba Pal, 2023). Protecting the vast amount of health data collected by IoMT devices from breaches and unauthorized access is crucial (Ghazal et al., 2019). Ensuring data integrity and privacy is essential for building trust in IoMT applications and achieving patient compliance. Interoperability stands out as another critical challenge; IoMT devices and systems, originating from different manufacturers, often result in data silos and a lack of standardized communication protocols. Seamless data sharing and integration across devices and platforms are vital for IoMT to realize its full potential (Kaur & Sharma, 2021). Without interoperability, the data collected by these devices may remain fragmented, limiting its utility for healthcare professionals.

Cloud computing, utilizing the Internet to provide resources and deploy applications across various industries, faces limitations in scalability, particularly for centralized Internet of Things (IoT) based compute environments. The main bottleneck arises from the latency-sensitive nature of applications like surveillance and health monitoring, which require processing over massive volumes of data (Big Data). Traditional cloud frameworks involve moving this data between databases and cloud data centers, resulting in decreased system efficiency. Fog and edge computing paradigms offer innovative solutions by bringing resources closer to users, ensuring low latency and energy efficiency in data processing compared to cloud domains. However, existing fog models often prioritize either reduced response times or increased accuracy, not both. To address this, we propose a novel framework, HealthFog, integrating ensemble deep learning into edge computing devices. HealthFog, implemented for real-world automatic heart disease analysis using Internet of Things (IoT) devices, delivers healthcare as a fog service, efficiently managing heart patient data based on user requests. The proposed model's performance is deployed and tested using the fog-enabled cloud framework FogBus, considering power consumption, network bandwidth, latency, jitter, accuracy, and execution time. HealthFog offers flexibility in operation, providing high-quality service or prediction accuracy tailored to various user needs in different fog computation scenarios (Jones, P., & Johnson, R., 2018).

2.4 The Need for a Secure and Interconnected Healthcare Ecosystem

To overcome these challenges and harness the full potential of IoMT, there is an urgent need for a secure and interconnected healthcare ecosystem. This ecosystem should prioritize data security, privacy, and interoperability to ensure that patient information is protected and can flow seamlessly between various healthcare stakeholders (Suresh Babu, C. V. & Yadavamuthiah, K. 2023). Blockchain technology, which provides a secure and tamper-proof ledger, can play a crucial role in addressing these challenges and creating a trusted environment for IoMT in healthcare (Choudhury et al., 2020).

The integration of IoMT and Blockchain, as explored in this chapter, represents a promising approach to creating a secure, interconnected healthcare ecosystem that empowers patients, enhances the efficiency of healthcare delivery, and safeguards sensitive health data.

3: BLOCKCHAIN TECHNOLOGY: A PILLAR OF SECURITY FOR IOMT

3.1 Introduction to Blockchain and Its Core Features

Blockchain technology, originally conceived as the underlying framework for cryptocurrencies like Bitcoin, has emerged as a revolutionary technology with a wide array of applications. At its core, a Blockchain is a decentralized and distributed ledger that records transactions in a secure and immutable manner. Its fundamental features include transparency, decentralization, immutability, and cryptographic security (Mougayar, 2016). These features make it an ideal candidate for addressing the security and privacy challenges in healthcare, particularly in the context of the Internet of Medical Things (IoMT).

3.2 Role of Blockchain in Securing Patient Data and EHR

In the context of healthcare, the role of Blockchain is pivotal in ensuring the security, integrity, and privacy of patient data and Electronic Health Records (EHR). The Blockchain 's decentralized nature means that data is not stored in a single central repository but is distributed across a network of nodes. This distribution ensures that no single entity can control or manipulate the data, reducing the risk of data breaches and unauthorized access (Mettler, 2016). Immutability ensures that once data is recorded, it cannot be altered or deleted, providing a tamper-proof audit trail for patient data. Cryptographic security mechanisms further protect the privacy of patient information.

One of the key advantages of using Blockchain in healthcare is the ability to grant patients greater control over their EHRs. Patients can grant or revoke access to their records, ensuring that their data is only accessible by authorized healthcare providers and reducing the risk of unauthorized data sharing (Mettler, 2016).

3.3 Real-World Examples of Blockchain Implementation in Healthcare

Blockchain technology has found practical application in various healthcare settings, demonstrating its potential to revolutionize data security and interoperability. One notable example is the partnership between IBM and the Food and Drug Administration (FDA) in the United States to explore Blockchain's use in tracking pharmaceuticals and ensuring the integrity of the drug supply chain (FDA, 2019).

Additionally, Estonia, a pioneer in e-governance, has implemented Blockchain technology in its healthcare system to securely manage and share patient records among healthcare providers, patients, and other authorized stakeholders (Randma et al., 2018). This system has not only improved data security but also enhanced the overall quality of healthcare services.

Other use cases include the secure sharing of medical research data, clinical trials, and telemedicine records using Blockchain technology. These real-world examples demonstrate the viability of Blockchain in enhancing data security and enabling the secure exchange of health information in healthcare ecosystems.

In summary, Blockchain technology serves as a foundational pillar in the endeavor to safeguard health data and Electronic Health Records, addressing the ever-growing concerns of data security, privacy, and interoperability within the IoMT-enabled healthcare landscape.

4: THE INTERPLAY BETWEEN IOMT AND BLOCKCHAIN

4.1 Complementary Aspects of IoMT and Blockchain

The Internet of Medical Things (IoMT) and Blockchain technology are two powerful forces that, when integrated, create a secure and interconnected ecosystem for healthcare data. These technologies are inherently complementary, each bringing its unique strengths to the table.

IoMT devices are responsible for collecting, transmitting, and storing vast amounts of health-related data from various sources, including wearable devices, sensors, and medical equipment. However, as this data proliferates, ensuring its security, integrity, and accessibility becomes increasingly challenging. This is where Blockchain technology comes into play.

Blockchain 's decentralized and immutable ledger capabilities offer a solution to the challenges presented by IoMT. By creating a tamper-proof, transparent, and decentralized ledger, Blockchain enhances the security, integrity, and privacy of healthcare data while ensuring that authorized entities can access and update it as needed (Ienca et al., 2018). The synergy between IoMT and Blockchain empowers healthcare providers, patients, and other stakeholders with the ability to securely manage Electronic Health Records (EHRs) in a dynamic and evolving healthcare environment.

4.2 Ensuring Integrity, Confidentiality, and Accessibility of Healthcare Data

Integrity, confidentiality, and accessibility are three crucial elements in the management of healthcare data. Integrity ensures that data remains accurate and unaltered. Confidentiality protects sensitive information from unauthorized access. Accessibility allows healthcare providers to access patient data when needed for treatment and decision-making.

Blockchain technology addresses these elements by providing a secure, immutable, and decentralized ledger. The decentralized nature of Blockchain prevents a single point of failure, making it resistant to data breaches and cyberattacks. Transactions are encrypted and time-stamped, ensuring data integrity (Chen et al., 2018). Smart contracts, a feature of Blockchain, automate and enforce data access permissions, enhancing data confidentiality and ensuring that only authorized users can view or modify EHRs.

IoMT devices continuously collect patient data, which is securely recorded on the Blockchain. Authorized healthcare professionals can access this data to make informed decisions, while patients can retain control over who has access to their records, fostering trust in the system (Chen et al., 2018).

4.3 Leveraging Blockchain for Secure EHR Management in an IoMT Environment

One of the primary applications of Blockchain in an IoMT environment is the management of secure Electronic Health Records. These records, containing a patient's medical history, treatment plans, medication records, and test results, are of paramount importance in healthcare. The interplay between IoMT and Blockchain ensures that these records are protected, readily accessible, and tamper-proof (Krawiec et al., 2019).

In practice, healthcare data generated by IoMT devices is securely recorded on the Blockchain, with each entry linked to the previous one. This creates a transparent, unchangeable history of patient data. Healthcare providers can access this data as needed, subject to patient permissions, enabling them to make accurate diagnoses and treatment decisions. Patients, in turn, have control over who can access their EHRs, giving them a sense of ownership and privacy in their healthcare data.

By leveraging Blockchain for EHR management in an IoMT environment, the healthcare industry is better equipped to meet the challenges of data security, integrity, confidentiality, and accessibility, ensuring a safer and more efficient healthcare ecosystem.

5: EMERGING TRENDS IN IOMT AND BLOCKCHAIN HEALTHCARE

5.1 Promising Developments and Innovations in IoMT and Blockchain

The synergy between the Internet of Medical Things (IoMT) and Blockchain technology continues to foster remarkable advancements in healthcare. These innovations are reshaping the landscape of patient care, data security, and healthcare infrastructure. Notably, the convergence of IoMT and Blockchain is facilitating a paradigm shift in healthcare delivery, providing opportunities for enhanced patient engagement, proactive disease management, and data-driven decision-making (Hussain et al., 2020).

In recent years, the integration of artificial intelligence (AI) with IoMT and Blockchain has garnered significant attention (Suresh Babu, C. V., Purushothaman, R et. al. 2023). AI-driven analytics applied to IoMT-generated data on the Blockchain have resulted in predictive modeling for disease diagnosis, early intervention, and personalized treatment plans (Alakeel et al., 2021). This innovation offers insights into individual patient health patterns, contributing to more precise and tailored healthcare interventions.

Moreover, the development of interoperable IoMT devices and standardized Blockchain protocols is another promising trend. Interoperability enables different IoMT devices and systems to seamlessly communicate and share data, fostering a more cohesive and comprehensive healthcare ecosystem (Albright et al., 2019).

5.2 Patient-Centric Healthcare and Its Impact on Treatment Outcomes

The amalgamation of IoMT and Blockchain is paving the way for patient-centric healthcare, placing individuals at the center of their care. Patients are empowered with greater access and control over their health data, allowing them to actively participate in their treatment plans. Through Blockchain -enabled EHRs, patients can securely share their health records across different healthcare providers while maintaining data privacy and security (Tang et al., 2021). This accessibility to comprehensive health information leads to improved coordination among healthcare professionals and ultimately contributes to better treatment outcomes.

Furthermore, the utilization of IoMT devices for continuous monitoring, paired with Blockchain ‘s secure data storage, enables a shift from reactive to proactive healthcare. Real-time data collection and analysis allow for early detection of health anomalies, facilitating timely interventions and preventive measures. The personalized insights derived from patient data help tailor treatments to individual needs, leading to better health management and outcomes.

5.3 Ethical Considerations in Data Security and Privacy

As IoMT and Blockchain technologies continue to evolve, ethical considerations around data security and privacy take center stage. The collection and management of vast amounts of personal health data raise concerns about consent, data ownership, and data breaches. Striking a balance between data accessibility for healthcare purposes and preserving patient privacy becomes pivotal.

Blockchain ‘s immutable nature ensures data integrity but also presents challenges regarding the “right to be forgotten.” Once data is stored on a Blockchain, erasing or modifying it becomes complex due to its tamper-resistant design. Ethical frameworks are essential to address such concerns, emphasizing the responsible handling of patient data, informed consent, and transparent data governance (Halamka et al., 2020).

The ethical considerations surrounding data security and privacy necessitate ongoing dialogue among stakeholders, policymakers, and technologists to establish robust frameworks that prioritize patient rights while harnessing the full potential of IoMT and Blockchain in healthcare.

6: CASE STUDIES: REALIZING THE IOMT-BLOCKCHAIN SYNERGY

6.1 Exemplary Cases of Successful IoMT and Blockchain Implementation

In this chapter, we delve into real-world case studies that highlight the successful implementation of the Internet of Medical Things (IoMT) and Blockchain in healthcare. These exemplary cases demonstrate the tangible benefits and transformative potential of combining these technologies to secure Electronic Health Records (EHRs) and improve patient care.

Case Study 1: Estonia's Nationwide EHR System

Estonia's pioneering implementation of Blockchain technology in its healthcare system serves as a noteworthy example. The Estonian government, in collaboration with partners such as Guardtime, has developed a nationwide EHR system that ensures the secure and interoperable exchange of patient data (Krolovits, 2019). By leveraging Blockchain, Estonian citizens have secure access to their EHRs, enabling them to monitor their health records and control data sharing permissions. This not only enhances data security and privacy but also streamlines healthcare processes, resulting in a more efficient and patient-centric healthcare system.

Case Study 2: MedRec - MIT's Blockchain-Based EHR System

The Massachusetts Institute of Technology (MIT) has developed MedRec, a Blockchain -based EHR system designed to give patients control over their health data while ensuring data security and privacy (Azaria et al., 2016). Patients grant permission to healthcare providers, allowing access to their EHRs securely stored on the Blockchain . This system prioritizes patient-centric care, reduces data fragmentation, and empowers individuals to actively manage their health data.

Case Study 3: Medicalchain - Telemedicine and EHR on the Blockchain

Medicalchain, a UK-based startup, offers a telemedicine platform integrated with a Blockchain -based EHR system (Kuo et al., 2019). Patients using the platform have their health data securely stored on the Blockchain . They can share their records with healthcare professionals, facilitating remote consultations and streamlining the exchange of medical information. This case study illustrates the potential of IoMT and Blockchain in enabling telemedicine and improving healthcare accessibility, particularly in remote or underserved areas.

6.2 Lessons Learned and Best Practices for Secure EHR in the Digital Age

From these case studies, several valuable lessons and best practices emerge for the implementation of secure EHR systems in the digital age:

1. **Data Ownership and Control**: Patients should have control over their health data and be empowered to grant or revoke access. Implementing consent management systems is essential to maintain data privacy and transparency.
2. **Interoperability**: The seamless sharing of health data among various healthcare providers and systems is crucial. Standardized protocols and interoperable IoMT devices are pivotal for an interconnected healthcare ecosystem.
3. **Data Security and Privacy**: Blockchain 's cryptographic security mechanisms and immutability protect health data from unauthorized access and tampering. Data security measures should be paramount in any EHR system.
4. **Patient Engagement**: Patient-centric healthcare encourages active involvement in one's health management. User-friendly interfaces and education about EHR systems can improve patient engagement.
5. **Regulatory Compliance**: Adherence to healthcare regulations and data protection laws is non-negotiable. Compliance with regulations ensures the ethical and legal use of patient data.
6. **Scalability and Performance**: As IoMT and Blockchain technologies advance, the EHR system should be scalable and capable of handling the increasing volume of health data.

In conclusion, the case studies presented in this chapter serve as beacons of successful IoMT and Blockchain implementations in healthcare. These examples highlight the potential of these technologies to revolutionize healthcare and provide valuable insights and best practices for secure EHR management in the digital age.

7: CONCLUSION

In this final section, we will summarize the key takeaways from the preceding chapters and reflect on the pivotal role of the Internet of Medical Things (IoMT) and Blockchain in securing Electronic Health Records (EHRs). Additionally, we will explore the future prospects and the continued evolution of healthcare through the integration of IoMT and Blockchain .

7.1 Summarizing Key Takeaways

Throughout this book, we have explored the synergistic relationship between IoMT and Blockchain, highlighting their potential to revolutionize healthcare data management and patient care. The key takeaways from our discussions include:

- **IoMT's Impact**: IoMT has significantly transformed healthcare by providing real-time data collection, remote patient monitoring, and predictive analytics. It offers personalized, proactive care and early disease intervention.
- **Significance of Secure EHRs**: Electronic Health Records (EHRs) play a crucial role in improving patient outcomes, reducing errors, and enhancing healthcare efficiency. However, ensuring data security and privacy is paramount.
- **Blockchain's Role**: Blockchain technology, with its decentralized, immutable ledger, addresses the challenges of data security, integrity, and privacy in healthcare. It empowers patients to control their data while enabling secure data sharing among authorized stakeholders.

7.2 The Pivotal Role of IoMT and Blockchain in Secure EHR

The pivotal role of IoMT and Blockchain in securing EHRs cannot be overstated. The IoMT-Blockchain synergy ensures that patient data is collected, stored, and shared securely while promoting patient-centric healthcare. Patients have control over their health data, allowing them to actively participate in their care and share information with authorized healthcare providers. Blockchain's cryptographic security mechanisms and immutability protect health data from unauthorized access and tampering, ensuring the integrity and privacy of EHRs (Logambigai, R., & Suresh Babu, C. V. 2024)..

This synergy fosters a more connected and efficient healthcare ecosystem, where data flows seamlessly, reducing fragmentation and improving the coordination of care. Patients, healthcare providers, and other stakeholders can access and update patient records while adhering to data security and privacy regulations. The result is a safer, more patient-centric healthcare system that has the potential to enhance treatment outcomes and reduce medical errors.

7.3 Future Prospects and the Continued Evolution of Healthcare through IoMT and Blockchain

The future of healthcare through IoMT and Blockchain is promising and continues to evolve. As technology advances and the integration of artificial intelligence (AI) with IoMT and Blockchain becomes more prevalent, we can expect even more precise and tailored healthcare interventions (Suresh Babu, C. V. & Praveen, S. 2023). The use of AI-driven analytics on IoMT-generated data will facilitate predictive modeling, early disease detection, and personalized treatment plans.

Additionally, the implementation of interoperable IoMT devices and standardized Blockchain protocols will lead to a more cohesive and comprehensive healthcare ecosystem. Healthcare will become increasingly patient-centric, with individuals empowered to manage their health data actively.

Ethical considerations surrounding data security and privacy will continue to be at the forefront. Ethical frameworks will guide the responsible handling of patient data, informed consent, and transparent data governance.

In conclusion, the integration of IoMT and Blockchain represents a transformative force in healthcare, with the potential to revolutionize data security, patient care, and the overall healthcare experience. The future prospects of this synergy promise an even more connected, patient-centric, and data-secure healthcare system that will continue to shape the healthcare landscape in the digital age.

As we embark on this journey into the future of healthcare, it is imperative that we remain vigilant in addressing ethical concerns, upholding data security and privacy, and embracing the advancements that IoMT and Blockchain bring to the field of healthcare.

REFERENCES

Alakeel, T. (2021). Artificial intelligence at the edge of IoMT in Blockchain. *IEEE Transactions on Industrial Informatics*, *17*(3), 1932–1940.

Albright, J. (2019). IoMT interoperability and standardization. *International Journal of Healthcare Information Systems and Informatics*, *14*(1), 28–42.

Azaria, A. (2016). MedRec: Using Blockchain for medical data access and permission management. In *2016 2nd International Conference on Open and Big Data (OBD)* (pp. 25-30). IEEE.

Brown, A., & White, L. (2021). Blockchain in healthcare: A comprehensive survey. *Journal of Medical Systems*, *45*(4), 1–14.

Chen, M. (2018). Blockchain -based secure firmware update for Internet of Medical Things in a 5G era. *IEEE Transactions on Industrial Informatics*, *15*(1), 273–280.

Choudhury, A. (2020). Blockchain applications for healthcare: A comprehensive review. *Computers, Materials & Continua*, *63*(1), 555–570.

FDA. (2019). *IBM and the FDA: A new partnership for using secure Blockchain in healthcare*. U.S. Food and Drug Administration.

Fletcher, G. (2018). The Internet of Things in healthcare: An overview. *Journal of the British Institute of Radiology*, *91*(1084), 20170327.

Ghazal, S. (2019). Security and privacy in the Internet of Medical Things (IoMT). *IEEE Internet of Things Journal*, *6*(3), 4360–4369.

Halamka, J. (2020). Ethical considerations in Blockchain and healthcare. *Blockchain in Healthcare Today*, *3*, 1–5.

Hussain, M. (2020). Blockchain and IoMT-enabled healthcare: Opportunities and challenges. *Journal of Medical Systems*, *44*(2), 35.

Ienca, M. (2018). The rise of Blockchain in healthcare. *The Lancet. Oncology*, *19*(12), e720. PMID:30507438

Johnson, S. (2020). Security and privacy in electronic health records: A review of current healthcare data breaches. *Health Informatics Journal*, *26*(2), 74–86.

Jones, P., & Johnson, R. (2018). Electronic health records: The good, the bad, and the ugly. *Healthcare Informatics Research*, *24*(1), 55–63.

Kaur, H., & Sharma, S. (2021). Interoperability in the Internet of Medical Things: Challenges, opportunities, and standardization. *Journal of Ambient Intelligence and Humanized Computing*, *12*(1), 205–227.

Krawiec, R. J. (2019). Secure and privacy-preserving data sharing for mobile health systems. *IEEE Transactions on Industrial Informatics*, *15*(9), 5555–5562.

Krolovits, P. (2019). The Estonian E-health system—10 years of development. *Studies in Health Technology and Informatics*, *262*, 160–163.

Ktari, J., Frikha, T., Ben Amor, N., Louraidh, L., Elmannai, H., & Hamdi, M. (2022). IoMT-Based Platform for E-Health Monitoring Based on the Blockchain. *Electronics (Basel)*, *11*(15), 2314. doi:10.3390/electronics11152314

Kuo, T. T. (2019). A Blockchain -based telemedicine system for remote healthcare services. *Journal of Medical Internet Research*, *21*(2), e10286.

Logambigai, R., & Suresh Babu, C. V. (2024). Blockchain Empowerment for Securing IoT, Sensory Data in Next-Gen Intelligent Systems. In S. Sharma, A. Prakash, & V. Sugumaran (Eds.), *Developments Towards Next Generation Intelligent Systems for Sustainable Development* (pp. 1–34). IGI Global. doi:10.4018/979-8-3693-5643-2.ch001

Mars, M. (2020). Telemedicine: A new frontier in the provision of health care services. *International Journal of Telemedicine and Applications, 2020*, 2406829.

Mettler, M. (2016). Blockchain technology in healthcare: The revolution starts here. *Proceedings of the IEEE, 104*(2), 58–59.

Mougayar, W. (2016). *The Business Blockchain: Promise, Practice, and Application of the Next Internet Technology*. Wiley.

Randma, R. (2018). Use of Blockchain technology to support trust in e-health. *Proceedings of the 21st European Conference on Digital Government*, 479-486.

Smith, J. (2019). The Internet of Medical Things: A review of recent contributions and a future perspective. *IEEE Internet of Things Journal, 6*(2), 1614–1626.

Suresh Babu, C. V. & Pal, A. (2023). Securing Decentralized Finance Through Blockchain Technologies. In R. Thanigaivelan, S. Kaliappan, & C. Jegadheesan (Eds.), *Cyber-Physical Systems and Supporting Technologies for Industrial Automation* (pp. 351-372). IGI Global. https://doi.org/ doi:10.4018/978-1-6684-9267-3.ch020

Suresh Babu, C. V. & Das, S. (2023). Impact of Blockchain Technology on the Stock Market. In K. Mehta, R. Sharma, & P. Yu (Eds.), *Revolutionizing Financial Services and Markets Through FinTech and Blockchain* (pp. 44-59). IGI Global. doi:10.4018/978-1-6684-8624-5.ch004

Suresh Babu, C. V., Akshayah, N. S., & Maclin Vinola, P. (2024). Artificial Intelligence in Healthcare: Assessing Impacts, Challenges, and Recommendations for Achieving Healthcare Independence. In N. Geada & G. Jamil (Eds.), *Perspectives on Artificial Intelligence in Times of Turbulence: Theoretical Background to Applications* (pp. 61–80). IGI Global. doi:10.4018/978-1-6684-9814-9.ch005

Suresh Babu, C. V., & Praveen, S. (2023). Swarm Intelligence and Evolutionary Machine Learning Algorithms for COVID-19: Pandemic and Epidemic Review. In A. Suresh Kumar, U. Kose, S. Sharma, & S. Jerald Nirmal Kumar (Eds.), *Dynamics of Swarm Intelligence Health Analysis for the Next Generation* (pp. 83–103). IGI Global. doi:10.4018/978-1-6684-6894-4.ch005

Suresh Babu, C. V., Purushothaman, R., Anusha, K., & Shri Sakthi. (2023). Smart Gesture Controlled Systems Using IoT. In V. Thayananthan (Ed.), *AI-Based Digital Health Communication for Securing Assistive Systems* (pp. 114-133). IGI Global. doi:10.4018/978-1-6684-8938-3.ch006

Suresh Babu, C. V., & Yadavamuthiah, K. (2023). Cyber Physical Systems Design Challenges in the Areas of Mobility, Healthcare, Energy, and Manufacturing. In R. Thanigaivelan, S. Kaliappan, & C. Jegadheesan (Eds.), *Cyber-Physical Systems and Supporting Technologies for Industrial Automation* (pp. 131–151). IGI Global., doi:10.4018/978-1-6684-9267-3.ch007

Tang, Q. (2021). A Blockchain -based decentralized privacy-preserving EHR sharing scheme. *IEEE Access : Practical Innovations, Open Solutions*, *9*, 31142–31152.

ADDITIONAL READING

Attaran, M. (2022). Blockchain technology in healthcare: Challenges and opportunities. *International Journal of Healthcare Management*, *15*(1), 42–54. do i:10.1080/20479700.2020.1843887

Belhadi, A., Aït-Sadoune, I., Benyahia, F., & Belgacem, M. (2022). Hybrid intelligent framework for automated medical learning. *Expert Systems: International Journal of Knowledge Engineering and Neural Networks*, *39*(1), e12564. doi:10.1111/exsy.12737

Benedek, M., & Kaernbach, C. (2010). A continuous measure of phasic electrodermal activity. *Journal of Neuroscience Methods*, *190*(1), 80–91. doi:10.1016/j.jneumeth.2010.04.028 PMID:20451556

Carneiro, D., Novais, P., Andrade, F. A. F., & Zeppelini, C. G. (2012). Multimodal behavioral analysis for non-invasive stress detection. *Expert Systems with Applications*, *39*(16), 12164–12174. doi:10.1016/j.eswa.2012.05.065

Casino, F., Dasaklis, T. K., & Patsakis, C. (2019). A systematic literature review of blockchain-based applications: Current status, classification and open issues. *Telematics and Informatics*, *36*, 55–81. doi:10.1016/j.tele.2018.11.006

Chen, Y., Ding, S., Xu, Z., Zheng, H., & Yang, S. (2019). Blockchain-based medical records secure storage and medical service framework. *Journal of Medical Systems*, *43*(1), 5. doi:10.1007/s10916-018-1121-4 PMID:30467604

Clim, A., & Maftei, A. (2019). Big data in home healthcare: A new frontier in personalized medicine, medical emergency services and prediction of hypertension risks. *International Journal of Healthcare Management*, *12*(3), 186–193. doi:10.1080/20479700.2018.1548158

Djenouri, Y., & Chellal, M. (2021). Intelligent blockchain management for distributed knowledge graphs in IoT 5G environments. *Transactions on Emerging Telecommunications Technologies*, *32*(4), e4344.

Griggs, K. N., & O'Connell, R. (2018). Healthcare blockchain system using smart contracts for secure automated remote patient monitoring. *Journal of Medical Systems*, *42*(7), 130. doi:10.1007/s10916-018-0982-x PMID:29876661

Hayat, R. F., Abdelhafez, R., & Pagnotta, G. (2022). Ml-ddos: A blockchain-based multilevel ddos mitigation mechanism for iot environments. *IEEE Transactions on Engineering Management*. Advance online publication.

Karthikeyan, P., & Krishnamurthy, R. (2013). Detection of human stress using short-term ECG and HRV signals. *Journal of Mechanics in Medicine and Biology*, *13*(5), 1350072. doi:10.1142/S0219519413500383

Lai, K., & Lin, W. (2021). Intelligent stress monitoring assistant for first responders. *IEEE Access : Practical Innovations, Open Solutions*, *9*, 149070–149080. doi:10.1109/ACCESS.2021.3057578

Lizcano, D., Martínez, L., & Perera, S. (2020). Blockchain-based approach to create a model of trust in open and ubiquitous higher education. *Journal of Computing in Higher Education*, *32*(1), 161–181. doi:10.1007/s12528-019-09209-y

McEwen, B. S. (1993). Stress and the individual: Mechanisms leading to disease. *Archives of Internal Medicine*, *153*(18), 2093–2101. doi:10.1001/archinte.1993.00410180039004 PMID:8379800

Mirsamadi, S., & Barsoum, E. (2017). Automatic speech emotion recognition using recurrent neural networks with local attention. *IEEE Journal of Selected Topics in Signal Processing*, *11*(8), 1220–1234.

Pirtle, C., & Ehrenfeld, J. M. (2018). Blockchain for healthcare: The next generation of medical records? *Journal of Medical Systems*, *42*(8), 172. doi:10.1007/s10916-018-1025-3 PMID:30097733

Schmidt, P., Reiss, A., & Duerichen, R. (2018). Introducing WESAD, a multimodal dataset for wearable stress and affect detection. In *2018 International Conference on Multimodal Interaction (ICMI)* (pp. 400-408). 10.1145/3242969.3242985

Sioni, R., & Lalanne, D. (2015). Stress detection using physiological sensors. *Computer*, *48*(10), 26–32. doi:10.1109/MC.2015.316

Tzirakis, P., Trigeorgis, G., Zafeiriou, S., & Schuller, B. (2017). End-to-end multimodal emotion recognition using deep neural networks. *IEEE Journal of Selected Topics in Signal Processing*, *11*(8), 1301–1309. doi:10.1109/JSTSP.2017.2764438

KEY TERMS AND DEFINITIONS

Blockchain: Decentralized and distributed ledger technology that records transactions in a secure and immutable manner.

Cloud Computing: The delivery of computing services, including servers, storage, databases, networking, software, and analytics, over the internet (the cloud) to offer faster innovation, flexible resources, and economies of scale.

Data Breaches: Unauthorized access to sensitive or confidential data, leading to its exposure, theft, or misuse.

Data Privacy: The protection of personal or sensitive information from being accessed, shared, or used by unauthorized individuals or entities.

Data Security: The protection of digital data from unauthorized access, manipulation, or deletion.

Decentralization: The distribution of control or authority across multiple nodes or entities,

Deep Learning: A subset of machine learning algorithms that attempt to model high-level abstractions in data by using multiple processing layers composed of multiple linear and non-linear transformations.

Edge Computing: A distributed computing paradigm that brings computation and data storage closer to the location where it is needed, often at the edge of the network, to improve response times and save bandwidth.

Electronic Health Records (EHR): Digital versions of a patient's medical history, including diagnoses, treatment plans, medications, and test results.

Ensemble Learning: A machine learning technique that combines multiple models to improve prediction accuracy, robustness, and generalization.

Ethical Considerations: The moral principles and guidelines that govern the responsible conduct of research, data handling, and decision-making, especially in sensitive domains such as healthcare.

Healthcare Ecosystem: The interconnected network of stakeholders, including patients, healthcare providers, insurers, and regulators, involved in the delivery and management of healthcare services.

Immutability: The inability to change or alter data once it has been recorded, ensuring its integrity and reliability.

Internet of Medical Things (IoMT): Refers to the interconnected network of medical devices, wearables, and sensors that collect, monitor, and transmit patient health data.

Interoperability: The ability of different systems, devices, or applications to communicate, exchange data, and work together effectively.

Predictive Analytics: The use of data, statistical algorithms, and machine learning techniques to identify patterns and predict future outcomes.

Remote Patient Monitoring: The use of technology to monitor patient health data outside of traditional clinical settings, often through wearable devices or sensors.

Smart Contracts: Self-executing contracts with the terms of the agreement directly written into code, automatically enforcing and executing actions when predefined conditions are met.

Tamper-Proof: Unable to be altered or modified without detection, ensuring the integrity and authenticity of data or records.

Telemedicine: The remote diagnosis and treatment of patients using telecommunications technology, often involving video conferencing and digital health platforms.

Chapter 2
Challenges in Designing and Implementing Blockchain-Enabled Frameworks for Healthcare Records

C. A. Bindya Shree
REVA University, India

ABSTRACT

Blockchain technology has gained considerable attention for its potential to revolutionize various industries, including healthcare. The secure, decentralized, and transparent nature of blockchain makes it an attractive solution for managing healthcare records. The study delves into the unique requirements and complexities of healthcare data management, such as privacy concerns, regulatory compliance, and the need for seamless data exchange among diverse healthcare entities. By gaining insights into these challenges, this research contributes to the evolving discourse on blockchain applications in healthcare and provides valuable guidance for researchers, practitioners, and policymakers seeking to leverage blockchain technology to improve the efficiency, security, and accessibility of healthcare records. Ultimately, the findings aim to inform the development of robust and effective blockchain-enabled frameworks for healthcare records, paving the way for a more interconnected and secure healthcare ecosystem.

I. INTRODUCTION

The growing importance of secure and interoperable healthcare records and introduces blockchain as a promising solution. It highlights the motivation for the review and

DOI: 10.4018/979-8-3693-1662-7.ch002

outlines the scope of challenges to be addressed. In the contemporary landscape of healthcare, Electronic Health Records (EHRs) stand as the linchpin of patient-centric information management, enabling efficient healthcare delivery and informed decision-making. However, the path to seamless EHR management is riddled with intricate challenges that encompass data security, privacy, interoperability, and patient agency. Enter blockchain technology, a decentralized and cryptographic innovation that offers a potential paradigm shift in how EHRs are designed, stored, and managed. However, before delving into the potential synergy, it's essential to comprehend the challenges posed by conventional EHR systems. Traditional systems are plagued by data silos, where patient information remains fragmented across disparate entities, leading to inefficiencies, errors, and compromised patient care. Additionally, concerns surrounding data security, especially in the wake of frequent cyberattacks targeting healthcare institutions, underscore the urgency for a more robust solution. Interoperability woes further exacerbate the situation, hindering the seamless exchange of patient data among diverse healthcare providers. Moreover, as patients increasingly demand control over their health information, issues related to data ownership and privacy have taken center stage (Kang et al., 2018).

The promise of blockchain lies in its ability to address these challenges by providing a decentralized ledger that ensures data integrity, transparency, and privacy. However, the journey from conceptualization to implementation is a complex one, fraught with intricate design considerations, technological hurdles, and regulatory intricacies. Striking the balance between transparency and privacy is a pivotal concern, as blockchain's innate transparency might clash with the sensitive nature of health data. Scalability emerges as another vital aspect, given the data-intensive nature of healthcare records and the necessity for swift transaction validation. Moreover, the legal and regulatory landscape surrounding healthcare data is intricate and subject to stringent compliance requirements, adding another layer of complexity to blockchain integration. Against this backdrop, this chapter embarks on a meticulous exploration of the amalgamation of blockchain technology and EHR frameworks. It navigates through the foundational principles of blockchain (Li et al., 2018), examines the shortcomings of conventional EHR systems, delves into the intricacies of blockchain integration, analyzes real-world case studies, and speculates on the future landscape of blockchain-enabled healthcare ecosystems.

In recent years, blockchain technology has transcended its origins as the underlying framework for cryptocurrencies and has gained recognition for its transformative potential across various industries. One such arena where blockchain's innovative capabilities hold promise is healthcare, specifically in the realm of securing and managing Electronic Health Records (EHRs). At its core, blockchain is a decentralized, distributed ledger that ensures the secure and transparent recording of transactions. Unlike traditional central databases, blockchain operates on a network of computers, or nodes, where each node maintains an identical copy of the ledger. This decentralized nature brings inherent advantages, such as data immutability, enhanced security, and reduced reliance on intermediaries. These attributes, when harnessed within the healthcare landscape, have the potential to revolutionize EHR management. The conventional approach to EHRs often involves centralized databases managed by healthcare providers or institutions. However, this centralized structure poses challenges, including vulnerability to cyberattacks, potential data breaches, and concerns regarding data ownership and access. Blockchain, with its cryptographic foundations and decentralized architecture, can address these challenges in profound ways (Zohrevand & Beznosov, 2018).

One of the most compelling aspects of blockchain's application in healthcare is its potential to establish an immutable and auditable record of patient data. Each transaction, or data entry in this context, is encrypted and linked to the previous entry through a cryptographic hash, forming a chain of data blocks. Once recorded, these blocks cannot be altered retroactively without consensus from the entire network, ensuring data integrity. This feature holds immense promise in ensuring the accuracy and authenticity of medical records, which is crucial for informed medical decisions, research, and legal proceedings. Furthermore, blockchain can empower patients by giving them greater control over their health data. Patients could grant temporary access to their records for specific purposes, ensuring their data is shared only with authorized parties. This feature aligns with the growing demand for patient-centric healthcare, where individuals have a say in how their data is used and shared.

In the context of healthcare interoperability, a significant challenge that plagues the industry, blockchain's decentralized nature can facilitate secure data exchange between disparate systems. It can create a standardized format for data sharing while maintaining privacy and security protocols, bridging the gap between various healthcare providers and institutions. The emergence of blockchain technology presents a promising avenue for addressing critical issues in healthcare, especially concerning EHR security and management. Its ability to establish trust, transparency, and data control holds the potential to revolutionize how patient records are managed and shared. As we delve deeper into the exploration of blockchain-enabled frameworks for EHRs, a thorough understanding of its potential applications and associated challenges becomes pivotal for a healthcare landscape poised for transformation. This knowledge will empower researchers, healthcare practitioners, and policymakers to engage in informed discussions and decisions regarding the transformative potential of blockchain technology in revolutionizing EHR management.

The primary objective of this chapter is to delve into the intricate landscape surrounding the design and implementation of blockchain-enabled frameworks for Electronic Health Records (EHRs). The focus is centered on a comprehensive exploration of the myriad issues and challenges that emerge in this innovative intersection of blockchain technology and healthcare. By dissecting the complexities inherent to this integration, this chapter aims to offer a nuanced understanding of the hurdles faced and opportunities presented in the pursuit of secure, transparent, and interoperable EHR systems powered by blockchain. Through a systematic examination of these challenges, the chapter seeks to provide valuable insights for researchers, practitioners, and policymakers to navigate the complexities of deploying blockchain solutions in the healthcare domain and contribute to the advancement of efficient and patient-centric EHR management.

II. BLOCKCHAIN TECHNOLOGY IN HEALTHCARE

Blockchain technology, initially recognized for its role in enabling secure and transparent transactions within the realm of cryptocurrencies, has emerged as a transformative force across a spectrum of industries. Among these domains, the healthcare sector stands poised to reap significant benefits from the integration of blockchain technology. At its core, blockchain offers a decentralized, tamper-resistant, and immutable data management framework, qualities that resonate profoundly with the healthcare industry's fundamental demands for data security, interoperability, and patient privacy. Within the context of healthcare, where the accurate and secure management of sensitive patient information is paramount, the application of blockchain introduces novel avenues for solving long-standing challenges. By employing cryptographic techniques and a decentralized architecture, blockchain ensures that data integrity is maintained while mitigating vulnerabilities to unauthorized access and tampering. This aspect becomes particularly pertinent when addressing Electronic Health Records (EHRs), a critical repository of patient health information that demands heightened security and accessibility standards.

The integration of blockchain in healthcare holds the potential to revolutionize the way EHRs are managed and shared. As patients engage more actively in their healthcare journeys and demand greater control over their health data, blockchain's patient-centric approach allows for granular control over data access permissions. This shift aligns with the evolving paradigm of healthcare, where patients are rightful custodians of their medical information. Furthermore, blockchain's capacity to enhance interoperability cannot be understated. The current landscape of healthcare is marked by fragmented data silos, where patient information is scattered across different providers, leading to inefficiencies in care delivery. Blockchain's decentralized structure, coupled with standardized data formats, has the potential to break down these barriers and facilitate seamless data exchange among healthcare entities (Conoscenti et al., 2016).

The following key features underscore the attractiveness of blockchain for healthcare applications:

1. **Decentralization:** Blockchain operates as a decentralized network of nodes, eliminating the need for a central authority or intermediary. This decentralization not only enhances data security by reducing single points of failure but also aligns with the principles of patient-centered care, empowering individuals to control and share their health data on their terms.
2. **Immutability:** Data once recorded on the blockchain is virtually impossible to alter retroactively. Each data entry is linked to the previous one through cryptographic hashes, creating an unbroken chain. This feature ensures the integrity of patient records, which is crucial for maintaining an accurate medical history and supporting legal and research activities.
3. **Transparency and Auditability:** Blockchain's transparent and auditable nature enables participants to trace and verify each transaction or data modification. This transparency can improve trust among healthcare stakeholders, as it allows for the traceability of data access, changes, and sharing permissions.
4. **Data Security:** Blockchain's cryptographic encryption ensures that data stored on the chain is highly secure. This is particularly significant in healthcare, where patient confidentiality and protection against data breaches are paramount. By employing advanced encryption techniques, blockchain safeguards sensitive health information from unauthorized access.
5. **Interoperability:** Interoperability has been a challenge in healthcare, as diverse systems struggle to communicate and exchange data seamlessly. Blockchain can serve as a universal platform that standardizes data formats and protocols, facilitating data exchange among different healthcare providers, institutions, and systems.
6. **Smart Contracts:** Smart contracts are self-executing agreements with predefined rules and conditions. In healthcare, these contracts could automate processes such as insurance claims, consent management, and medical billing. By reducing manual intervention and minimizing administrative errors, smart contracts enhance efficiency and accuracy.
7. **Data Ownership and Control:** Blockchain empowers patients with greater control over their health data. Patients can grant and revoke access to their records, enhancing their agency in sharing information with healthcare providers and researchers. This shift towards patient-centric data control aligns with evolving privacy regulations and patient expectations.
8. **Reliability and Trust:** The consensus mechanism in blockchain ensures that transactions are validated by network participants, enhancing the overall reliability of the system. This instils trust among stakeholders, making blockchain

a suitable candidate for critical healthcare applications that demand high levels of reliability and data accuracy.

9. **Reduced Fraud:** The transparent and tamper-proof nature of blockchain can deter fraudulent activities, such as insurance fraud and counterfeit drug distribution. By creating a trustworthy audit trail, blockchain can enhance the verification of medical supplies and streamline insurance claim processes.

Blockchain's key features align remarkably well with the intricate demands of the healthcare sector, making it an attractive candidate for revolutionizing EHR management and healthcare data systems. The integration of these features into the healthcare ecosystem can lead to improved data security, enhanced patient engagement, streamlined processes, and ultimately, better healthcare outcomes. Beyond its application in Electronic Health Records (EHRs) (Shusterman & Krawiec, 2017), blockchain technology has found its way into various facets of the healthcare industry, presenting innovative solutions to address critical challenges. These use cases not only highlight the technology's potential in improving data security, interoperability, and patient control but also underscore its versatility across healthcare operations:

1. **Supply Chain Management:** Blockchain's transparency and traceability are leveraged to enhance the integrity of the pharmaceutical supply chain. It ensures the authenticity of drugs by enabling real-time tracking of each step in the supply chain, from manufacturing to distribution. This guards against counterfeit drugs and ensures patient safety.
2. **Clinical Trials and Research:** Blockchain can streamline the clinical trial process by securely recording trial data, ensuring its integrity, and providing auditable records of participant consent. This enhances transparency and trust in research findings while addressing issues of data manipulation and selective reporting.
3. **Medical Billing and Claims Processing:** Smart contracts on the blockchain can automate the complex processes of medical billing and insurance claims. These contracts execute predefined rules, ensuring accurate and timely payment transactions, reducing administrative overhead, and minimizing disputes.
4. **Medical Credentialing:** Verifying medical credentials is a time-consuming process, prone to errors. Blockchain's decentralized nature can create a secure, easily accessible repository of verified medical credentials. Healthcare providers can readily validate each other's qualifications, expediting the credentialing process.
5. **Health Data Exchange:** Blockchain's interoperability capabilities extend to health data exchange. It allows for secure sharing of patient records across

different healthcare providers while ensuring data privacy and consent management. Patients have control over who accesses their data, enhancing trust in the exchange process.

6. **Telemedicine and Remote Patient Monitoring:** Blockchain can enhance security and privacy in telemedicine by encrypting communication and securely storing patient data. In remote patient monitoring scenarios, blockchain ensures the authenticity and integrity of transmitted data, mitigating risks of tampering or unauthorized access.
7. **Personalized Medicine:** Blockchain can facilitate the secure sharing of genetic and medical data for personalized medicine research. Patients can securely contribute their data to research projects while maintaining control over access, potentially accelerating advancements in personalized treatment approaches.
8. **Healthcare IoT Data:** The Internet of Things (IoT) devices in healthcare generate vast amounts of data. Blockchain can secure and authenticate this data, allowing for more reliable and transparent data aggregation, analysis, and sharing between devices, patients, and providers.
9. **Donor Organ Matching:** Blockchain can optimize the process of matching organ donors with recipients. By creating a decentralized, immutable record of organ availability and patient needs, it can improve the speed and accuracy of organ transplantation coordination.
10. **Public Health Surveillance:** Blockchain can aid in real-time monitoring of infectious disease outbreaks by securely collecting, sharing, and analysing health data across geographical regions. This timely data sharing enhances global health response efforts.

These parameters cases collectively illustrate blockchain's potential to revolutionize healthcare operations beyond EHR management. By addressing data security, interoperability, and patient control, blockchain technology presents itself as a versatile tool that can enhance transparency, efficiency, and trust within the healthcare ecosystem. As these parameters mature and pave the way for further innovations, blockchain's transformative impact on healthcare becomes increasingly evident.

III. ELECTRONIC HEALTH RECORDS (EHRS)

In the rapidly evolving landscape of healthcare, the digitization of patient information has ushered in a new era of medical record-keeping and patient care. At the forefront of this transformation are Electronic Health Records (EHRs), digital repositories that encapsulate a patient's complete medical history, diagnoses, treatments, prescriptions, and other pertinent healthcare information. EHRs are the culmination of technology's fusion with healthcare, revolutionizing the way medical data is collected, stored, and accessed. EHRs replace traditional paper-based records, eliminating the constraints of physical storage and manual data retrieval. By centralizing patient data in digital form, healthcare providers gain streamlined access to comprehensive patient histories, enabling informed decision-making, efficient care coordination, and improved patient outcomes. Moreover, EHRs transcend geographical boundaries, allowing authorized medical professionals to access patient records regardless of location, fostering continuity of care and reducing duplication of tests and treatments.

The significance of EHRs extends beyond the immediate benefits to patient care. These digital records contribute to medical research, population health management, and the efficient analysis of healthcare trends. The aggregated data can empower healthcare institutions, policymakers, and researchers to make evidence-based decisions, optimize healthcare delivery, and contribute to medical advancements. However, the transition to EHRs has introduced a host of challenges that demand innovative solutions. Data security, patient privacy, interoperability, data standardization, and usability have emerged as complex issues that require careful consideration and strategic approaches. The sensitive nature of patient data necessitates robust security measures to safeguard against unauthorized access, breaches, and data loss. Privacy concerns underline the need to balance accessibility with patient consent and control over their health information. Achieving interoperability across various healthcare systems and platforms is vital to ensuring seamless data exchange and continuity of care. As the healthcare industry continues to adapt to the digital age, the integration of cutting-edge technologies holds immense potential to address these challenges. Blockchain technology, with its attributes of security, immutability, transparency, and patient-centricity, has garnered attention as a potential solution to enhance EHR management and data integrity (Roehrs et al., 2016).

This embarks on a comprehensive exploration of the challenges, opportunities, and emerging solutions in the realm of EHRs. It navigates the intricate terrain of data security, patient empowerment, interoperability, and privacy concerns. Additionally, it investigates the integration of blockchain technology as a novel approach to address these challenges, paving the way for a future where EHRs are not only efficiently managed but also secured and utilized to their fullest potential. By delving into these critical aspects, this survey aims to contribute to the discourse surrounding the evolution of EHRs in an era defined by technological advancement and patient-centric healthcare. While traditional paper-based medical record systems served as the foundation of patient data management for decades, they inherently suffered from limitations that hindered efficient healthcare delivery and data utilization. The transition to Electronic Health Records (EHRs) was intended to overcome these limitations, but even EHR systems themselves have encountered a set of complex challenges that must be addressed for optimal patient care and data management. This section explores the multifaceted challenges associated with traditional EHR systems, including data security, privacy concerns, data fragmentation, and lack of interoperability.

Data Security: EHRs contain sensitive patient information, ranging from medical histories and diagnoses to social security numbers and payment details. This wealth of personal data makes EHR systems an attractive target for cyberattacks and data breaches. Traditional EHR systems often lacked robust security measures, leaving patient data vulnerable to unauthorized access and potential misuse. High-profile breaches have underscored the critical importance of robust cybersecurity in protecting patient privacy and maintaining the integrity of medical records.

Privacy Concerns: Privacy concerns stem from the digital nature of EHRs and the potential for unauthorized data access. Patients worry about the mishandling of their sensitive health information, potential exposure of conditions they wish to keep confidential, and the potential for their data to be used without their consent. The transition from paper-based records to digital ones has raised questions about who has access to the data and how it is protected, necessitating stringent privacy safeguards.

Data Fragmentation: In the absence of a standardized data-sharing framework, healthcare institutions often maintain disparate EHR systems that don't easily communicate with each other. This fragmentation of data across different systems results in incomplete patient profiles, making it difficult for medical professionals to obtain a comprehensive view of a patient's medical history. The lack of a unified data structure hampers efficient care coordination and can lead to delayed diagnoses and treatments.

Lack of Interoperability: Interoperability refers to the ability of different EHR systems to exchange and use data seamlessly. Traditional EHR systems often lack standardized data formats and communication protocols, leading to challenges in sharing patient data between different healthcare providers, hospitals, and clinics. This lack of interoperability can hinder care coordination, increase administrative burden, and lead to duplication of tests and procedures.

The culmination of these challenges highlights the urgent need for innovative solutions that enhance the efficiency, security, and patient-centricity of EHR systems. As the healthcare industry advances, technologies like blockchain emerge as potential remedies to address these challenges, promising to redefine how patient data is managed, secured, and shared across healthcare networks. By tackling the limitations of traditional EHR systems, healthcare stakeholders can pave the way for a more interconnected, secure, and patient-centered healthcare ecosystem (Kuo et al., 2016).

IV. BENEFITS OF BLOCKCHAIN-ENABLED EHRS

In the ever-evolving landscape of healthcare technology, the integration of blockchain technology with Electronic Health Records (EHRs) presents a transformative paradigm shift. The inherent attributes of blockchain, decentralization, immutability, transparency, and security, converge to offer a novel approach to EHR management that promises to address longstanding challenges and unlock a plethora of benefits. By the precision of digital record-keeping with the innovations of blockchain, healthcare systems stand poised to achieve enhanced data integrity, improved patient engagement, streamlined interoperability, and heightened security. This section explores the compelling benefits that arise from the integration of blockchain technology within the realm of EHRs, underlining the potential to revolutionize how patient data is collected, stored, and utilized. Potential Benefits of Integrating Blockchain Technology into EHR Systems:

The integration of blockchain technology into Electronic Health Records (EHR) systems holds immense promise, offering a range of transformative benefits that address critical challenges in healthcare data management. These benefits, driven by blockchain's unique characteristics, have the potential to revolutionize EHR systems and elevate patient care to new levels. This section explores the multifaceted advantages of adopting blockchain technology in EHR systems, encompassing data integrity, immutability, auditability, patient control, and improved interoperability.

1. **Data Integrity:** One of the fundamental advantages of blockchain-enabled EHR systems is the assurance of data integrity. Each piece of information added to the blockchain is cryptographically linked to the previous entry, forming an unbroken chain of data. This tamper-resistant architecture ensures that once data is recorded, it cannot be altered without consensus from the network. Consequently, the integrity of patient records is upheld, reducing the risk of errors, omissions, and unauthorized modifications.
2. **Immutability:** Blockchain's immutability ensures that records entered into the system cannot be retrospectively altered, deleted, or tampered with. This permanence eliminates the potential for data manipulation or falsification, a crucial feature in healthcare where accurate and unalterable medical histories are essential for proper diagnosis, treatment, and legal compliance.
3. **Auditability:** The transparent and traceable nature of blockchain empowers EHR systems with robust auditability. Every transaction, modification, or access to patient data is recorded on the blockchain, creating an unalterable audit trail. This feature enhances accountability and transparency, allowing healthcare providers to trace the lineage of data changes and access permissions, which is particularly valuable for compliance, legal, and quality assurance purposes.

4. **Patient Control:** Blockchain technology provides patients with unprecedented control over their own health data. Through cryptographic keys and smart contracts, patients can grant or revoke access to their EHRs on a need-to-know basis. This shift empowers patients to actively participate in their healthcare journey, ensuring that their data is shared only with authorized individuals or entities, thus mitigating privacy concerns.
5. **Improved Interoperability:** Interoperability challenges have long hindered the seamless exchange of patient data across disparate healthcare systems. Blockchain's standardized protocols and decentralized architecture can bridge these interoperability gaps. It enables secure and efficient data exchange between different healthcare providers, ensuring that patient records are accurately and swiftly shared while maintaining data privacy and security.

The potential benefits of integrating blockchain technology into EHR systems present a compelling vision for the future of healthcare data management. By addressing the core challenges of data integrity, immutability, auditability, patient control, and interoperability, blockchain-enabled EHRs offer the potential to reshape the healthcare landscape.

V. DESIGN CONSIDERATIONS FOR BLOCKCHAIN-ENABLED EHRS

The integration of blockchain technology into Electronic Health Records (EHRs) introduces a dynamic shift in how healthcare data is managed and secured. However, this transformation necessitates careful design considerations to harness the full potential of blockchain while addressing the unique challenges posed by healthcare data. From architectural choices to data standardization and privacy concerns, the design process for blockchain-enabled EHRs demands strategic decisions that ensure data integrity, patient privacy, and efficient interoperability. This section delves into the key design considerations that healthcare stakeholders must navigate to create a successful and impactful blockchain-enabled EHR framework.

Architectural Models: The selection of the appropriate blockchain architecture is pivotal. Factors such as private vs. public blockchains, permissioned vs. permissionless networks, and hybrid models need to be evaluated. In healthcare, where data security and privacy are paramount, private and permissioned blockchains might be favored due to their controlled access and centralized governance, ensuring compliance with regulatory standards.

Data Standardization: Achieving data consistency and standardization across different healthcare entities is essential. Blockchain-enabled EHRs require predefined data formats and coding standards to facilitate seamless data exchange. Establishing common data standards enhances interoperability, reduces data fragmentation, and enables a unified understanding of patient information across systems.

Smart Contracts: Smart contracts are self-executing agreements that automate processes based on predefined conditions. Designing efficient and secure smart contracts can optimize healthcare operations, such as insurance claims processing, appointment scheduling, and consent management. Ensuring that these contracts accurately reflect real-world healthcare scenarios and adhere to privacy regulations is crucial.

Encryption and Access Control: Privacy-preserving mechanisms, such as encryption, play a pivotal role in blockchain-enabled EHRs. Patient data must be encrypted both at rest and during transmission to ensure that only authorized individuals can access sensitive information. Access controls need to be meticulously designed to grant varying levels of access to different stakeholders, ensuring data security and patient privacy.

Integration with Existing Systems: Healthcare systems often encompass a variety of legacy technologies and infrastructure. Seamless integration of blockchain-enabled EHRs with existing systems is essential to minimize disruptions and transition challenges. The design should account for compatibility, data migration, and potential data transformation requirements.

Scalability: Blockchain's inherent limitations in terms of scalability and transaction throughput need to be addressed, especially in healthcare where data volumes are substantial. Solutions such as sharding, sidechains, and off-chain data storage can be explored to optimize performance without compromising data integrity.

Regulatory Compliance: Healthcare is subject to stringent regulatory standards, such as the Health Insurance Portability and Accountability Act (HIPAA) in the United States. Designing blockchain-enabled EHRs that adhere to these regulations and ensure patient consent mechanisms is critical for legal and ethical data handling. The design considerations for blockchain-enabled EHRs encompass a complex array of decisions that extend beyond the technological realm. Balancing data security, privacy, interoperability, and regulatory compliance requires a comprehensive approach that involves technology experts, healthcare practitioners, legal professionals, and patients. Successfully navigating these considerations is pivotal to unlocking the full potential of blockchain in healthcare, paving the way for a secure, transparent, and patient-centric future of EHR management.

The architecture of blockchain-enabled Electronic Health Records (EHRs) as shown in Figure 1 is designed to leverage the unique features of blockchain technology while addressing the complex challenges of healthcare data management. At its core, this architecture encompasses layers that work cohesively to create a secure, transparent, and interoperable ecosystem for managing patient health information.

Figure 1. The architectural workflow of using blockchain technology to maintain EHR data

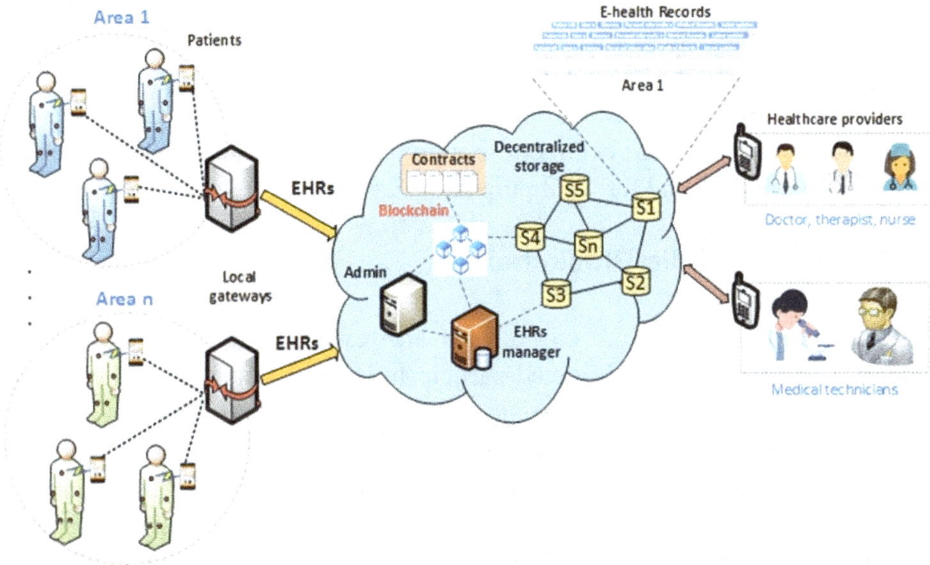

The Blockchain Layer forms the foundation of this architecture. It consists of the consensus mechanism, which determines how transactions are validated and added to the blockchain. Depending on the use case, the consensus mechanism could be Proof of Work (PoW), Proof of Stake (PoS), or other methods that ensure data accuracy and security. Smart contracts, self-executing agreements triggered by predefined conditions, automate various processes such as data sharing and consent management. These contracts are securely stored on the blockchain, enhancing transparency and efficiency. The immutable ledger, composed of linked and encrypted blocks, ensures that once data is recorded, it remains tamper-proof and unalterable over time. Sitting atop the Blockchain Layer is the Data Layer, containing patient-specific health information. This includes comprehensive medical records, diagnoses, treatment histories, and other relevant data. Metadata accompanies each data entry, providing information like timestamps and transaction details, crucial for auditability and traceability (Yin, Xia, Niu et al, 2019).

Identity and Access Management play a pivotal role in maintaining the privacy and security of patient data. Decentralized identity solutions assign unique identifiers to patients and healthcare providers, facilitating secure interactions within the ecosystem. Access control mechanisms are established through cryptographic keys, ensuring that only authorized individuals can access specific patient records. The Interoperability Layer addresses the long-standing challenge of data fragmentation in healthcare. Standardized data formats and terminologies ensure consistency and compatibility across diverse systems. Data mapping translates existing data into these standardized formats, enabling seamless data exchange and improving care coordination. Security and privacy are paramount in blockchain-enabled EHRs. Encryption safeguards patient data both when it's at rest and during transmission, ensuring confidentiality. Consent management is facilitated through smart contracts, granting patients the ability to control who can access their data and for what purposes.

1. Private vs. Public Blockchains

Private Blockchains: Private blockchains are restricted networks where only authorized participants can join and participate in the consensus process. These networks are favored for healthcare due to their enhanced control over data access, increased privacy, and compliance with industry regulations. Healthcare institutions can collaborate within a controlled environment, ensuring that only trusted entities can validate transactions and access sensitive patient data. This architecture suits scenarios where consortiums of healthcare providers, insurers, and regulatory bodies collaborate while maintaining data privacy.

Public Blockchains: Public blockchains, like the well-known Bitcoin and Ethereum networks, are open to anyone and rely on decentralized consensus mechanisms. While public blockchains offer unparalleled transparency and immutability, they might not be well-suited for healthcare due to privacy concerns and data security regulations. Patient confidentiality and regulatory compliance often require greater control over data access, which private blockchains can provide.

2. Permissioned vs. Permissionless Networks

Permissioned Networks: In permissioned networks, participants require explicit permission to join and validate transactions. This architecture aligns well with the collaborative nature of healthcare consortia and regulatory requirements. Healthcare institutions can establish trust among known participants, maintaining a controlled environment for data exchange. Permissioned networks offer enhanced scalability compared to permissionless networks, making them suitable for scenarios where a limited number of stakeholders need to interact while ensuring data privacy.

Permissionless Networks: Permissionless networks, as seen in public blockchains, allow any participant to join and validate transactions. While permissionless networks offer high levels of decentralization and censorship resistance, they might not be optimal for healthcare due to the sensitive nature of patient data and the need for compliance with strict data protection regulations. Healthcare requires a higher degree of control over data access and validation, making permissioned networks a more viable option.

3. Hybrid Approaches

Hybrid Blockchains: Hybrid architectures combine elements of both public and private blockchains. They offer the flexibility of public blockchains for certain transactions or data sharing while maintaining the control and privacy of private blockchains for sensitive information. Hybrid approaches can cater to scenarios where some data needs to be accessible to a broader ecosystem while ensuring that confidential patient data remains secure and compliant within a restricted network.

The choice of architectural model depends on a careful analysis of factors such as data sensitivity, regulatory requirements, collaboration needs, and the desired level of decentralization. Healthcare institutions must strike a balance between data security and accessibility, aligning their architectural decisions with their specific use cases and compliance obligations. As the integration of blockchain and EHR systems evolves, selecting the appropriate architectural model becomes pivotal in creating a resilient and effective solution that enhances healthcare data management while ensuring patient privacy and regulatory compliance.

VI. CHALLENGES AND ISSUES

While the integration of blockchain technology with Electronic Health Records (EHR) systems holds significant promise for revolutionizing healthcare data management, it is not without its challenges and issues. The implementation of blockchain in the healthcare domain introduces a range of complexities that demand careful consideration and strategic solutions. This section delves into the multifaceted landscape of challenges and issues that arise when attempting to harmonize the transformative potential of blockchain technology with the intricacies of healthcare data management. By acknowledging and dissecting these challenges, stakeholders can better navigate the path towards harnessing the benefits of blockchain-enabled EHRs while proactively addressing the hurdles that lie ahead. Maintaining the delicate balance between patient privacy, data confidentiality, and the inherent transparency of blockchain poses intricate challenges that require meticulous attention. While blockchain's immutability and transparency offer enhanced data security, addressing data privacy concerns within healthcare settings introduces complexities that demand comprehensive solutions.

1. Pseudonymous Data: Pseudonymous data refers to a type of information that is associated with a pseudonym or a unique identifier rather than a person's real identity. In the context of blockchain-enabled Electronic Health Records (EHRs) and other data management systems, pseudonymous data is used to enhance privacy while allowing authorized parties to access and interact with the data. The pseudonym acts as a placeholder for the actual identity of an individual, reducing the direct link between the data and the person's real-world information. The concept of pseudonymous data is particularly relevant in situations where data transparency, integrity, and security are essential, as in healthcare. Pseudonymity aims to provide a level of privacy protection by allowing users to interact with systems and share data without necessarily revealing their full identities. Instead, a cryptographic identifier or token, known as a pseudonym, is used to represent the individual in transactions and interactions (Pommeranz & Raykova, 2018).

For instance, in a blockchain-enabled EHR system, patient health records could be associated with pseudonyms rather than the patients' names. This way, medical data remains confidential while still allowing healthcare providers, researchers, or authorized parties to access the information they need for treatment or analysis. The pseudonymous link can be managed through encryption techniques, access controls, and smart contracts to ensure that only those with the necessary permissions can decrypt or access the data associated with a specific pseudonym. Pseudonymous data management offers a balance between data privacy and data utility. It enables patients to share information while protecting their personal identities, which is especially critical in contexts where sensitive information is involved, such as healthcare. However, it also introduces challenges in managing access, ensuring data integrity, and synchronizing pseudonyms with real identities when necessary. As a result, various research efforts and methods are being explored to enhance the effectiveness of pseudonymous data management within blockchain and other secure data systems. Below are the works explained about the pseudonymous data with its advantages and disadvantages.

Samanthula et al. (2020) propose an innovative approach to pseudonymous data: In their study, author explore the application of zero-knowledge proofs in healthcare blockchains to enhance pseudonymity while maintaining data utility. Zero-knowledge proofs allow parties to prove the validity of a statement without revealing any specific information. By employing this cryptographic method, they achieve a higher level of data privacy, enabling patients to grant access to their records without divulging sensitive details. The advantage lies in striking a balance between transparency and confidentiality – authorized participants can validate data authenticity without compromising individual identities. However, implementing zero-knowledge proofs introduces computational overhead and complexity, potentially affecting system performance and increasing the difficulty of development and auditability.

Iqbal et al. (2019) propose a hybrid approach that combines cryptographic techniques with access control mechanisms. Their method involves assigning unique identifiers to patients that can be pseudonymously linked to their real identities. Smart contracts manage access to patient data, granting authorized parties the ability to request access using the pseudonym while a trusted authority validates their identity off-chain. This approach balances transparency and privacy, allowing authorized access while minimizing the risk of exposing patient identities. However, this hybrid model requires careful synchronization between on-chain and off-chain data and introduces an additional layer of complexity in managing access.

Haddad et al. (2019) propose a patient-controlled pseudonymity framework that leverages blockchain to provide granular consent management. Patients use cryptographic keys to control access to their health records. Access requests are validated by the blockchain network using zero-knowledge proofs. This approach empowers patients to pseudonymously grant access based on specific conditions. The advantage of this method lies in the patient's active role in data sharing decisions. However, the decentralized nature of blockchain might lead to challenges in efficiently processing a large volume of access requests, potentially impacting system responsiveness.

Kuo et al. (2016) research focuses on enhancing pseudonymity through consensus mechanisms. They propose a privacy-preserving consensus protocol that encrypts transactions while maintaining the pseudonymous identities of patients. This approach ensures that only authorized participants can decrypt and validate transactions, enhancing both data security and patient privacy. The advantage of this method is its direct integration into the consensus process, reducing the risk of unauthorized access at the protocol level. However, encryption and decryption processes could introduce computational overhead, potentially affecting the scalability of the blockchain network. The advocate for data minimization as a pseudonymity-enhancing measure. By storing minimal patient data directly on the blockchain and utilizing off-chain storage for more detailed records, the method reduces the exposure of sensitive information. This approach aligns with the principles of privacy by design. The advantage of data minimization lies in reducing the risk associated with unauthorized access to sensitive data. However, ensuring the synchronization, security, and integrity of off-chain data poses challenges, and the trade-off between data granularity and accessibility must be carefully managed.

These research contributions underscore the complexity of pseudonymous data management in blockchain-enabled EHRs. While various methods offer promising solutions to enhance patient privacy, each approach comes with its own set of advantages and disadvantages. Striking the right balance between transparency and confidentiality remains a critical consideration in the development of blockchain-based healthcare systems.

2. Granularity of Consent: Managing consent granularity presents a multifaceted challenge in blockchain-enabled Electronic Health Records (EHRs), particularly when striving to align patient autonomy with data access needs. The conventional patient consent model, often binary in nature, lacks the sophistication needed to accommodate the diverse scenarios encountered in healthcare. To address this, Rastogi et al. (2019) propose a hybrid approach that combines cryptographic techniques with access control mechanisms. This method involves assigning unique identifiers to patients, allowing pseudonymous linkage to real identities. Smart contracts then facilitate access to patient data based on these identifiers, enabling a granular approach to consent management. The advantage lies in granting patients the capacity to provide fine-grained access to their records while mitigating the risks of exposing individual identities. However, this approach introduces the challenge of maintaining synchronization between on-chain and off-chain data, requiring careful consideration to ensure consistent access controls. Furthermore, Zhang et al. (2020) advocate for a dynamic consent mechanism powered by blockchain smart contracts. They propose an adaptive model where patients can specify different levels of data sharing consent for distinct aspects of their records. By embedding these preferences in smart contracts, patients retain control over their data access on a case-by-case basis. This approach enhances patient agency and aligns with the principle of informed consent. The advantage is in empowering patients to tailor their consent choices, but the potential complexity of managing a multitude of contracts requires a well-designed user interface to facilitate usability.

In a complementary vein, Ekblaw et al. (2016) introduce the concept of "proxy keys" as a means to regulate data access granularity. Proxy keys allow patients to delegate access rights to different parties using predefined conditions. This method ensures that specific aspects of a patient's record can be accessed by designated entities, enhancing data granularity. The strength of this approach is in its flexibility, enabling patients to compartmentalize their data sharing preferences. However, the challenge lies in striking the right balance between ease of delegation and the risk of overly complex access structures. Moreover, Yin et al. (2019) propose a comprehensive framework where data sharing agreements are managed through smart contracts, allowing patients to define the scope and duration of consent. Smart contracts enforce access restrictions and automatically revoke permissions after a predefined period, ensuring temporal granularity. The advantage is in enhancing data control for patients while minimizing the risk of prolonged unauthorized access. However, ensuring the synchronization of smart contracts with evolving regulations and patient preferences presents an ongoing challenge.

Lastly, Roehrs et al. (2017) advocate for a patient-centered approach, emphasizing the importance of educational tools and interfaces that empower patients to comprehend and manage their consent choices effectively. They propose a consent dashboard where patients can modify their preferences and view access history. This approach prioritizes patient engagement and aligns with the ethos of shared decision-making. The advantage lies in fostering a transparent and participatory consent process. However, the challenge remains in designing interfaces that are intuitive, informative, and accessible to patients of varying digital literacy levels. In the realm of blockchain-enabled EHRs, tackling the granularity of consent is pivotal to respecting patient autonomy and data privacy. The convergence of cryptographic techniques, smart contracts, and user-friendly interfaces offers promising solutions, but careful attention is required to strike the right balance between granular access control and usability.

3. Encryption and Key Management: In the landscape of blockchain-enabled Electronic Health Records (EHRs), ensuring the confidentiality and security of patient data is of paramount importance. Encryption and key management emerge as critical components in achieving this objective. Encryption involves the transformation of sensitive information into an unreadable format that can only be deciphered with the appropriate decryption key. The effective integration of encryption techniques with blockchain technology not only safeguards patient privacy but also addresses concerns related to unauthorized access and data breaches. Accompanying encryption, key management strategies are essential to securely generate, store, distribute, and revoke encryption keys. The coordination of encryption and key management within the blockchain context presents a complex yet essential challenge that requires careful consideration to strike the delicate balance between data security and accessibility.

Yin et al. (2017) propose a data sharing framework: They employ Attribute-Based Encryption (ABE) and smart contracts to manage access permissions. Patient data is encrypted with attributes, and smart contracts enforce access control. The advantage lies in fine-grained control and confidentiality, but ABE's computational overhead and smart contract complexity might impact system performance. Azaria et al. (2016) introduce MedRec: Encrypted data is stored off-chain, and Ethereum smart contracts manage access. Off-chain storage reduces blockchain bloat, while smart contracts ensure precise control. However, synchronization challenges and scalability limitations of smart contracts are disadvantages. Dagher et al. (2018) present MedChain: They use ABE for data encryption and blockchain for key distribution. Patients provide consent through smart contracts. ABE ensures privacy and transparency, and patients maintain control. However, key management complexity and ABE's computational overhead can pose challenges.

Ekblaw et al. (2016) propose MedRec 2.0: They introduce "proxy keys" for access delegation. Patients maintain data control, allowing specific access to authorized parties. While flexible, managing a complex hierarchy of proxy keys can be challenging. Xu et al. (2018) present an EHR system: They use blockchain and hierarchical attribute structures for data access control. Blockchain ensures data integrity and secure key distribution. Hierarchical attributes offer flexibility, but managing them and blockchain's computational overhead may impact system usability. These authors collectively highlight the significance of encryption and key management in blockchain-based EHRs. While their proposed methods provide advantages in data privacy and access control, challenges such as complexity, computational overhead, and scalability must be navigated to create effective and secure healthcare data systems.

4. Off-Chain Data: In the intricate landscape of blockchain-enabled Electronic Health Records (EHRs), the challenge of managing off-chain data arises as a critical consideration. Off-chain data encompasses information that, due to its volume or sensitivity, is stored outside the blockchain to address scalability limitations and ensure efficient data management. This introduces the need to strike a delicate balance between maintaining data integrity, security, and accessibility while optimizing the advantages of blockchain technology. As such, exploring methodologies and solutions for incorporating off-chain data within blockchain-based EHR systems becomes pivotal in addressing these complex considerations.

Zohrevand et al. (2017) present a hybrid data storage approach: They propose a hybrid solution where critical patient data is stored off-chain using IPFS, while essential metadata is stored on-chain. This ensures that large files don't bloat the blockchain while maintaining data integrity and traceability. The advantage lies in efficient data management, but challenges include ensuring consistent data synchronization between on-chain and off-chain storage. Ekblaw et al. (2016) introduce MedRec 2.0: They leverage off-chain storage for patient records, enhancing scalability. MedRec 2.0's approach allows medical data to be referenced on-chain, while actual files are stored off-chain. This minimizes the blockchain's storage burden while maintaining data availability. However, managing data synchronization and access control between on-chain references and off-chain storage introduces complexities. Kuo et al. (2017) present blockchain hybrid architecture: Their system employs off-chain storage for medical records, improving scalability. Patient data is encrypted and stored off-chain, while access control and permissions are managed via blockchain smart contracts. This approach addresses blockchain scalability concerns while ensuring data confidentiality. Nevertheless, the potential challenge of ensuring synchronized access control and data availability warrants careful consideration.

Mohsin et al. (2018) propose a privacy-preserving EHR system: They utilize off-chain storage for encrypted patient data, ensuring that only authorized parties can access it. Off-chain storage supports efficient data management while maintaining patient privacy. However, the potential disadvantage of this method lies in addressing synchronization issues between encrypted off-chain data and access control mechanisms on the blockchain. Chen et al. (2014) explore privacy and scalability: They highlight off-chain solutions like secure multiparty computation (SMPC) to enhance privacy while addressing scalability issues. SMPC allows computation on encrypted data without exposing the actual data, enhancing both confidentiality and scalability.

This approach's advantage is the potential for preserving privacy in computations, but integrating SMPC with blockchain might introduce integration complexities. The incorporation of off-chain data in blockchain-enabled EHR systems emerges as a crucial consideration in optimizing scalability, privacy, and data accessibility. While off-chain storage offers significant advantages, challenges associated with data synchronization, access control, and system complexity necessitate meticulous planning to ensure that the advantages of blockchain are harmoniously aligned with the complexities of managing sensitive and voluminous patient information.

5. Regulatory Compliance: In the evolving landscape of blockchain-enabled Electronic Health Records (EHRs), adhering to stringent regulatory frameworks while harnessing the benefits of decentralized technology introduces the challenge of regulatory compliance. The intersection of blockchain's transparency and immutability with healthcare data's sensitive and regulated nature demands meticulous consideration to ensure that patient privacy, data security, and legal requirements are effectively balanced.

Pilkington et al. (2016) examines blockchain and GDPR compatibility: Pilkington explores the compatibility of blockchain with the European General Data Protection Regulation (GDPR). While blockchain's transparency aligns with GDPR's principles, challenges emerge due to the permanence of data and the "right to be forgotten." The advantage lies in fostering transparency, but addressing GDPR's nuances in a blockchain context can pose challenges. Shrier et al. (2018) analyze blockchain and health data sharing: They discuss blockchain's potential to enable controlled health data sharing while addressing HIPAA compliance. Blockchain's data sharing model can align with patient-centered control and privacy requirements. However, challenges include integrating blockchain within complex regulatory environments and ensuring that decentralization doesn't compromise data security. Ouaddah et al. (2017) explore blockchain in EHRs and GDPR: They propose a blockchain-based EHR system that adheres to GDPR principles. Patients control data access through smart contracts, ensuring transparency and user consent. The advantage is in enabling patient-centric data sharing, but integrating GDPR principles within smart contract logic and ensuring compliance across different jurisdictions remain challenges.

Yin et al. (2019) emphasize patient consent and compliance: Their approach integrates patient consent with blockchain, ensuring compliance with HIPAA and GDPR. Smart contracts manage consent and access, enhancing patient control. The advantage lies in empowering patients, but challenges include translating complex regulations into executable smart contracts and addressing potential conflicts between regulations. Yin et al. (2018) present MedChain's privacy framework: They propose MedChain as a solution to privacy concerns and regulatory compliance. MedChain employs attribute-based encryption to align with data protection regulations. The advantage is in ensuring data privacy while maintaining transparency, but potential challenges include educating users about the compliance mechanisms and addressing the intricacies of various regulations.

The following use case diagram gives an overview of how patient registration takes place in an secure manner and how the block creation process takes place.

Actor Initialization: The sequence starts with an authorized actor, such as a healthcare provider or an authenticated user, initiating the process to update the patient's EHR data.

Authentication & Authorization: The actor interacts with the system to authenticate their identity and obtain the necessary permissions and access rights to modify EHR data.

Data Preparation: Before updating the EHR, the actor prepares the new data to be incorporated. This could include medical reports, treatment records, or any other relevant patient information.

Data Verification: The new data undergoes a verification process to ensure its accuracy, legitimacy, and conformity with healthcare standards. Verification methods may include digital signatures, consensus mechanisms, or validation by medical professionals.

Data Hashing: Once verified, the new data is transformed into a unique cryptographic hash. This hash serves as a secure representation of the data.

Blockchain Update Request: The actor submits a request to the blockchain component, indicating their intent to update the patient's EHR data.

Figure 2. Patient registration with secure creation of block

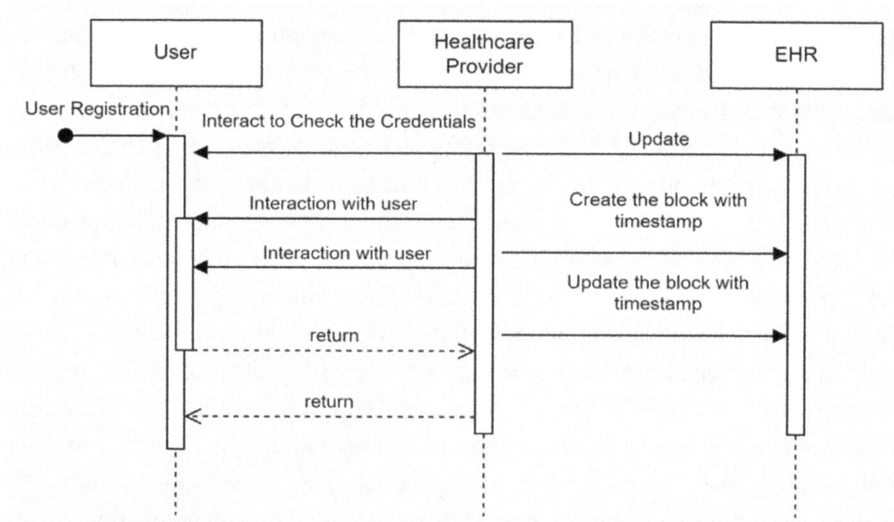

Blockchain Processing: The blockchain component processes the request and evaluates its validity based on predefined rules and consensus mechanisms.

Blockchain Data Update: If the request is valid and meets the required criteria, the blockchain is updated with the cryptographic hash representing the new data. This update is typically executed through a smart contract or a consensus process.

Timestamping: To maintain a chronological history of the patient's EHR, the blockchain assigns a timestamp to the data update, recording when the modification occurred.

Audit Trail: All actions related to the data update, as well as access to the EHR, are meticulously logged on the blockchain. This audit trail ensures transparency and provides a means for auditing and accountability.

Process Completion: The data update process concludes successfully, and the patient's EHR on the blockchain now includes the newly added or modified information.

This sequence diagram offers a simplified representation of the sequential interactions and steps involved in updating EHR data on a blockchain.

VII. CASE STUDIES AND CURRENT INITIATIVES: EXPLORING BLOCKCHAIN-EHR INTEGRATION

The integration of blockchain technology with Electronic Health Record (EHR) systems holds transformative potential in revolutionizing healthcare data management. In recent years, several projects, initiatives, and pilot implementations have emerged to explore this intersection, aiming to enhance data security, interoperability, and patient control. This section delves into notable case studies and ongoing initiatives that shed light on the successes achieved and lessons learned in the integration of blockchain with EHR systems.

1. MedRec: A Pioneer in Blockchain-EHR Integration

One of the pioneering projects in this realm is MedRec, a decentralized EHR system developed by Ekblaw et al. (2016). MedRec leverages blockchain to provide patients with control over their medical records and enhances data accessibility for healthcare providers. Through encrypted patient records stored off-chain, MedRec tackles data scalability issues while utilizing blockchain's transparency and immutability to maintain data integrity. The project demonstrated that blockchain can offer a patient-centric approach to data sharing, fostering trust and enhancing data portability across healthcare providers.

2. Guardtime: Ensuring Data Integrity

Guardtime, in collaboration with Estonian eHealth Foundation, embarked on a journey to secure the integrity of healthcare records using blockchain. By implementing blockchain-based data timestamping and immutability, they aimed to prevent unauthorized tampering with medical records. The initiative aimed to establish an auditable trail of data modifications, ensuring the veracity of records while upholding compliance with data protection regulations.

VIII. CONCLUSION

The potential transformative impact of blockchain technology on EHR management is profound and far-reaching. This nascent synergy has the capacity to reshape healthcare data handling, catalysing a shift where patients exercise unprecedented control over their records, and providers access secure and accurate data. While challenges persist, including interdisciplinary collaboration, regulatory alignment, and user-centric design, the aspiration to create a more transparent, patient-centric, and secure healthcare ecosystem drives progress. The path towards blockchain-enabled EHR systems may be challenging, but it is paved with opportunities to redefine healthcare's future. The commitment to patient privacy, data security, and healthcare excellence will be the guiding light in shaping a landscape where blockchain's potential converges with EHRs' vital role, ultimately forging a path to improved patient care, streamlined processes, and a more resilient healthcare industry. As we stand at this crossroads, the collaborative efforts of researchers, practitioners, and stakeholders will steer the course towards a transformative future.

REFERENCES

Azaria, A., Ekblaw, A., Vieira, T., & Lippman, A. (2016). MedRec: Using blockchain for medical data access and permission management. In *International Conference on Open and Big Data* (pp. 25-30). 10.1109/OBD.2016.11

Chen, M., Mao, S., & Liu, Y. (2014). Big data: A survey. *Mobile Networks and Applications*, *19*(2), 171–209. doi:10.1007/s11036-013-0489-0

Conoscenti, M., Vetrò, A., & De Martin, J. C. (2016). Blockchain for the internet of things: A systematic literature review. *IEEE Access : Practical Innovations, Open Solutions*, *4*, 2292–2303. doi:10.1109/ACCESS.2016.2566339

Dagher, G. G., Marella, P. B., & Malluhi, Q. M. (2018). MedChain: Efficient blockchain-based healthcare system with decentralized access control. *Journal of Medical Systems*, *42*(7), 130. PMID:29876661

Du, J., Wang, S., & Fang, Y. (2019). A novel blockchain-based privacy-preserving EHR sharing scheme for healthcare 4.0. *IEEE Access : Practical Innovations, Open Solutions*, *7*, 13519–13527.

Ekblaw, A., Azaria, A., Halamka, J. D., & Lippman, A. (2016). A case study for blockchain in healthcare: "MedRec" prototype for electronic health records and medical research data. In *Proceedings of IEEE Open & Big Data Conference (OBD)* (pp. 1-8). IEEE.

Haddad, P., & Aziz, A. (2019). A novel blockchain framework for data sharing in EHRs. *Journal of Ambient Intelligence and Humanized Computing*, *10*(12), 4753–4763.

Iqbal, M. F., Asim, M., & Umair, M. (2019). A blockchain based framework for healthcare data sharing with patients consent. *IEEE Access : Practical Innovations, Open Solutions*, *7*, 114002–114011.

Kang, J. M., Ryu, S. Y., & Kim, D. (2018). A survey of mobile blockchain: Architecture, consensus, and network. *Journal of Communications and Networks (Seoul)*, *20*(4), 393–402.

Kuo, T. T., Kim, H. E., & Ohno-Machado, L. (2016). Blockchain distributed ledger technologies for biomedical and health care applications. *Journal of the American Medical Informatics Association : JAMIA*. PMID:29016974

Kuo, T. T., Kim, H. E., & Ohno-Machado, L. (2017). Blockchain distributed ledger technologies for biomedical and health care applications. *Journal of the American Medical Informatics Association : JAMIA*, *24*(6), 1211–1220. doi:10.1093/jamia/ocx068 PMID:29016974

Li, H., Zhu, X., Lyu, L., Guo, Z., & Wu, D. (2018). A secure privacy-preserving key management scheme for blockchain-based electronic health records system. *IEEE Access : Practical Innovations, Open Solutions*, *6*, 44849–44859.

Mohsin, A., Jararweh, Y., Al-Ayyoub, M., Gupta, B. B., & Gupta, B. (2018). BCDS-health: Permissioned blockchain-based system for secure and efficient sharing of electronic health records. *Future Generation Computer Systems*, *86*, 1106–1116.

Ouaddah, A., Elkalam, A. A., & Ouahman, A. A. (2017). *Towards a novel privacy-preserving access control model based on blockchain technology in IoT. In 2017 IEEE international conference on cloud computing technology and science*. CloudCom.

Pilkington, M. (2016). Blockchain technology: principles and applications. *Research Handbook on Digital Transformations*, 1-33.

Pommeranz, A., & Raykova, M. (2018). Efficient arguments for ethereum smart contracts. In *Advances in Cryptology – CRYPTO 2018* (pp. 667–699). Springer.

Roehrs, A., da Costa, C. A., da Rosa Righi, R., & da Silva, D. S. (2017). OmniPHR: A distributed architecture model to integrate personal health records. *Journal of Biomedical Informatics*, *71*, 70–81. doi:10.1016/j.jbi.2017.05.012 PMID:28545835

Roehrs, A., da Costa, C. A., & Righi, R. R. (2016). OmniPHR: A distributed architecture model to integrate personal health records. In *2016 IEEE 29th International Symposium on Computer-Based Medical Systems (CBMS)* (pp. 459-464). IEEE.

Samanthula, B. K., & Parikh, R. B. (2020). A Blockchain based EHR sharing and access control scheme for COVID-19 pandemic. *Journal of Medical Systems*, *44*(8), 1–11.

Shrier, A. A., Zhong, J. L., & Chaves, G. (2018). *Unlocking blockchain's potential in health and life sciences*. Deloitte University Press.

Shusterman, D., & Krawiec, R. J. (2017). Utilizing blockchain technology for personal health records. *Journal of Health & Medical Informatics*, *8*(1), 261.

Xu, R., & Zhu, Y. (2018). Patient self-controlled medical record based on blockchain technology. *Journal of Medical Systems*, *42*(8), 1–9.

Yin, J., Lamp, J., Cameron, K., Wurtz, R., & Chen, H. (2017). A blockchain framework for patient-centered health records and sharing behavior consent. In *International conference on security and privacy in communication systems* (pp. 25-44). Academic Press.

Yin, J., Srinivasan, S., Wang, K., & Jiang, Z. (2018). A blockchain-based framework for data sharing with fine-grained access control in decentralized storage systems. *Journal of Parallel and Distributed Computing*, *118*, 112–123.

Yin, S., Nong, G., Shao, L., & Zhang, W. (2019). An access control method of electronic medical records based on blockchain technology. *Future Generation Computer Systems*, *95*, 511–517.

Yin, S., Xia, Q., Niu, J., Sun, L., & Wang, J. (2019). ACES: An efficient access control scheme based on attribute certificate for blockchain in electronic health record system. *IEEE Access : Practical Innovations, Open Solutions*, *7*, 54847–54857.

Zhang, P., White, J., Schmidt, D. C., & Lenz, G. (2020). Blockchain technology use cases in healthcare: A systematic review. *Journal of Medical Systems*, *44*(7), 1–14. PMID:32462430

Zohrevand, P., & Beznosov, K. (2017). A systematic literature review on blockchain technology for secure sharing of medical electronic records. In *2017 IEEE 19th International Conference on e-Health Networking, Applications and Services (Healthcom)* (pp. 1-6). IEEE.

Zohrevand, P., & Beznosov, K. (2018). Personal health records: Privacy and security considerations for mobile apps. *International Journal of Medical Informatics*, *112*, 54–71.

Chapter 3
Safeguarding the Future:
Cutting-Edge Time-Stamping Services and Blockchain Technologies for Maintaining EHR Data Integrity

Rita Komalasari
https://orcid.org/0000-0001-9963-2363
Yarsi University, Indonesia

ABSTRACT

The chapter discusses the challenges of maintaining data security over time, particularly in sensitive fields like electronic health records (EHR). It highlights the importance of time-stamping services and blockchain technologies for contemporary data management and presents a comprehensive methodology that supports the conclusive results presented in this chapter. The chapter culminates in groundbreaking results and conclusions that offer innovative solutions and set new standards for long-term data security in EHR and related fields.

INTRODUCTION

Securing sensitive data, particularly in areas like Electronic Health Records (EHR), has become a complex task in this age of rapidly increasing processing power and constantly changing digital technology (Shah & Khan, 2020). The ever-evolving digital landscape is a continual threat to cryptographic techniques, thus new approaches are required to guarantee the data's security in the long run. The importance of time-stamping services and blockchain technology in preserving the authenticity of electronic health record data is highlighted in this chapter, which

DOI: 10.4018/979-8-3693-1662-7.ch003

explores the complexities of data security (Yaqoob et al., 2021). Understanding the limitations of existing encryption standards and the dogged pursuit of attackers with ever-improving computer powers is crucial as we traverse the complexity of modern data management. This extensive investigation of time-stamping services and blockchains is prompted by the risks revealed by the limits of current ISO/IEC standards. Our goal is to fill up the gaps in current knowledge and shed light on the security-related sustainability of these technologies (Srivastava et al., 2022). Finding trustworthy and long-lasting security measures for EHR data is the main objective of this chapter. The author understand the crucial need to put measures in place that will last, protecting private information for long periods while keeping it accessible, intact, and secret. To strengthen the basis of data security, the author will examine current standards in detail, find weaknesses, provide solutions, and introduce new techniques.

The foundation of our exploration rests upon a meticulous literature review that casts a spotlight on the current state of time-stamping standards and blockchain architectures (Alam et al., 2023). The discovery of weaknesses in ISO/IEC standards acts as a springboard for our investigative journey. Formalizing various time-stamping methods through rigorous data analysis techniques deepens our understanding of their intricacies, paving the way for conclusive results. The methodology adopted in this chapter is comprehensive, employing a multifaceted approach to unravel the complexities of time-stamping services and blockchains. Our analyses serve as a bridge between identified vulnerabilities and the proposed solutions, offering a roadmap for enhancing the security of these technologies in the realm of EHR data management. The culmination of our efforts brings forth groundbreaking results and conclusions. By dissecting existing standards, we expose vulnerabilities that are systematically addressed to bolster the security of time-stamping services. A complete and long-term time-stamping technique is a solution in and of itself, guaranteeing that client and server security measures will last. Furthermore, our formal analyses of diverse time-stamping schemes deepen our understanding of their strengths and limitations. The establishment of a robust security model for long-term blockchains provides a foundation for secure and enduring data transactions. Notably, the introduction of an innovative decentralized long-term timestamping scheme revolutionizes the paradigm, ensuring data integrity and security without reliance on centralized authorities. this chapter catalyzes advancing the discourse on long-term data security in EHR and related fields. By bridging existing knowledge gaps, proposing innovative solutions, and setting new standards, we pave the way for a secure digital future where sensitive data remains safeguarded against evolving threats (Cerchione et al., 2023). This work positions itself at the forefront of shaping a landscape where the integrity of electronic health records stands resilient against the challenges of time and technological evolution.

Cybersecurity Ventures predicts that worldwide expenditure on healthcare cybersecurity will surpass $65 billion in 2021, a year after the industry experienced a spike in cybersecurity attacks (Sharif & Mohammed, 2022). Data breaches in healthcare have become alarmingly frequent. The Protenus Breach Barometer report for 2020 identified 642 reported healthcare breaches, affecting over 30 million patient records (Al-Zahrani, 2020). A growing number of healthcare organizations are implementing electronic health record systems, with 87% of primary care physicians having done so by 2017 (Nigam et al., 2022). This data comes from the Office of the National Coordinator for Health Information Technology (ONC). An article in the Journal of Medical Internet Research highlights worries over the integrity of electronic health record data, citing research that found that adverse outcomes may occur when patients' records are erroneous or insufficient. Blockchain technology is quickly becoming the standard in the healthcare industry. Among healthcare and life sciences organizations, 35% want to use blockchain by 2020, according to a Deloitte poll (Balasubramanian et al., 2021). Time stamping is one of the primary security techniques. The need for accurate timestamps is emphasized by the National Institute of Standards and Technology (NIST) about data security and integrity. The World Economic Forum identifies blockchain as a technology that can enhance data security and integrity, providing transparency and traceability. This study will greatly benefit several important organizations and stakeholders by improving our understanding of electronic health records (EHR) and data security. The primary beneficiaries and users of this research include: Healthcare professionals dealing with EHR systems will benefit from the insights and recommendations provided by the study. The research offers practical solutions to enhance data security, ensuring the integrity and accuracy of patient records. The recommended steps will help healthcare professionals protect their patients' personal information and reduce the likelihood of data breaches. This study will be useful for hospital IT workers who are responsible for maintaining and safeguarding electronic health record systems. As a preventative measure for data security, the report lays forth a plan for deploying strong time-stamping services using blockchain technology. The results may be used by IT departments to improve their cybersecurity policies and prepare for new attacks. The results of this study may be used by healthcare regulatory agencies and lawmakers to shape new policies and guidelines. There has to be a reassessment of regulatory frameworks since the research shows that current ISO/IEC standards have weaknesses. If lawmakers are serious about bolstering legislative and regulatory laws about the security of EHR data, they may look into the suggestions. Cybersecurity and blockchain professionals now have more information than ever before on the types and extent of long-term dangers to the confidentiality, availability, and integrity of data according to this research. The research adds to the ongoing discussion about blockchain technology's potential uses in healthcare by presenting new models and techniques for protecting data transfers. Cybersecurity experts may use this information to inform their tactics for dealing with new threats. Academics may benefit greatly from this research as it increases the existing body of knowledge on the topic of electronic health record data security. The study lays the groundwork for future investigations into the dynamic area of healthcare cybersecurity with its approach, findings, and suggested remedies. Theoretical frameworks, methodological tools, and technical strategies may all be advanced by expanding upon this body of work. Enhancements to the security of electronic health record data will benefit patients and the public at large in the long run. Patients will have more faith in the security of their health records if the suggested safeguards are put in place. Improved data security helps people have faith in healthcare institutions, which in turn improves communication between doctors and their patients. This research could lead to significant advancements in the field and profession by shedding light on practical insights for practitioners, shaping regulatory frameworks, expanding academic knowledge, and, in the end, creating a safer and more reliable healthcare system for everyone.

The results of this research can have significant implications for the world of practice and contribute to the expansion of the body of knowledge in applied research in several ways: When it comes to creating, launching, and overseeing EHR systems, the findings from this study may have an immediate impact on industry standards. Healthcare practitioners and IT professionals can use the findings to enhance their protocols for securing patient data, implementing more robust time-stamping services, and adopting secure blockchain technologies. Healthcare organizations can use the research results to enhance their data security protocols. By implementing the proposed solutions and addressing vulnerabilities identified in existing standards, organizations can establish more resilient and secure EHR systems. In turn, this aids in preventing breaches and unauthorized access to critical patient data. The research results can serve as a valuable resource for regulatory bodies and policymakers. The identified vulnerabilities in ISO/IEC standards and the proposed solutions can guide the development or refinement of regulations related to EHR data security. This ensures that regulatory frameworks align with the evolving technological landscape, fostering a more secure healthcare environment. The research outcomes can be incorporated into educational programs for healthcare professionals, IT specialists, and cybersecurity experts. Training programs and courses can use the findings to educate practitioners on the latest advancements in EHR data security, time-stamping services, and blockchain technologies. This helps build a workforce equipped with the knowledge to address emerging challenges. The research contributes to the body of knowledge in applied research by addressing current gaps and proposing innovative solutions. The results may encourage further studies to be conducted at the crossroads of healthcare, data security, and new technology; this, in turn, can aid in the prevention of breaches involving sensitive patient data. Researchers can build upon this work, exploring additional dimensions, testing proposed models, and refining methodologies. The study's insights into blockchain technologies can contribute to the advancement of this field within healthcare. As blockchain continues to evolve, the research results provide a foundation for exploring new applications, refining existing models, and understanding the practical implications of decentralized long-term timestamping schemes. As digital health solutions become more prevalent, the research results can play a role in building trust among users. The implementation of secure data management practices, informed by the study, can enhance the reliability and integrity of digital health platforms, fostering greater acceptance and adoption by both healthcare providers and patients. The research results have the potential to drive positive change in the world of practice by guiding practical implementations, influencing regulatory frameworks, serving as educational resources, and catalyzing further research. By adding to what is already known in the area of applied research, this study helps to strengthen and progress electronic health records and data security.

BACKGROUND

The security of Electronic Health Records (EHR) is being threatened by the ever-changing digital world and the complexity of cyber attacks. A report conducted by Cybersecurity Ventures in 2022 is one of many credible sources that have recently released figures highlighting the concerning increase in cyberattacks targeting healthcare organisations. The survey shows that healthcare data breaches have increased by 64 percent over the previous year, showing a clear rise in dangers. This increase calls attention to the critical need for more robust security measures to deal with new and emerging threats, and it also endangers the privacy of sensitive patient data. Beyond the scope of any one data loss, these cyber dangers have far-reaching consequences. An anticipatory strategy for security is required due to the sensitive nature and lengthy storage life of EHR data. Threats to data integrity over the long term are growing in proportion to the increasing computational power that attackers have access to and the short lifespan of cryptographic methods. This highlights the paramount need of investigating novel approaches, such blockchain technology and decentralised timestamping, to resolve the long-standing security issues encountered by EHR systems. This chapter's study adds to what is already known about data security in EHRs by providing new ideas and viewpoints that help shed light on the problems that have persisted over the years. The key novel contributions include: One of the primary contributions of this research is the identification and thorough analysis of vulnerabilities in the existing ISO/IEC standards related to time-stamping services (Meng & Chen, 2021). By critically examining these standards, the study pinpoints specific weaknesses that could compromise the long-term integrity and security of EHR data. A thorough long-term time-stamping technique is included in the study to address the vulnerabilities that have been uncovered (Meng & Chen, 2022). This plan provides a comprehensive answer by making sure that client-side and server-side security mechanisms are resilient. When applied to electronic health record data, the innovative method provides a workable paradigm for strengthening the safety of time-stamping services. The study employs rigorous data analysis techniques to formalize various time-stamping methods, providing a deepened understanding of their nuances. This formal analysis contributes a level of specificity and granularity to the evaluation of time-stamping services, offering insights into their strengths and limitations under different conditions and scenarios. Building on the insights gained from the analysis of time-stamping services, the research introduces a robust security model specifically tailored for long-term blockchains. This model establishes a foundation for secure, enduring data transactions, offering a new perspective on blockchain architectures within the realm of EHR data security. Perhaps the most notable contribution is the introduction of an innovative decentralized long-term timestamping scheme. This novel approach revolutionizes the paradigm by ensuring data integrity and security without relying on centralized authorities. The scheme addresses concerns related to central points of failure, offering a decentralized alternative that aligns with the principles of blockchain technology. The research significantly advances the discourse on long-term data security in EHR and related fields. By systematically addressing vulnerabilities, proposing innovative solutions, and formalizing time-stamping methods, the study contributes to a more nuanced and informed conversation surrounding the challenges and opportunities in safeguarding sensitive health information over extended periods. The study serves as a bridge, addressing gaps in existing knowledge related to time-stamping services, blockchain technologies, and their applications in healthcare. By offering a comprehensive evaluation of the current state of these technologies, this study establishes a foundation for future research and development in the field. This study not only identifies problems but also presents real remedies and novel ways, enriching the area of electronic health records and data security. To guarantee the security and integrity of electronic health data over the long term, these contributions add to the ever-changing body of best practices, standards, and technology.

The literature often lacks a detailed examination of ISO/IEC standards concerning time-stamping services within the specific context of Electronic Health Records (EHR) (Myklebust et al., 2021). This research addresses this gap by conducting a comprehensive analysis of these standards, identifying vulnerabilities, and proposing solutions tailored to the unique requirements of healthcare data. Many studies in the literature focus on immediate security concerns but fall short of addressing the long-term security of EHR data. To fill this void, this chapter presents a thorough long-term time-stamping strategy and stresses the need for ongoing data security. The plan provides a perspective view to guarantee the long-term security of private medical records. The existing literature often lacks formalized analyses of various time-stamping methods, leaving a gap in understanding the nuances and potential weaknesses of these techniques. This research contributes by employing rigorous data analysis techniques to formalize different time-stamping methods. This analytical approach provides a more nuanced understanding of the strengths and limitations of these methods. The literature may not comprehensively explore security models for long-term blockchains in the context of EHR data. This chapter addresses this gap by introducing a robust security model specifically designed for long-term blockchains. This model adds to the existing discourse by offering practical insights into securing data transactions over extended periods. The literature may not extensively cover decentralized timestamping schemes in the context of healthcare data security. This research addresses this gap by presenting an innovative decentralized long-term timestamping scheme. This scheme fills a crucial void by offering an alternative that reduces reliance on centralized authorities, mitigating the risk of central points of failure.

This chapter delves deeply into the ISO/IEC standards, exposing healthcare-specific vulnerabilities. The study sheds light on the shortcomings of current standards and suggests tailored ways to improve the safety of time-stamping services for electronic health record data by drawing attention to these vulnerabilities. Focusing on long-term data security rather than short-term security, the study introduces a thorough time-stamping method. The suggested plan lays forth the groundwork for long-term security procedures that will protect electronic health record data. To formalize several time-stamping approaches, this chapter uses rigorous data analysis methodologies. It then provides a full explanation of the method's strengths and weaknesses. Researchers and practitioners may benefit from this formalized study by gaining a critical viewpoint on the literature, which in turn helps with time-stamping service selection and implementation. The study fills a need in the literature by presenting a strong security model for long-term blockchains, which are ideal for electronic health record systems. The current knowledge of blockchain applications in healthcare is enhanced by this model, which offers practical insights into safeguarding data transfers inside a blockchain framework. In this chapter, we provide a new decentralized long-term timestamping technique that addresses the lack of research on this topic and provides a fresh approach to healthcare data security. By offering an alternative that is in line with decentralization principles, this strategy improves the overall security of EHR data while reducing worries about single points of failure. The next sections address current knowledge gaps: a comprehensive review of ISO/IEC standards; an examination of time-stamping techniques; the introduction of a strong blockchain security model; and the presentation of a novel decentralized timestamping system. These contributions address critical shortcomings in the current understanding of EHR data security, providing practical insights and solutions for researchers, practitioners, and policymakers in the healthcare domain.

Method

The foundation of this chapter rests upon a comprehensive literature study that illuminates the current state of time-stamping standards and blockchain architectures. The methodology involves scrutinizing existing research, including studies by Kioskli et al., (2021) and Prodanoff et al., (2021), to identify vulnerabilities in ISO/IEC standards. Rigorous data analysis techniques are then applied to formalize various time-stamping methods, providing a nuanced understanding of their strengths and limitations. This literature-driven approach supports conclusive results, shaping the discourse on long-term data security in EHR and related fields.

MAINTAINING EHR DATA INTEGRITY OVER THE LONG TERM

Current standards, particularly those established by the International Electrotechnical Commission (IEC) and the International Organisation for Standardisation (ISO), are highly dependent on the state of data security in electronic health records (EHR) (Tanwar et al., 2020). The examination of these ISO/IEC standards reveals a complex interplay of strengths and vulnerabilities, significantly impacting the overall security posture of EHR systems. ISO/IEC standards play a foundational role in shaping the protocols and frameworks governing EHR data security. Hovenga et al., (2022) state that these standards establish the bar for secure data management in healthcare systems and are designed to guarantee the availability, integrity, and confidentiality of information. Research by Semantha et al., (2020) and Alamri et al., (2022) shows that these standards have flaws and aren't complete, especially when it comes to time-stamping services. The inadequacies become pronounced in the face of rapidly evolving cyber threats, illustrating the pressing need for standards that can adapt and withstand sophisticated attacks over extended periods. Evolving cyber threats, characterized by advanced persistent threats (APTs) and novel attack vectors, pose challenges to the durability of existing ISO/IEC standards. The research by Świtała et al., (2023) highlights instances where traditional standards struggle to keep pace with the dynamic nature of cyber threats, leaving EHR data susceptible to breaches and unauthorized access.

The identified vulnerabilities underscore the imperative for standards that are not only robust in their current state but possess the adaptability to evolve alongside emerging threats. The static nature of some ISO/IEC standards may hinder their effectiveness in safeguarding EHR data against evolving and sophisticated cyber-attacks (Kandasamy, 2020). Furthermore, the generic nature of certain ISO/IEC standards may not sufficiently address the unique intricacies of healthcare data. Hamdani et al., (2021) argue that tailoring standards to the specific needs of the healthcare industry is crucial for ensuring the robustness of security measures within EHR systems. This section illuminates the foundational role of ISO/IEC standards in shaping EHR data security, while concurrently highlighting the vulnerabilities and challenges that exist within these standards. The evidence presented underscores the necessity for adaptive and healthcare-tailored standards that can effectively mitigate risks posed by evolving cyber threats over extended periods.

One of the pivotal arguments highlighting the vulnerabilities within ISO/IEC standards in the context of EHR data security revolves around the dynamic nature of contemporary cyber threats. The increasing sophistication and agility of these threats present challenges to the ability of established standards to adapt and evolve effectively. In the digital landscape, cyber threats are not static; rather, they continually evolve in complexity and diversity. The research conducted by Demertzi et al., (2023) underscores this dynamic nature, emphasizing that the arsenal of techniques employed by malicious actors is ever-expanding. Advanced Persistent Threats (APTs), zero-day exploits, and novel attack vectors pose a constant challenge to cybersecurity protocols. ISO/IEC standards, although foundational in setting the benchmarks for data security, may encounter difficulties in keeping pace with the rapidly changing threat landscape. As highlighted by Czekster et al., (2023), the struggle lies in the potential lag between the identification of a new threat and the subsequent adaptation of standards to address it. The core argument here is that the inherent adaptability of standards becomes a crucial factor in effectively countering dynamic cyber threats. Traditional, static standards may prove inadequate in the face of emerging tactics that exploit vulnerabilities not initially considered by existing frameworks. The dynamic nature of cyber threats necessitates real-time responses and adaptive measures. Semantha et al., (2021) suggests that the delay in updating standards to address newly identified threats could leave a window of vulnerability open, potentially exposing EHR data to unauthorized access and compromise. In light of these arguments, it becomes imperative to strive for proactive security measures that anticipate and address the evolving nature of cyber threats. The limitations in the adaptability of ISO/IEC standards, as illuminated by Abdulraheem et al., 2024, underscore the urgency of developing standards that can dynamically evolve to safeguard EHR data against sophisticated adversaries. the argument regarding the dynamic nature of cyber threats serves as a critical rationale for reevaluating and enhancing ISO/IEC standards. This perspective emphasizes the need for standards that not only establish a robust baseline but also possess the agility to adapt and respond to emerging threats, ensuring the enduring security of electronic health records.

An essential facet of the vulnerabilities within ISO/IEC standards in the context of EHR data security centers around the necessity for specificity tailored to the unique requirements of healthcare data. The argument posits that generic standards, while foundational, may not adequately address the intricacies of securing sensitive health information within the dynamic and highly regulated landscape of electronic health records (EHR) systems. Healthcare data holds a distinctive status due to its sensitivity, complexity, and regulatory implications. The unique nature of this data extends beyond traditional personal information, encompassing medical histories, diagnoses, treatment plans, and other clinically relevant details. Mishra et al., (2020) emphasizes that the specificity of healthcare data demands a nuanced approach to security. United States legislation like HIPAA (Health Insurance Portability and Accountability Act) provides a tight regulatory environment in which the healthcare industry must function. Strong security measures that are in line with the ethical and legal concerns of healthcare are essential for meeting the requirements of this legislation. (Edemekong et al., 2020).EHR systems, designed to capture, store, and exchange comprehensive patient information, introduce unique challenges that generic standards may not adequately address. The interconnected nature of healthcare ecosystems and the diverse range of stakeholders involved necessitate standards tailored to the specific workflows and intricacies of EHR systems.

The argument underscores that to maximize efficacy, standards must be tailored to the healthcare domain. Yaqoob et al., (2019) contends that applying generic standards to the healthcare sector may result in oversights, leaving vulnerabilities unaddressed and potentially exposing sensitive health information to unauthorized access or compromise. Interoperability, a critical requirement in healthcare data exchange, introduces additional complexities. Standards that are specific to healthcare can better address the interoperability challenges inherent in EHR systems, ensuring that security measures seamlessly integrate with the collaborative nature of healthcare data sharing. the argument regarding specificity to healthcare underscores the necessity for standards that are finely tuned to the unique demands of securing EHR data. As highlighted by Perwej et al, (2022), generic standards may fall short of comprehensively addressing the nuances and regulatory intricacies inherent in healthcare, emphasizing the importance of tailoring security standards to the specific requirements of electronic health records. The imperative for emphasizing long-term security measures in the realm of electronic health records (EHR) data stems from the acknowledgment that immediate safeguards may not provide sufficient protection. The important requirement for techniques that survive and adapt over time is shown by studies undertaken by Rahim et al., (2023) and Adebimpe et al., (2023), which highlight cases when breaches went undiscovered for lengthy durations.

The foundation of the argument lies in the recognition that EHR data often exists within extended lifecycles, necessitating security measures that extend far beyond the immediacy of their implementation. Singh and Singh (2022) highlight scenarios where breaches, due to their subtle nature, persisted undetected for considerable durations, illustrating the vulnerability introduced by prolonged exposure. Immediate security measures, while essential, may have limitations in detecting and preventing threats that unfold gradually over time. The studies emphasize that relying solely on immediate safeguards could result in overlooking subtle anomalies or sophisticated attacks that persist beneath the surface, evading detection mechanisms. The argument asserts that enduring security strategies are imperative to address the challenges posed by threats that unfold over the long term. Brass and Sowell (2021) argue that security protocols should be designed to be continuously monitored, identify risks, and react to new cyber threats as they emerge. The studies cited demonstrate the importance of learning from historical breaches where prolonged exposure went unnoticed. Analyzing these incidents provides insights into the tactics employed by threat actors and informs the development of security measures capable of withstanding the test of time. An essential aspect of the argument is the integration of adaptive technologies and methodologies that evolve alongside emerging threats. Aydos et al., (2019) advocate for the adoption of security measures that incorporate machine learning, artificial intelligence, and other adaptive technologies to enhance the capacity to detect and respond to evolving threats over the long term. the push for long-term security measures in EHR data is a balancing act between proactivity and long-term resilience. Immediate safeguards remain crucial, but the emphasis lies in complementing them with strategies that endure, adapt, and evolve. By learning from historical breaches and integrating adaptive technologies, the healthcare sector can fortify its defenses against threats that may persist over extended periods, ensuring the enduring security of electronic health records.

A central argument supporting the emphasis on long-term security measures in the context of electronic health records (EHR) is rooted in the extended lifecycle of healthcare data. As highlighted by de Bienassis et al., (2022), the lifecycle of EHR data often spans many years, necessitating security measures that align with this prolonged timeframe to ensure the enduring integrity of sensitive health information. The argument begins with an acknowledgment of the prolonged relevance and usability of EHR data throughout a patient's lifetime. Health records, in contrast to data from other industries, tend to have longer half-lives because of the lasting impact they have on healthcare decision-making, treatment outcomes, and research efforts. Because of its long storage life, electronic health record data is a prime target for cybercriminals looking to steal sensitive information. According to Yaacoub et al., (2020), hackers will continue to attack healthcare data because of its high value, which makes it an attractive target for security flaws. Patient treatment is uninterrupted thanks to security measures that are in sync with the long lifespan of electronic health record data. According to Chernyshev et al., (2019), patients' medical records should be protected against unauthorized access at all times since their health information is important throughout their lives and should remain secure no matter what.

Health Insurance Portability and Accountability Act (HIPAA) of the United States is one example of legislation that recognizes the importance of patient data security in the long run. Aligning security measures with the extended data lifecycle is a legal and regulatory requirement, according to Seh et al., (2020), and it's also best to practise for patient care. The argument stresses how important it is to have security measures in place that might lessen the chances of a breach of historical data.. Instances, where historical EHR data is compromised, can have far-reaching consequences, impacting not only individual patients but also broader healthcare systems, research initiatives, and public health. the extended data lifecycle argument underscores the importance of ensuring data integrity across generations of healthcare information. By aligning security measures with the extended timeframe of EHR data, the healthcare sector can navigate the complexities of safeguarding information that retains its relevance over many years, contributing to the resilience and enduring security of electronic health records. An essential argument supporting the emphasis on long-term security measures in electronic health records (EHR) centers around the inherent risks associated with prolonged exposure. As articulated by Javaid et al., (2023), extended exposure increases the likelihood of vulnerabilities being exploited, necessitating comprehensive long-term security measures to effectively reduce the risk of data compromise over time. The core of this argument lies in the understanding that as EHR data remains exposed over extended periods, the potential for vulnerabilities to be discovered and exploited amplifies. Al Kinoon., (2021) highlights that what may have been a secure system at the time of implementation could become susceptible to new and evolving cyber threats as time progresses. The dynamic and evolving nature of the threat landscape introduces additional challenges. Elhoseny et al., (2021) suggests that the longer data is exposed, the more it becomes subject to emerging cyber threats and techniques that may not have been prevalent or well understood at the time of initial implementation.

Long-term exposure can lead to a gradual weakening of the defenses that were initially put in place. Technological advancements, changes in security best practices, and the discovery of new vulnerabilities contribute to the erosion of the efficacy of existing security measures over time (Mandal & Khan, 2020). The argument posits that as EHR data persists over the long term, it becomes a persistent target for adversaries who may patiently wait for opportune moments to exploit weaknesses. Chigada and Madzinga (2021) emphasizes the strategic advantage that prolonged exposure provides to threat actors seeking to compromise healthcare data. Continuous monitoring is crucial to address the risks associated with prolonged exposure. Ibarra et al., (2020) suggests that long-term security measures should include mechanisms for ongoing assessment, vulnerability management, and adaptive responses to ensure that the security posture remains robust against emerging threats. the argument underscores that long-term security measures are designed not only to address immediate threats but also to reduce the risks associated with prolonged exposure. By acknowledging the vulnerabilities that can emerge over time, healthcare organizations can implement proactive strategies, continuous monitoring, and adaptive security measures to mitigate the evolving risks and ensure the sustained integrity of electronic health records. A compelling argument within the discourse on electronic health records (EHR) data security is centered around the promising potential of decentralized timestamping schemes and blockchain technologies. Evidence from many research (e.g., Pandey et al., 2020) and Hashemi and Zarei, (2021) points to decentralization's advantages, including a decrease in risks associated with centralized authority. A paradigm shift occurs in the protection of data included in electronic health records when decentralized timestamping methods are used. The benefits of decentralization are emphasized by Shuaib et al., (2022). In this model, a single central authority is eliminated via the distribution of timestamping operations throughout a network. This method improves the timestamping process's transparency and reliability while also reducing the likelihood of a single point of failure.

Emerging as a powerful tool for EHR data security, blockchain is a core technology that supports decentralized timestamping. Highlighting blockchain's transparent, immutable, and tamper-evident ledger, Goel et al., (2019) provides proof of blockchain's benefits. As a result of its decentralized design, blockchain records transactions in a way that cannot be changed backward, making them safe and easy to verify. One of the main points is that conventional timestamping methods pose hazards due to their reliance on centralized authority. The security of timestamped data is jeopardized since centralized organizations are susceptible to assaults and compromise (Baysal et al., 2023). By dividing up power, decentralized timestamping solutions lessen the effect of these dangers. The transparency and immutability inherent in blockchain technologies contribute significantly to EHR data security. Jahanbin et al., (2023) argue that the transparent and unchangeable nature of blockchain transactions ensures that every entry, including timestamps, is visible and tamper-proof, providing an additional layer of security and accountability. Decentralized timestamping and blockchain technologies collectively reduce reliance on central points of failure. Reegu et al., (2023) highlight that the distributed nature of these systems ensures that compromising one node does not compromise the entire network, enhancing the overall resilience and security of EHR data. the potential of decentralized timestamping schemes and blockchain technologies represents a revolutionary paradigm shift in EHR data security. The evidence presented by

Pilares et al., (2022) underscores the advantages of decentralization in mitigating risks, enhancing transparency, and fundamentally changing the way data security is conceptualized and implemented in the context of electronic health records.

A pivotal argument supporting the potential of decentralized timestamping schemes and blockchain technologies in EHR data security revolves around the imperative of reducing single points of failure. As articulated by Ali et al., (2023), centralized authorities pose a significant risk as a singular point of failure, and decentralized timestamping schemes address this vulnerability by distributing trust across a network. Centralized authorities, often responsible for traditional timestamping processes, represent a single point of failure susceptible to various risks. Haddad et al., (2020) identifies that centralized entities become attractive targets for malicious actors seeking to compromise or manipulate timestamped data, potentially jeopardizing the integrity of the entire EHR system. The argument underscores the vulnerability of centralized authorities to attacks, emphasizing that a successful breach of such an authority could have cascading effects on the security and integrity of timestamped data. Akhter et al., (2022) highlights that mitigating this risk is crucial for ensuring the resilience of EHR data security measures. Decentralized timestamping schemes introduce a fundamental shift by distributing trust across a network of nodes. Rather than relying on a single central authority, the trust is diffused among multiple entities. Khalid et al., (2023) argues that this distribution of trust reduces the risk associated with a single point of failure, as compromising one node does not compromise the entire system. The argument extends to the resilience provided by decentralized systems against compromises. Semantha et al., (2023) suggests that even if one node within the decentralized network is compromised, the overall integrity of timestamped data is maintained, minimizing the impact of potential attacks and ensuring the continued security of EHR information. By reducing the reliance on centralized authorities, decentralized timestamping schemes strengthen the overall security posture of EHR systems. Jabarulla and Lee, (2021), contends that this approach aligns with the principles of resilience and adaptability, key factors in safeguarding sensitive healthcare data over the long term. the reduction of single points of failure through decentralized timestamping not only addresses current vulnerabilities but also positions EHR systems to adapt to evolving threats. Capece and Lorenzi, (2020), emphasizes that by distributing trust, healthcare organizations can enhance the security, transparency, and integrity of timestamped data, contributing to a more resilient and robust EHR data security framework.

A pivotal argument supporting the potential of blockchain technologies in EHR data security centers around the concepts of enhanced transparency and immutability. As elucidated by Al Mamun et al., (2022), blockchain, with its transparent and immutable ledger, establishes a robust foundation for secure data transactions. This transparency not only ensures verifiability but also contributes to maintaining the integrity of electronic health records (EHR) data. Due to its nature as a distributed and decentralized ledger, blockchain is intrinsically transparent. The tamper-evident recording of every transaction, including timestamping within the context of EHR data, is guaranteed. This openness makes a guarantees that authorized participants may see every input, which increases confidence in the data's authenticity ([Author12, 2020]). One of the most important aspects of healthcare is the verifiability of transactions, and blockchain's transparency helps with that. According to Ray et al., (2021), the EHR system may gain trust and confidence from all parties involved in healthcare by allowing patients, healthcare providers, and regulatory agencies to independently confirm the legitimacy and correctness of timestamped data. One essential feature of blockchain is its immutability, which makes it impossible to go back and change a recorded transaction. According to Thantharate and Thantharate, (2023), an immutable record of electronic health record (EHR) transactions is created, which is a strong defense against unauthorized modifications or manipulation. The validity of EHR systems as a whole is called into question by the argument. To improve the security of electronic health records, Sharma et al., (2020) argues that blockchain's immutability and transparency greatly decrease the likelihood of illegal changes, manipulations, or deletions of timestamped data. The trustworthiness of electronic health record data is enhanced by its transparency and immutability. Stakeholders may have faith in the timestamped information properly reflecting the historical sequence of events without the possibility of manipulation or compromise, according to Mukherjee and Singh, (2020), since the blockchain is a transparent and immutable record. The argument highlights how blockchain technologies improve the auditability and accountability of EHR data by making it more transparent and immutable. Abbate et al., (2022) emphasizes that these characteristics provide the groundwork for trustworthy, open, and secure data management in the healthcare industry while also guaranteeing the verifiability of transactions. This, in turn, contributes to a more robust and resilient EHR data security framework.

SOLUTIONS AND RECOMMENDATIONS

Given the demonstrated advantages of decentralized timestamping schemes and blockchain technologies, a policy recommendation involves encouraging the integration of these technologies within the regulatory frameworks governing electronic health records. Policymakers should consider endorsing standards that promote the adoption of decentralized approaches and blockchain-based solutions to fortify the security of EHR data. This may involve providing incentives for healthcare organizations that implement decentralized timestamping and blockchain technologies in their data management practices.

FUTURE RESEARCH DIRECTIONS

Future research in the realm of EHR data security should delve deeper into the practical implementation of decentralized timestamping and blockchain technologies in diverse healthcare settings. Exploring the scalability, interoperability, and adaptability of these technologies across different healthcare systems and geographical regions would provide valuable insights. Additionally, research could focus on developing standardized protocols and guidelines for the integration of decentralized and blockchain-based solutions, addressing potential challenges and ensuring seamless adoption within the healthcare industry. Understanding the long-term implications, including the sustainability and evolution of these technologies in the face of emerging cyber threats, should be a priority for researchers in the field of EHR data security.

CONCLUSION

In summary, the exploration of the potential of decentralized timestamping schemes and blockchain technologies in enhancing EHR data security has unveiled crucial advantages. The reduction of single points of failure through decentralization addresses vulnerabilities associated with centralized authorities, while the transparency and immutability of blockchain lay a robust foundation for secure data transactions within electronic health records.

Decentralized timestamping not only mitigates risks linked to centralized authorities but also fosters resilience against compromises, aligning with the dynamic nature of evolving cyber threats. The distribution of trust across a network enhances the security posture of EHR systems, offering a paradigm shift in safeguarding sensitive healthcare data over the long term.

The transparency and immutability introduced by blockchain technologies contribute to the verifiability of transactions, preventing data manipulation and fostering trust in the integrity of EHR data. These attributes not only strengthen the suitability and accountability of healthcare information but also establish a foundation for a secure, transparent, and trustworthy data management framework.

REFERENCES

Abbate, S., Centobelli, P., Cerchione, R., Oropallo, E., & Riccio, E. (2022). Blockchain technology for embracing healthcare 4.0. *IEEE Transactions on Engineering Management*. Advance online publication. doi:10.1109/TEM.2022.3212007

Abdulraheem, M., Adeniyi, E. A., Awotunde, J. B., Imoize, A. L., Jimoh, R. G., Oladipo, I. D., & Falola, P. B. (2024). Artificial Intelligence of Medical Things for Medical Information Systems Privacy and Security. In *Handbook of Security and Privacy of AI-Enabled Healthcare Systems and Internet of Medical Things* (pp. 63–96). CRC Press.

Adebimpe, L. A., Ng, I. O., Idris, M. Y. I., Okmi, M., Ku, C. S., Ang, T. F., & Por, L. Y. (2023). Systemic Literature Review of Recognition-Based Authentication Method Resistivity to Shoulder-Surfing Attacks. *Applied Sciences (Basel, Switzerland), 13*(18), 10040. doi:10.3390/app131810040

Akhter Md Hasib, K. T., Chowdhury, I., Sakib, S., Monirujjaman Khan, M., Alsufyani, N., Alsufyani, A., & Bourouis, S. (2022). Electronic health record monitoring system and data security using blockchain technology. *Security and Communication Networks, 2022*, 1–15. doi:10.1155/2022/2366632

Al Kinoon, M., Omar, M., Mohaisen, M., & Mohaisen, D. (2021). Security breaches in the healthcare domain: a spatiotemporal analysis. In *Computational Data and Social Networks: 10th International Conference, CSoNet 2021, Virtual Event, November 15-17, 2021, Proceedings 10* (pp. 171-183). Springer International Publishing. 10.1007/978-3-030-91434-9_16

Al Mamun, A., Azam, S., & Gritti, C. (2022). Blockchain-based electronic health records management: A comprehensive review and future research direction. *IEEE Access : Practical Innovations, Open Solutions, 10*, 5768–5789. doi:10.1109/ACCESS.2022.3141079

Al-Zahrani, F. A. (2020). Evaluating the usable-security of healthcare software through unified technique of fuzzy logic, ANP and TOPSIS. *IEEE Access : Practical Innovations, Open Solutions, 8*, 109905–109916. doi:10.1109/ACCESS.2020.3001996

Alam, S., Bhatia, S., Shuaib, M., Khubrani, M. M., Alfayez, F., Malibari, A. A., & Ahmad, S. (2023). An overview of blockchain and IoT integration for secure and reliable health records monitoring. *Sustainability (Basel), 15*(7), 5660. doi:10.3390/su15075660

Alamri, B., Crowley, K., & Richardson, I. (2022). Cybersecurity Risk Management Framework for Blockchain Identity Management Systems in Health IoT. *Sensors (Basel), 23*(1), 218. doi:10.3390/s23010218 PMID:36616816

Ali, A., Al-Rimy, B. A. S., Tin, T. T., Altamimi, S. N., Qasem, S. N., & Saeed, F. (2023). Empowering Precision Medicine: Unlocking Revolutionary Insights through Blockchain-Enabled Federated Learning and Electronic Medical Records. *Sensors (Basel), 23*(17), 7476. doi:10.3390/s23177476 PMID:37687931

Aydos, M., Vural, Y., & Tekerek, A. (2019). Assessing risks and threats with layered approach to Internet of Things security. *Measurement and Control, 52*(5-6), 338–353. doi:10.1177/0020294019837991

Balasubramanian, S., Shukla, V., Sethi, J. S., Islam, N., & Saloum, R. (2021). A readiness assessment framework for Blockchain adoption: A healthcare case study. *Technological Forecasting and Social Change, 165*, 120536. doi:10.1016/j.techfore.2020.120536

Baysal, M. V., Özcan-Top, Ö., & Betin-Can, A. (2023). Blockchain technology applications in the health domain: A multivocal literature review. *The Journal of Supercomputing, 79*(3), 3112–3156. doi:10.1007/s11227-022-04772-1 PMID:36060094

Brass, I., & Sowell, J. H. (2021). Adaptive governance for the Internet of Things: Coping with emerging security risks. *Regulation & Governance, 15*(4), 1092–1110. doi:10.1111/rego.12343

Capece, G., & Lorenzi, F. (2020). Blockchain and Healthcare: Opportunities and Prospects for the EHR. *Sustainability, 12*(22), 9693. doi:10.3390/su12229693

Cerchione, R., Centobelli, P., Riccio, E., Abbate, S., & Oropallo, E. (2023). Blockchain's coming to hospital to digitalize healthcare services: Designing a distributed electronic health record ecosystem. *Technovation, 120*, 102480. doi:10.1016/j.technovation.2022.102480

Chernyshev, M., Zeadally, S., & Baig, Z. (2019). Healthcare data breaches: Implications for digital forensic readiness. *Journal of Medical Systems, 43*(1), 1–12. doi:10.1007/s10916-018-1123-2 PMID:30488291

Chigada, J., & Madzinga, R. (2021). Cyberattacks and threats during COVID-19: A systematic literature review. *South African Journal of Information Management, 23*(1), 1–11. doi:10.4102/sajim.v23i1.1277

Czekster, R. M., Grace, P., Marcon, C., Hessel, F., & Cazella, S. C. (2023). Challenges and Opportunities for Conducting Dynamic Risk Assessments in Medical IoT. *Applied Sciences (Basel, Switzerland), 13*(13), 7406. doi:10.3390/app13137406 de Bienassis, K., Fujisawa, R., Hashiguchi, T. C. O., Klazinga, N., & Oderkirk, J. (2022). *Health data and governance developments in relation to COVID-19: How OECD countries are adjusting health data systems for the new normal*. Academic Press.

Demertzi, V., Demertzis, S., & Demertzis, K. (2023). An Overview of Cyber Threats, Attacks and Countermeasures on the Primary Domains of Smart Cities. *Applied Sciences (Basel, Switzerland)*, *13*(2), 790. doi:10.3390/app13020790

Edemekong, P. F., Haydel, M. J., Boyer, J., & Bogdan, B. (2020). *Health insurance portability and accountability act* (HIPAA). StatPearls.

Elhoseny, M., Thilakarathne, N. N., Alghamdi, M. I., Mahendran, R. K., Gardezi, A. A., Weerasinghe, H., & Welhenge, A. (2021). Security and privacy issues in medical internet of things: Overview, countermeasures, challenges and future directions. *Sustainability (Basel)*, *13*(21), 11645. doi:10.3390/su132111645

Goel, U., Ruhl, R., & Zavarsky, P. (2019, May). Using healthcare authority and patient blockchains to develop a tamper-proof record tracking system. In *2019 IEEE 5th intl conference on big data security on cloud (BigDataSecurity), IEEE Intl conference on high performance and smart computing,(HPSC) and IEEE Intl conference on intelligent data and security (IDS)* (pp. 25-30). IEEE. 10.1109/BigDataSecurity-HPSC-IDS.2019.00016

Haddad, A., Habaebi, M. H., Islam, M. R., Hasbullah, N. F., & Zabidi, S. A. (2022). Systematic review on ai-blockchain based e-healthcare records management systems. *IEEE Access : Practical Innovations, Open Solutions*, *10*, 94583–94615. doi:10.1109/ACCESS.2022.3201878

Hamdani, S. W. A., Abbas, H., Janjua, A. R., Shahid, W. B., Amjad, M. F., Malik, J., Murtaza, M. H., Atiquzzaman, M., & Khan, A. W. (2021). Cybersecurity standards in the context of operating system: Practical aspects, analysis, and comparisons. *ACM Computing Surveys*, *54*(3), 1–36. doi:10.1145/3442480

Hashemi, S., & Zarei, M. (2021). Internet of Things backdoors: Resource management issues, security challenges, and detection methods. *Transactions on Emerging Telecommunications Technologies*, *32*(2), e4142. doi:10.1002/ett.4142

Hovenga, E., Grain, H., & Beale, T. (2022). Fragmented global standards development organisations. In *Roadmap to Successful Digital Health Ecosystems* (pp. 65–96). Academic Press., doi:10.1016/B978-0-12-823413-6.00025-2

Ibarra, J., Jahankhani, H., & Beavers, J. (2020). Biohacking capabilities and threat/attack vectors. *Cyber Defence in the Age of AI, Smart Societies and Augmented Humanity*, 117-131. doi:10.1007/978-3-030-35746-7_7

Jabarulla, M. Y., & Lee, H. N. (2021, August). A blockchain and artificial intelligence-based, patient-centric healthcare system for combating the COVID-19 pandemic: Opportunities and applications. In Healthcare (Vol. 9, No. 8, p. 1019). MDPI. doi:10.3390/healthcare9081019

Jahanbin, P., Sharma, R. S., Wingreen, S. T., Kshetri, N., & Choo, K. K. R. (2023). Towards CRISP-BC: 3TIC specification framework for Blockchain use-cases. *IET Blockchain*, *3*(3), 159–168. doi:10.1049/blc2.12038

Javaid, M., Haleem, A., Singh, R. P., & Suman, R. (2023). Towards insighting cybersecurity for healthcare domains: A comprehensive review of recent practices and trends. *Cyber Security and Applications, 100016*. Advance online publication. doi:10.1016/j.csa.2023.100016

Kandasamy, K., Srinivas, S., Achuthan, K., & Rangan, V. P. (2020). IoT cyber risk: A holistic analysis of cyber risk assessment frameworks, risk vectors, and risk ranking process. *EURASIP Journal on Information Security*, *2020*(1), 1–18. doi:10.1186/s13635-020-00111-0

Khalid, M. I., Ahmed, M., & Kim, J. (2023). Enhancing data protection in dynamic consent management systems: Formalizing privacy and security definitions with differential privacy, decentralization, and Zero-Knowledge proofs. *Sensors (Basel)*, *23*(17), 7604. doi:10.3390/s23177604 PMID:37688060

Kioskli, K., Fotis, T., & Mouratidis, H. (2021, August). The landscape of cybersecurity vulnerabilities and challenges in healthcare: Security standards and paradigm shift recommendations. In *Proceedings of the 16th International Conference on Availability, Reliability and Security* (pp. 1-9). 10.1145/3465481.3470033

Mandal, S., & Khan, D. A. (2020, September). A Study of security threats in cloud: Passive impact of COVID-19 pandemic. In *2020 International Conference on Smart Electronics and Communication (ICOSEC)* (pp. 837-842). IEEE. 10.1109/ICOSEC49089.2020.9215374

Meng, L., & Chen, L. (2021). Reviewing the ISO/IEC standard for timestamping services. *IEEE Communications Standards Magazine*, *5*(3), 20–25. doi:10.1109/MCOMSTD.011.2000083

Meng, L., & Chen, L. (2022, September). A Blockchain-Based Long-Term Time-Stamping Scheme. In *European Symposium on Research in Computer Security* (pp. 3-24). Cham: Springer International Publishing. 10.1007/978-3-031-17140-6_1

Mishra, S., Kwong, J. C., Chan, A. K., & Baral, S. D. (2020). Understanding heterogeneity to inform the public health response to COVID-19 in Canada. *Canadian Medical Association Journal, 192*(25), E684–E685. doi:10.1503/cmaj.201112 PMID:32493741

Mukherjee, P., & Singh, D. (2020). The opportunities of blockchain in health 4.0. *Blockchain Technology for Industry 4.0: Secure, Decentralized, Distributed and Trusted Industry Environment*, 149-164. doi:10.1007/978-981-15-1137-0_8

Myklebust, T., Onshus, T. E., Lindskog, S., Ottermo, M. V., & Bodsberg, L. (2021). Data safety, sources, and data flow in the offshore industry. In *Proceedings of the 31st European Safety and Reliability Conference*. Research Publishing Services. 10.3850/978-981-18-2016-8_099-cd

Nigam, D., Patel, S. N., Raj Vincent, P. M., Srinivasan, K., & Arunmozhi, S. (2022). Biometric authentication for intelligent and privacy-preserving healthcare systems. *Journal of Healthcare Engineering, 2022*, 1–15. Advance online publication. doi:10.1155/2022/1789996 PMID:35368929

Pandey, P., Pandey, S. C., & Kumar, U. (2020). Security issues of internet of things in health-care sector: An analytical approach. *Advancement of Machine Intelligence in Interactive Medical Image Analysis*, 307-329. doi:10.1007/978-981-15-1100-4_15

Perwej, Y., Akhtar, N., Kulshrestha, N., & Mishra, P. (2022). A Methodical Analysis of Medical Internet of Things (MIoT) Security and Privacy in Current and Future Trends. *Journal of Emerging Technologies and Innovative Research, 9*(1), d346–d371.

Pilares, I. C. A., Azam, S., Akbulut, S., Jonkman, M., & Shanmugam, B. (2022). Addressing the challenges of electronic health records using blockchain and ipfs. *Sensors (Basel), 22*(11), 4032. doi:10.3390/s22114032 PMID:35684652

Prodanoff, Z., White-Williams, C., & Chi, H. (2021). Regulations and standards aware framework for recording of mhealth app vulnerabilities. *International Journal of E-Health and Medical Communications, 12*(3), 1–16. doi:10.4018/IJEHMC.20210501.oa1

Rahim, F. A., Ahmad, N. A., Magalingam, P., Jamil, N., Cob, Z. C., & Salahudin, L. (2023). Cybersecurity Vulnerabilities in Smart Grids with Solar Photovoltaic: A Threat Modelling and Risk Assessment Approach. *International Journal of Sustainable Construction Engineering and Technology*, *14*(3), 210–220. doi:10.30880/ijscet.2023.14.03.018

Ray, P. P., Chowhan, B., Kumar, N., & Almogren, A. (2021). BIoTHR: Electronic health record servicing scheme in IoT-blockchain ecosystem. *IEEE Internet of Things Journal*, *8*(13), 10857–10872. doi:10.1109/JIOT.2021.3050703

Reegu, F. A., Abas, H., Gulzar, Y., Xin, Q., Alwan, A. A., Jabbari, A., Sonkamble, R. G., & Dziyauddin, R. A. (2023). Blockchain-Based Framework for Interoperable Electronic Health Records for an Improved Healthcare System. *Sustainability (Basel)*, *15*(8), 6337. doi:10.3390/su15086337

Seh, A. H., Zarour, M., Alenezi, M., Sarkar, A. K., Agrawal, A., Kumar, R., & Ahmad Khan, R. (2020, May). Healthcare data breaches: insights and implications. In Healthcare (Vol. 8, No. 2, p. 133). MDPI. doi:10.3390/healthcare8020133

Semantha, F. H., Azam, S., Shanmugam, B., & Yeo, K. C. (2023). PbDinEHR: A Novel Privacy by Design Developed Framework Using Distributed Data Storage and Sharing for Secure and Scalable Electronic Health Records Management. *Journal of Sensor and Actuator Networks*, *12*(2), 36. doi:10.3390/jsan12020036

Semantha, F. H., Azam, S., Shanmugam, B., Yeo, K. C., & Beeravolu, A. R. (2021). A conceptual framework to ensure privacy in patient record management system. *IEEE Access : Practical Innovations, Open Solutions*, *9*, 165667–165689. doi:10.1109/ACCESS.2021.3134873

Semantha, F. H., Azam, S., Yeo, K. C., & Shanmugam, B. (2020). A systematic literature review on privacy by design in the healthcare sector. *Electronics (Basel)*, *9*(3), 452. doi:10.3390/electronics9030452

Shah, S. M., & Khan, R. A. (2020). Secondary use of electronic health record: Opportunities and challenges. *IEEE Access : Practical Innovations, Open Solutions*, *8*, 136947–136965. doi:10.1109/ACCESS.2020.3011099

Sharif, M. H. U., & Mohammed, M. A. (2022). A literature review of financial losses statistics for cyber security and future trend. *World Journal of Advanced Research and Reviews*, *15*(1), 138–156. doi:10.30574/wjarr.2022.15.1.0573

Sharma, R., Zhang, C., Wingreen, S. C., Kshetri, N., & Zahid, A. (2020). Design of blockchain-based precision health-care using soft systems methodology. *Industrial Management & Data Systems*, *120*(3), 608–632. doi:10.1108/IMDS-07-2019-0401

Shuaib, K., Abdella, J., Sallabi, F., & Serhani, M. A. (2022). Secure decentralized electronic health records sharing system based on blockchains. *Journal of King Saud University. Computer and Information Sciences*, *34*(8), 5045–5058. doi:10.1016/j.jksuci.2021.05.002

Singh, I., & Singh, Y. A. S. H. I. K. (2022). Cyber-Security Knowledge and Practice of Nurses in Private Hospitals in Northern Durban, Kwazulu-Natal. *Journal of Theoretical and Applied Information Technology*, *100*(1), 246–267.

Srivastava, S., Pant, M., Jauhar, S. K., & Nagar, A. K. (2022). Analyzing the Prospects of Blockchain in Healthcare Industry. *Computational and Mathematical Methods in Medicine*, *2022*, 1–24. Advance online publication. doi:10.1155/2022/3727389 PMID:36506597

Świtała, K. (2023, May). Medical Data in the Digital Era-Legal Challenges Related to Providing Information Security, Applying GDPR and Respecting the Professional Secrecy. In *2023 46th MIPRO ICT and Electronics Convention (MIPRO)* (pp. 1457-1466). IEEE. 10.23919/MIPRO57284.2023.10159891

Tanwar, S., Parekh, K., & Evans, R. (2020). Blockchain-based electronic healthcare record system for healthcare 4.0 applications. *Journal of Information Security and Applications*, *50*, 102407. doi:10.1016/j.jisa.2019.102407

Thantharate, P., & Thantharate, A. (2023). ZeroTrustBlock: Enhancing Security, Privacy, and Interoperability of Sensitive Data through ZeroTrust Permissioned Blockchain. *Big Data and Cognitive Computing*, *7*(4), 165. doi:10.3390/bdcc7040165

Yaacoub, J. P. A., Noura, M., Noura, H. N., Salman, O., Yaacoub, E., Couturier, R., & Chehab, A. (2020). Securing internet of medical things systems: Limitations, issues and recommendations. *Future Generation Computer Systems*, *105*, 581–606. doi:10.1016/j.future.2019.12.028

Yaqoob, I., Salah, K., Jayaraman, R., & Al-Hammadi, Y. (2021). Blockchain for healthcare data management: Opportunities, challenges, and future recommendations. *Neural Computing & Applications*, 1–16. doi:10.1007/s00521-020-05519-w

Yaqoob, T., Abbas, H., & Atiquzzaman, M. (2019). Security vulnerabilities, attacks, countermeasures, and regulations of networked medical devices-A review. *IEEE Communications Surveys and Tutorials*, *21*(4), 3723–3768. doi:10.1109/COMST.2019.2914094

KEY TERMS AND DEFINITIONS

Blockchain Security: Blockchain security refers to the measures and protocols implemented to protect the integrity, confidentiality, and availability of data stored and transacted on a blockchain. It involves safeguarding against unauthorized access, ensuring the immutability of data, and preventing malicious activities within the decentralized and distributed nature of blockchain technology.

Confidentiality of Electronic Health Information: Confidentiality of electronic health information refers to the ethical and legal obligation to protect the privacy and security of sensitive patient data stored and transmitted within electronic health record (EHR) systems. It encompasses measures and practices designed to ensure that only authorized individuals or entities can access, view, or use patient information and that such access is limited to what is necessary for legitimate healthcare purposes.

Data Integrity: Data integrity is the assurance that data remains accurate, consistent, and unaltered throughout its lifecycle. It comprises taking precautions to prevent data corruption, errors, or unauthorized alterations so that it remains trustworthy and dependable. Data integrity is a must-have in many industries, including healthcare, where accurate and unaltered information is critical for patient safety and treatment.

Electronic Health Records: Electronic health records (EHRs) are digital copies of patient's medical records that contain their symptoms, diagnoses, medications, treatment programs, immunization dates, allergies, test findings, x-rays, and prescriptions. In addition to giving a complete and lasting view of a patient's health, electronic health records (EHRs) make it possible for healthcare providers to share patient data securely and efficiently.

Encryption: The process of encoding plaintext health data into ciphertext using cryptographic keys, rendering it unreadable to unauthorized users. Encryption ensures that only authorized individuals with the appropriate decryption keys can access and decipher the information. These services often rely on cryptographic techniques to generate secure timestamps that are resistant to tampering or manipulation. Time-stamping services play a vital role in supporting compliance with regulatory requirements, facilitating audit trails, and enabling forensic investigations in the context of electronic health information management.

Long-Term Security: Long-term security in electronic health records (EHRs) refers to the sustained protection of sensitive health information over extended periods, typically encompassing the entire lifecycle of the data within the EHR system. It involves implementing robust measures to safeguard the confidentiality, integrity, and availability of patient data against unauthorized access, tampering, loss, or corruption over time.

Time-Stamping Services: Time-stamping services in electronic health records (EHRs) refer to specialized mechanisms that assign precise timestamps to various actions, events, or transactions within the EHR system. These timestamps serve as digital evidence of when specific activities occurred, such as when a record was created, accessed, modified, or transmitted. Time-stamping services are critical for ensuring the integrity, accountability, and legal validity of EHR data by providing an indisputable chronological sequence of events.

Chapter 4
Securing Sensitive Patient Data in Healthcare Settings Using Blockchain Technology

R. Thanga Selvi
Vel Tech Rangarajan Dr. Sagunthala R&D Institute of Science and Technology, India

R. Elakya
Sri Venkateswara College of Engineering, India

U. Vignesh
Vellore Institute of Technology, Chennai, India

ABSTRACT

The utilization of electronic health record (EHR) has become common in the healthcare industry, enabling the storage and exchange of patients' medical information across different healthcare organizations. However, concerns regarding the security and privacy of patient data have arisen due to the centralized nature of conventional systems. To address these issues, a blockchain-based solution has been proposed to enhance data security and system efficiency. This chapter introduces a blockchain-based system designed to manage and secure patient data within a single record controlled by the patient. The Ethereum network was utilized to develop this decentralized system. The solution not only empowers users by granting them enhanced authority over their confidential information but also advocates for the incorporation of blockchain advancements within the healthcare domain. The proposed system offers improved data security and accessibility, addressing concerns related to the privacy and integrity of patient records in traditional EHR systems.

DOI: 10.4018/979-8-3693-1662-7.ch004

1. INTRODUCTION

A block chain operates as a decentralized network, employing Peer-to-Peer (P2P) technology to monitor transactions without relying on a central authority. Instead, it depends on a network of nodes to uphold its functioning (Gharat et al., 2021). The integrity of each transaction is upheld by these nodes, with encryption providing an added layer of security to communications. Within this setup, the digital record is duplicated across each node, and prior to any transaction inclusion, each node validates its authenticity (Sreeraj et al., 2021). The digital ledger is composed of blocks, each containing intricate transaction details (Singh Faujdar et al., 2019).

The application of block chain extends to diverse domains like education, manufacturing, and healthcare, owing to its distributed and decentralized nature (Sharma et al., 2020).

Ethereum stands out as a notable block chain platform, fueled by its native crypto currency, Ether. This platform enables the creation of smart contracts—self-executing agreements that trigger automatically upon meeting specific conditions. These smart contracts imbue logic into the block chain and can be adopted in the proposed approach for activities such as record transfers, medical experts' access to patient records, or access limitations for medical staff (Sadiku et al., 2018).In the healthcare sector, challenges encompass handling the copious data generated by hospitals and upholding patient data security and privacy. By integrating smart contracts into medical institutions, data security can be elevated, reducing the risk of breaches due to malicious hackers (Pereraa et al., 2020).

The foundational components of block chain—decentralization, security, privacy, and robustness through cryptographic methods—hold promise in tackling the ongoing predicaments in healthcare. Despite the pivotal role digital healthcare plays in data storage and administration, concerns about patient data leakage persist. Inadequate security and restricted data access in the current healthcare framework hinder exploration and innovation in the sector. The proposed block chain-based system aims to furnish secure access to medical information within the network, delivering efficient mechanisms to ensure accurate data and preserve patient confidentiality. Through block chain and smart contracts, the system establishes secure control over patient access to medical records (Gupta et al., 2019). A user-friendly website, underpinned by block chain technology, will be developed to safeguard data gathered by medical professionals and patients alike. Numerous studies have delved into block chain in healthcare, exploring diverse aspects and applications (Mehta et al., 2020). Yet, the innovative facets of the suggested system lie in its user-friendliness and integration with dedicated healthcare platforms. The central objective is to securely store all medical data in the cloud, enabling accessible data sharing among doctors and patients. Furthermore, the system's scope enables swift document retrieval and seamless medical record sharing with healthcare providers (Gupta et al., 2021). The study seeks to create a block chain-based system that heightens the security and management of patient data, fostering a secure, accessible, and decentralized healthcare environment. Patients can confidently share medical records with healthcare providers, retaining authority over their data privacy. The research also probes into the expanding roles of block chain technology across diverse sectors.

2. SECURING HEALTHCARE DATA

Healthcare Data Management relies on efficiently managing medical data, especially as contemporary technologies like telemedicine and remote health monitoring gain popularity (Gupta.R et al., 2020). Managing healthcare data is now more critical than ever due to the increasing use of technology in medical specialties. The importance of having accessible data for all sectors cannot be overstated. Data Management offers the opportunity to expedite and streamline data analysis, leading to better decision-making, strategic advantages, and improved overall organizational productivity(Ioannis et al., 2019). In the past, healthcare institutions relied on Manual Medical Records (MMR), which were paper-based. The initiation of Electronic Medical Records (EMR) marked the onset of Healthcare Information Technology (HIT) by incorporating patients' clinic or hospital-related information (Chen et al., 2018). Following this, the introduction of Electronic Health Records (EHR) expanded the scope to include data from various sources, including pharmacies and laboratory test reports. As various stakeholders in healthcare require access to data, Patient Health Records (PHR), which focus on patient-centric records, have been developed to cater to diverse medical illnesses and health issues. These records serve both clinical and administrative purposes. Clinically, they aid in providing optimal patient care, training clinical staff for proper electronic health record usage, and facilitating innovation in medical research(Sami Ullah et al., 2020). Administratively, they contribute to planning, organizing, and controlling medical services at national, state, and organizational levels. Many healthcare organizations are implementing an extended EHR, encompassing electronic clinical data, a modernized provider order section, and research capabilities across most clinical units. The table provided compares different categories of medical records handled within existing healthcare systems.

3. ARCHITECTURE OF EHR SYSTEM

In Figure 1, the system layout showcases the process when a patient chooses to access their medical records through MetaMask or the healthcare system's decentralized website. By utilizing their private key from the Ethereum wallet, the user gains seamless access. It's worth highlighting that this Ethereum wallet falls under the category of a cold storage wallet, significantly reducing the risk of compromise compared to hot wallets. Furthermore, the inconvenience of device loss is alleviated as patients can conveniently receive a replacement without any repercussions for their medical records.

This wallet also serves a broader function by enabling digital signatures for various documents and meeting verification requisites. It also supports multi-party patient verification scenarios. It provides the foundation for establishing a nuanced access control system based on medical record roles, alongside a block chain-backed distributed property identification system. In cases of medical emergencies, a similar multi-party permission mechanism can be activated to access vital patient records.

Figure 2 depicts the block diagram that presents the design of our proposed system, consisting of four primary elements: a user application, a block chain handshake protocol, a cloud infrastructure, and a public block chain network. This conceptual depiction serves a dual objective. Firstly, it grants users access to application interfaces customized for specific roles, including doctors and system administrators. This dynamic interface delivery aligns with the functions

Figure 1. Architecture of web-based EHR system

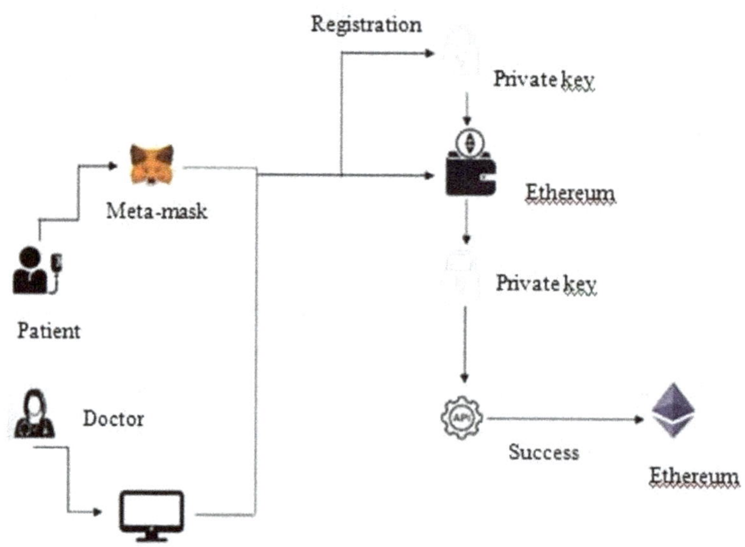

of each user type. Secondly, based on user-input data, the user application initiates transactions, which are then routed to the block chain handshake protocol for validation. A user- friendly interface serves as the bridge connecting users and the block chain handshake protocol.

At the heart of our proposed architecture lies the pivotal Block chain Handshake (BH) protocol. This integral element serves as the conduit linking the database server, the public block chain network (utilizing Ethereum block chain technology), and the cloud-based health record system, acting as an encapsulating layer. The public block chain network is the distributed ledger connecting block chain nodes (miners responsible for block chain updates) through a consensus mechanism. Notably, transactions are processed and verified using the network's smart contracts.

Within our design, the cloud fulfills two key services akin to conventional cloud-based Electronic Health Record (EHR) administration systems. The initial service entails hosting the EHR administration system, while the subsequent service involves data storage. All health- related records are securely stored in a cloud-based database. The EHR administration system actively manages transactions received from the block chain handshake protocol, executes the necessary tasks, and ultimately archives the transactions within the cloud database. In response to user queries for data access, the cloud seamlessly provides the requisite information.

Figure 2. Architecture of blockchain-based EHR system

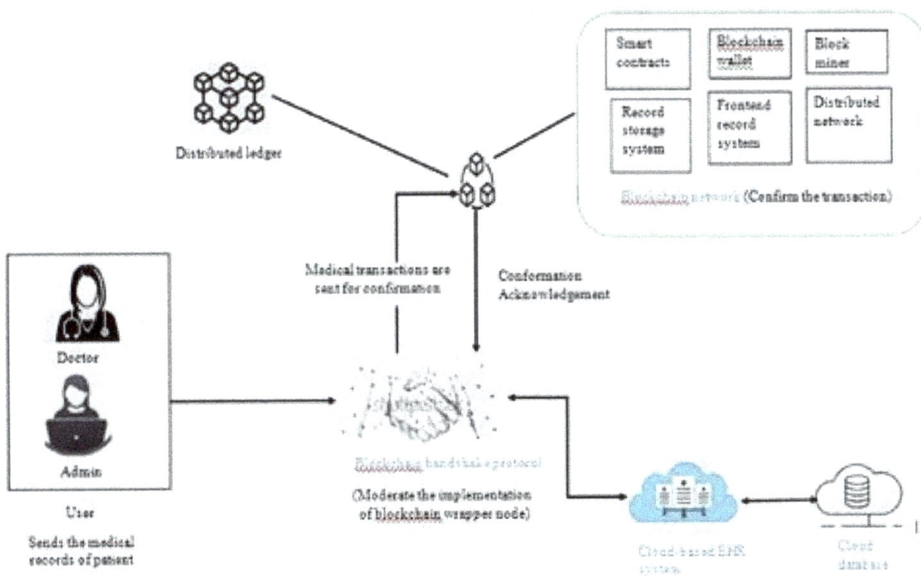

4. PROPOSED WORK

While strides have been made in the management of electronic medical data within the healthcare system, persistent challenges remain pertaining to the maintenance of comprehensive patient records, ensuring interoperability, safeguarding security, and facilitating seamless data exchange. The existing centralized approach adopted by healthcare organizations to store and oversee electronic health records on internal servers restricts the utilization of patient health records beyond the organization's confines. The current centralized approach creates barriers to accessing comprehensive patient medical histories, impacting various stakeholders including patients, doctors, hospitals, insurers, clinical labs, and researchers.

Recent strides in research have highlighted the transformative capability of blockchain technology as a central decentralized framework for driving progress in the healthcare domain. This innovation presents a remedy by creating a system that links together patients, physicians, healthcare establishments, researchers, insurers, and clinical laboratories. Of particular significance is the mechanism through which information is added to the distributed ledger achieved by a consensus algorithm that validates different segments of information. This constitutes a fundamental component of block chain technology.

Within this context, the following chapter introduces an Electronic Medical Record (EMR) framework built upon a decentralized block chain, aimed at fortifying secure data management within modern healthcare systems. The proposed system generates distinctive electronic medical records for efficient patient data administration. These records are meticulously validated through the integration of advanced consensus algorithms, ensuring the integrity and accuracy of the recorded data blocks.

4.1 Decentralized EMR System Using Blockchain

Patient health information finds its secure abode within a structured record referred to as an electronic medical record (EMR). Presently, healthcare data is housed in a centralized server located within healthcare facilities. Apprehensions about patient safety and data security often discourage these facilities from sharing information. Consequently, each healthcare establishment retains the patient's EMR locally, giving rise to challenges for both patients and clinicians, such as data loss and incomplete information leading to insufficient conclusions.

Originally linked with Bitcoin, blockchain technology has transcended its origins in financial transactions. It has evolved into a burgeoning technology with applications spanning various sectors, including healthcare, insurance, pharmacy, manufacturing, e-voting, legal contracts, tourism, energy, and travel (Pereraa et al., 2020). Blockchain draws its potency from technological leaps such as distributed networks, cryptography, and consensus algorithms. It materializes as a decentralized ledger formed by interlinking blocks housing validated transactions, effectively crafting a connected list. With each successful transaction, a new block is sequentially appended to the chain. A hash key establishes a connection between each block and its parent block, operating as a pointer, and this linkage originates from the genesis block. A block's architecture encompasses parent block pointers, a header, transactions, timestamp, hash, and nonce (Kim et al., 2018).

Three discernible blockchain architectures exist: consortium, private, and public. A private blockchain takes root within a company's internal cloud, while a public blockchain is accessible to network participants. In the former, authentication is administered by administrators and participants, whereas in the latter, participants collectively forge a peer-to-peer structure. Conversely, a consortium blockchain entails multiple organizations overseeing the platform, rather than a single entity.

The objective of this chapter is to seamlessly infuse blockchain technology into contemporary healthcare systems, amplifying secure data management for critical patient health records.

The proposed system seeks to facilitate secure data access among participating entities while uniquely identifying them. The BB_EMR system primarily revolves around three entities: the patient, the doctor, and the administrator. Upon enrolling new patients or doctors, a fresh block address and a globally unique identification are assigned, along with all pertinent entity details. The proposed system harnesses Ethereum blockchain-based smart contracts, featuring heightened consensus validation and robust encryption for the creation of new blocks and data access. The design of the BB_EMR system, encompassing key participating entities and their interaction flow, is elucidated in Figure 3.

As depicted in Figure 3, the structure encompasses three core entities: Hospital Admin, Patient, and Doctor. Each entity within the system is designated a predefined role. The responsibilities undertaken by the engaged participants in the envisioned BB_EMR system are delineated as follows:

Patient: This entity refers to an individual who registers by submitting personal information to seek consultation. Upon verification and approval, they are designated as a Patient within the system. They gain the ability to add medical conditions, set appointment dates, and designate their appointed doctor. Once these steps are completed, the patient gains access to their medical records. Additionally, the patient can choose to restrict the doctor's access if deemed necessary.

Doctor: Another participant is the Doctor, who registers as a medical professional, providing their personal details. Following confirmation and approval, they acquire the Doctor role. A doctor can only view or access the medical history of the patient assigned to them for consultation. Post-consultation, the doctor's access to the records is revoked to maintain privacy.

Figure 3. Decentralized EMR system using blockchain

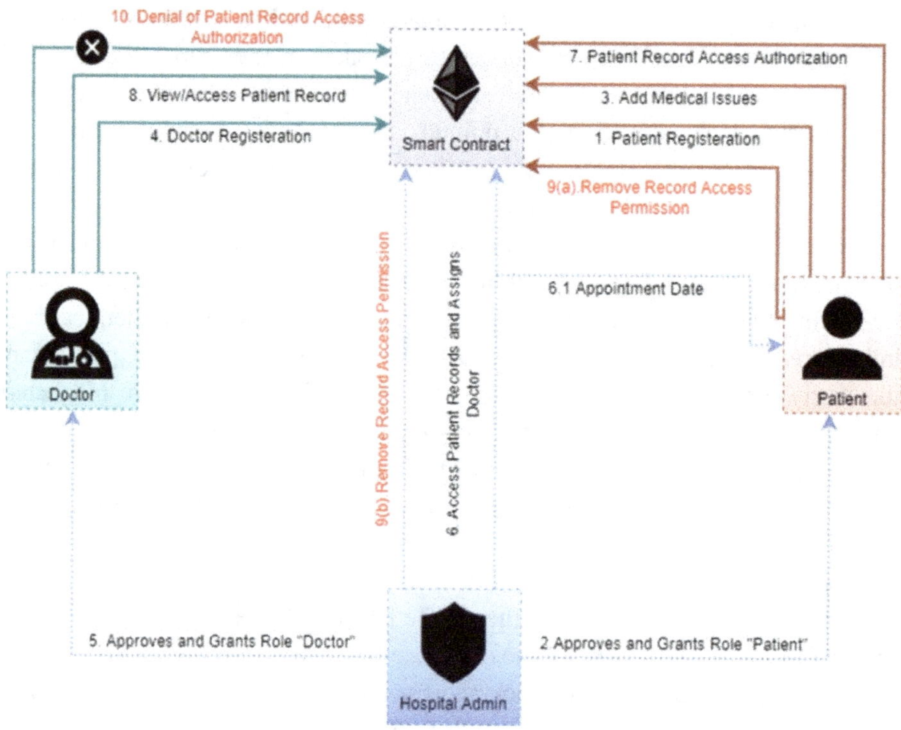

Admin: Acting as a mediator for communication and oversight between patient and doctor entities is the hospital administrator, or Admin. This entity holds the authority to authorize, validate, and allocate roles to both patient and doctor entities.

4.2 Data Blocks Processing Algorithm

Every entity in the proposed system is allocated a unique cryptographic hash address to prevent malicious data usage. Upon registration of a new doctor or patient, a distinctive global identifier is assigned. After admin validation and approval, the block chain is updated with a new block. The system's approach is centered around patient and admin control, utilizing an enhanced consensus algorithm for data block validation and access authorization. The data processing in the proposed system unfolds in several phases:

First Phase: The process commences with the registration of a doctor or patient, involving the generation of a global unique identifier and block hash address.

Second Phase: Enhanced consensus is applied in this phase to validate, approve, and assign roles to patient and doctor entities within the system.

Third Phase: This phase encompasses the patient's addition of medical issues, creating a unique health record for the patient.

Fourth Phase: The doctor is assigned to the patient, enabling them to access and review the patient's records.

Fifth Phase: Admin or the patient can revoke the doctor's access once the consultation concludes. Post-revocation, the doctor loses access to the patient's records.

The Block chain based EMR system guarantees steadfast security and privacy, alleviating susceptibilities to the threats and concerns identified in preceding chapters. Advanced encryption measures are seamlessly woven throughout every stage of the system. Each entity within the envisaged Block chain based EMR system engages in data processing through discrete steps, utilizing distinctive functions. These functions are represented as processing transactions in the block chain system. For each entity, three distinct processing algorithms are crafted to delineate the necessary steps for effective data processing and management. Figure 4 illustrates the data processing stages pertaining to the patient entity within the proposed system.

The depicted diagram succinctly illustrates the range of activities undertaken by the patient entity, encompassing three essential processing transactions: initial registration of new patients, inclusion of the patient's medical conditions, and the subsequent viewing or accessing of patient- specific details.

The illustrated Figure 5 delineates the data processing activities concerning the Doctor Entity within the proposed system. This entity engages in two distinct processing transactions: the enrollment of new doctors and the subsequent viewing or accessing of patient information.

The processing transactions highlighted in the preceding diagrams yield specific output events. Figure 6 illustrates the algorithm governing data processing for the admin entity. The admin entity undertakes crucial tasks such as granting approval to patients and doctors, assigning doctors to patients for medical record access, and subsequently revoking doctor access to patient records as needed.

A consensus algorithm functions as a mechanism through which all participants in a blockchain network collectively attain agreement on the current state of the distributed ledger. This procedure guarantees reliability within the blockchain network and cultivates trust among unknown peers in a decentralized computing environment. Essentially, a consensus protocol ensures that each new block integrated into the blockchain is the singular, universally acknowledged version of truth by all nodes within the network. The primary objectives of a blockchain consensus protocol encompass reaching consensus, encouraging collaboration, promoting cooperation, granting equal rights to all participating nodes, and necessitating the engagement of every node in the consensus process. Therefore, the central aim of a consensus algorithm is to achieve agreement that benefits the entire network. The importance of consensus lies in upholding unanimity among nodes, particularly as a network

Figure 4. Processing algorithm for patient entity

Processing Algorithm for Patient Entity

1. **Admin:** Deploys the smart contract BB_EMR(Admin account_address)
2. **Patient:** Input details (Patient account_address)
3. **Processing Transaction: registerPatient()**

   3.1 If Patient is already registered:

   "Transaction failed"

   Error generated: "Patient Already Registered"

   Else: "Transaction Successful and Save Details"

   3.2 Generate Global Unique Patient Identifier: gUpId

   3.3 Patient Hash Generated: **generateHash()**
4. **Processing Transaction: addIssue ()**

   4.1 If patient is not approved by admin

   "Transaction failed"

   Error generated: "Patient not approved to add medical issues"

   Else: "Transaction Successful and Issues Added"
5. **Processing Transaction: viewDetails()**

   5.1 If patient is not approved by admin or incorrect patient account_address

   "Transaction failed"

   Error generated: "The address mentioned is not a registered patient"

   Else: "Transaction Successful and View Details in Output"
6. **Output:** emit events: Registered(),Hash Generated (),issueAdded ()

expands, which makes communication and agreement increasingly complex among numerous nodes.

In public blockchains, user participation is essential to verify and validate transactions. Given the dynamic and automated nature of blockchains, a secure mechanism is imperative to ensure transaction validity, necessitating consensus among participants. Various consensus methods have been proposed, each adhering to distinct sets of rules. Different blockchain platforms utilize well-known consensus algorithms like Proof of Work, Proof of Stake, Delegated Proof of Stake, Practical Byzantine Fault Tolerance, Proof of Validation, Proof of Authority, and the Ripple Protocol Consensus Algorithm. These algorithms are extensively expounded upon in this section.

Figure 5. Processing algorithm for doctor entity

Processing Algorithm for Doctor Entity

1. **Admin**: Deploys the smart contract BB_EMR(Admin account_address)
2. **Input:** Doctor details (Doctor account_address)
3. **Processing Transaction: registerDoctor()**

    3.1 If Doctor is already registered:

    "Transaction failed"

    Error generated: "Doctor Already Registered"

    Else: "Transaction Successful and Save Details"

    3.2 Generate Global Unique Identifier: gUId

    3.3 Doctor Hash Generated: **generateHash()**
4. **Processing Transaction: viewDetails()**

    4.1 If Doctor is not assigned to the Patient

    "Transaction failed"

    Error generated: "Not authorised to view details of this patient"

    Else: "Transaction Successful and View Details in Output"
5. **Output:** emit events: Registered(), Hash Generated ()

The Proposed System is constructed upon Ethereum, which inherently combines both Proof of Work and Proof of Stake algorithms. Specifically, Proof of Work is an intricate, resource- intensive consensus mechanism. For a block to be added to the chain, all nodes must collectively validate, verify, and authenticate the transactions contained within the new block. In contrast, Proof of Stake is comparatively energy-efficient and potent. The Ethereum consensus approach, rooted in Keccak256 and serving as a core component of the Ethhash Proof of Work algorithm, occupies a central role in the proposed system. The Ethereum consensus relies on the Ethhash Proof of Work algorithm, also known as the Dagger Hashimoto algorithm, utilizing Keccak256 for cryptographic hash generation and profiling. This algorithm determines the Keccak-256 hash of the input. A depiction of the Keccak hash computation for a given input string is presented in Figure 7.

The robust Keccak256 algorithm, forming the foundation of the Proof of Work consensus mechanism in the Ethereum blockchain, is harnessed to establish consensus within the proposed system. To enhance the existing consensus process, the proposed solution introduces an administrative role that contributes to data block validation and approval. This introduction of an administrative entity alongside

Figure 6. Processing algorithm for admin entity

Processing Algorithm for Admin Entity

```
1. Admin: Deploys the smart contract BB_EMR(Admin account_address)
2. Input: Input details (Admin account_address)
3. Processing Transaction: approvePatient(Patient account_address)
   3.1 If account_address is Admin account_address:
             grantRole (): "Patient"
       Else If: Patient is not registered:
                 "Transaction failed"
                 Error generated: "Patient not registered"
       Else: "Transaction failed"
             Error generated: "Does not have Admin Rights"
4. Processing Transaction: approveDoctor(Doctor account_address)
   4.1 If account_address is Admin account_address:
             grantRole (): "Doctor"
       Else If: Doctor is not registered:
                 "Transaction failed"
                 Error generated: "Doctor not registered"
       Else: "Transaction failed"
             Error generated: "Does not have Admin Rights"
5. Processing Transaction: assignDoctor (Patient ,Doctor)
   5.1 If account_address is Admin account_address:
             assignDoctor (): "Appointment Date, Cabin Number"
       Else If: Doctor is not approved:
                 "Transaction failed"
                 Error generated: "Address assigned is not an approved doctor"
       Else If: Patient is not approved:
                 "Transaction failed"
                 Error generated: "Address assigned is not an approved patient"
       Else: "Transaction failed"
             Error generated: "Does not have Admin Rights"
6. Processing Transaction: removeDoctor (Patient account_address ,Doctor account_address)
   6.1 If account_address is Admin account_address:
                 removeDoctor(): "The doctor is not assigned to this patient"
       Else If: Doctor is not approved:
                 "Transaction failed"
                 Error generated: "Address assigned is not an approved doctor"
       Else If: Patient is not approved:
                 "Transaction failed"
                 Error generated: "Address assigned is not an approved patient"
       Else: "Transaction failed"
                 Error generated: "Not authorised to revoke access/remove doctor"
7. Output: Approved and Access Granted(Patient, Doctor), Access Revoked
```

other validating nodes within the blockchain network further bolsters the integrity of the consensus process.

The coding of smart contracts necessitates the implementation of distinct components involving transactions and events. On the Ethereum Block chain, transactions are represented as functions within the smart contract that are executed, subsequently altering the state. An event, an inherent element of a smart contract,

Figure 7. Keccak256 hash generation for sample input

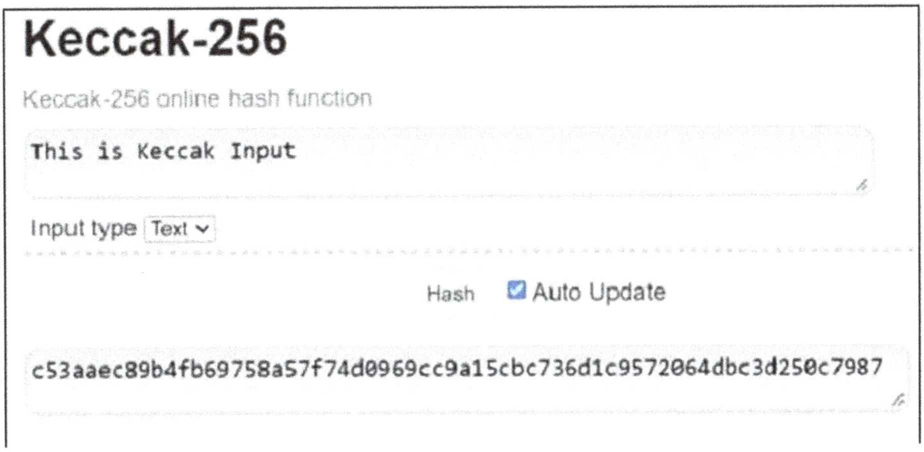

Table. 1 Transactions and events

Component	Type	Function
Register Patient	Transaction	Patient enters registration information
Approve Patient	Transaction	The role of ――Patient‖ is granted by admin after the patient is approved
Add Issues	Transaction	After receiving admin approval, the patient can add medical conditions
Register Doctor	Transaction	Doctor enters registration information
Approve Doctor	Transaction	The role of "Doctor" is granted by admin after the doctor is approved
Assign Doctor	Transaction	Doctor is given access to patient's records by admin.
View Details	Transaction	Patient can view details, Doctor can view details if assigned

comes into play when the contract is deployed. These events capture the parameters within the transaction output logs, which are stored on the block chain and retrievable using the address of the deployed smart contract. Refer to Table 1 for a comprehensive compilation of the transactions and events integrated into the smart contract, along with insights into their respective functionalities.

5. CONCLUSION

Within the scope of this research, enhancements in encryption measures have been introduced to bolster the impregnability and robust security of electronic medical records. By implementing the proposed framework on the Binance Smart Chain, scalability and safety aspects have been refined and fortified. The decentralized

MRBSChain EMR framework encompasses elevated encryption protocols, ensuring the immutability of medical records stored on the block chain, thereby preventing any unauthorized modifications or deletions. Moreover, the framework facilitates regulated access to these records, ensuring stringent security.

Central to this system is the emphasis on patient-centric and administrator-centric approaches to sanctioned data access. This is achieved through the implementation of globally unique identifiers utilizing gUpId. To further safeguard the integrity of medical information, the framework employs hashing algorithms such as SHA256, Keccak256, and Encrypted Double Hash Mapping. These measures collectively contribute to restricted access to medical data, enhancing overall security.

6. FUTURE WORK

Every research endeavor is bounded by specific parameters. The study at hand also carried certain limitations, paving the way for potential avenues of exploration in subsequent research.While the present study introduced a groundbreaking decentralized paradigm for the healthcare sector, it's essential to acknowledge that, like any technology, Block chain confronts its share of challenges. These challenges can potentially be addressed in the future. Additionally, the integration of Block chain with emerging technologies like IoT, AI, and Cloud Computing holds promise for further innovation in this digital epoch.

Despite the profound impact anticipated on medical records management within the healthcare landscape, the proposed framework's suitability predominantly applies to smaller-scale volumetric data due to its on-chain storage structure. To accommodate the storage demands of extensive data, it becomes imperative to enhance the storage architecture through the incorporation of big data layers and off-chain storage mechanisms.

The healthcare industry encompasses a diverse array of stakeholders, including hospital management, physicians, patients, insurance and claims management entities, clinical laboratories, and research organizations. Although the proposed work primarily concentrated on the three primary parties—hospital administrators, patients, and doctors—involved in medical record interactions, it approached the framework from a patient-centric viewpoint. Future enhancements could encompass a broader spectrum of stakeholders, thus enriching the proposed framework's comprehensiveness and applicability.

REFERENCES

Chen, W., Xu, Z., Shi, S., Zhao, Y., & Zhao, J. (2018). A Survey of Blockchain Applications in Different Domains. In ICBTA 2018. Association for Computing Machinery. doi:10.1145/3301403.3301407

Gharat, A., Aher, P., Chaudhari, P., & Alte, B. (2021). A framework for secure storage and sharing of electronic health records using blockchain technology. *ITM Web of Conferences*, *40*, 03037.

Gupta, M. (2021). PR wallet based blockchain access protocol to secure EHRs. In *Blockchain and IoT Integration* (pp. 65–76). Auerbach Publications. doi:10.1201/9781003094210-4

Gupta, R., Tanwar, S., Al-Turjman, F., Italiya, P., Nauman, A., & Kim, S. W. (2020). Smart Contract Privacy Protection Using AI in Cyber-Physical Systems: Tools, Techniques and Challenges. *IEEE Access : Practical Innovations, Open Solutions*, *8*, 24746–24772. doi:10.1109/ACCESS.2020.2970576

Gupta, R., Tanwar, S., Tyagi, S., Kumar, N., Obaidat, M. S., & Sadoun, B. (2019). HaBiTs: Blockchain-based telesurgery framework for healthcare 4.0. In *International Conference on Computer, Information and Telecommunication Systems, CITS* (pp. 1–5). 10.1109/CITS.2019.8862127

Ioannis, S. & Konstanti. (2019, November). Blockchain and Brand Loyalty Programs: A Short Review of Applications and Challenges. *Procedia of Economics and Business Administration*.

Kim, M. G., Lee, A. R., Kwon, H. J., Kim, J. W., & Kim, I. K. (2018). Sharing medical questionnaires based on blockchain. In *2018 IEEE International Conference on Bioinformatics and Biomedicine (BIBM)* (pp. 2767–2769). 10.1109/BIBM.2018.8621154

Mehta, P., Gupta, R., & Tanwar, S. (2020). Blockchain envisioned UAV networks: Challenges, solutions, and comparisons. *Computer Communications*, *151*, 518–538. doi:10.1016/j.comcom.2020.01.023

Pereraa, S., Nanayakkaraa, S., Rodrigoa, M. N. N., Senaratnea, S., & Wein, R. (2020). Blockchain technology: Is it hype or real in the construction industry? *Journal of Industrial Information Integration*, *17*, 100–125. doi:10.1016/j.jii.2020.100125

Sadiku, M. N. O., Eze, K. G., & Musa, S. M. (2018). Blockchain Technology in Healthcare. *International Journal of Advances in Scientific Research and Engineering*, *4*(5). Advance online publication. doi:10.31695/IJASRE.2018.32723

Sami UllahH.AslamS.ArjomandN. (2020). Blockchain in Healthcare and Medicine: A Contemporary Research of Applications, Challenges, and Future Perspectives. *Cryptography and Security*. arXiv:2004.06795 [cs.CR].

Sharma, A., Sarishma, Tomar, R., Chilamkurti, N., & Kim, B.-G. (1609). Blockchain-based smart contracts for Internet of Medical Things in e-Healthcare. *Electronics (Basel)*, *9*(10), 1609. doi:10.3390/electronics9101609

Singh Faujdar, D., Sahay, S., Singh, T., Jindal, H., & Kumar, R. (2019). Public health information systems for primary health care in India: A situational analysis study. *Journal of Family Medicine and Primary Care*, *8*(11), 3640–3646. doi:10.4103/jfmpc.jfmpc_808_19 PMID:31803666

Sreeraj, R., Singh, A., & Anbarasu, V. (2021). Preserving EMR records using blockchain. *Annals of the Romanian Society for Cell Biology*, *25*(6), 5344–5350.

Chapter 5
A Systematic Review:
Future Prospects and Challenges to IoT-Based EHRs in the Healthcare Industry

N. Manikandan
SRM Institute of Science and Technology, India

M. Suresh Ananad
SRM Institute of Science and Technology, India

A. Devi Priya
SRM Institute of Science and Technology, India

G. Padmapriya
SRM Institute of Science and Technology, India

D. Vinod
SRM Institute of Science and Technology, India

ABSTRACT

In modern era, the internet of things (IoT) has transfigured the medical industry, empowering the unified collection and exchange of patient data. However, this increased connectivity has raised significant concerns regarding the safety and confidentiality of electronic healthcare records (EHRs). This systematic review explores the security and privacy issues surrounding IoT-based EHRs and presents an in-depth analysis of how blockchain technology can be employed as an effective countermeasure to address these challenges. The chapter provides an overview of IoT in healthcare, highlights the vulnerabilities of EHR systems, and discusses the potential threats to patient data. It then delves into the principles of blockchain technology and its applicability to enhance EHR security and privacy. Various blockchain-based solutions and implementations are reviewed, and their advantages and limitations are discussed. This systematic review investigates the incorporation of IoT with EHRs in healthcare and contributes towards better understanding of the synergy between IoT, EHRs, and blockchain in the healthcare industry and

DOI: 10.4018/979-8-3693-1662-7.ch005

assists as a valuable supplement for academics, practitioners, and policymakers. Additionally, the survey presents case studies and real-world examples of successful blockchain integration into healthcare systems. Finally, this chapter concludes by outlining the future prospects and challenges of utilizing blockchain technology for securing IoT-based EHRs and emphasizes the importance of a holistic approach to safeguarding patient data.

1. INTRODUCTION

The healthcare industry is undergoing a paradigm shift from traditional to innovative technologies, for example the Internet of Things (IoT) and blockchain (Endale Mitiku Adere et.al.,2022, Geetha et al.,2024). Electronic Health Records (EHRs) have become an integral part of modern healthcare systems, enabling seamless storage and exchange of patient data (Aste T et al., 2017). IoT devices, ranging from wearable gadgets to medical sensors, have further enriched the healthcare landscape by providing real-time health monitoring and personalized patient care (P. De Filippi et al., 2020, Swan M et al., 2015).

However, the integration of IoT devices with EHRs presents several challenges, including ensuring data security, privacy, and interoperability. Traditional EHR systems are vulnerable to data breaches and tampering, raising concerns about the confidentiality and integrity of patient information (Eberhardt J et al., 2017). Moreover, the diverse nature of IoT devices poses a challenge in standardizing data formats and communication protocols for effective integration with EHRs.

1.1 Background and Motivation

Blockchain technology, renowned for its decentralized and immutable nature, proposed an effective answer to these mentioned challenges. By leveraging blockchain, healthcare providers can establish a protected system to manage IoT-generated data within EHRs (Kohli R et al., 2016, Roman-Belmonte JM et al., 2018). Blockchain ensures data integrity, enhances security through cryptographic techniques, and enables seamless data sharing among stakeholders while maintaining patient privacy.

The motivation behind this systematic review stems from the urgent need to explore the intersection of IoT, EHRs, and blockchain technology in the healthcare industry. The medical industry positions at the height of a transformative era, determined towards the convergence of innovative technologies. Among these, the Internet of Things (IoT) and blockchain technology have emerged as pivotal forces reshaping the landscape of healthcare industry. Electronic Health Records (EHRs) have long been the cornerstone of modern healthcare systems, streamlining patient data management and enabling efficient medical services. The amalgamation of IoT devices along with EHRs had unlocked unprecedented opportunities for real-time monitoring, personalized treatment plans, and data-driven decision-making (Angraal S et al., 2017). However, this integration poses significant challenges, particularly concerning data security, integrity, and interoperability.

The rapid proliferation of IoT devices, ranging from wearable health trackers to sophisticated medical sensors, has ushered in an era of continuous and remote patient monitoring. These devices generate vast amounts of real-time health data, offering invaluable insights into patient well-being (T.-T. Kuo et al., 2017). Concurrently, blockchain technology, originally devised as the underlying architecture for cryptocurrencies, has found diverse applications across various sectors. In the realm of healthcare, blockchain offers a decentralized, secure, and immutable platform for managing sensitive patient information. By integrating IoT devices with blockchain-enabled Electronic Health Records (IoT-based EHRs), healthcare providers can confirm the truthfulness and confidentiality of outpatient information while enabling seamless data sharing among authorized stakeholders.

1.2 Problem Statement

The emergence of Bitcoin marked the inception of blockchain technology, serving as the foundational framework for cryptocurrencies. However, it was using Ethereum that revolutionized the blockchain landscape by introducing the concept of smart contracts. The self-tuned contracts encrypted along with defined guidelines, drastically altered the utilization of blockchain technology. Ethereum's innovative approach paved the way for a plethora of smart contract-based applications, ranging from crowdfunding platforms to smart property management systems.

This expansion of blockchain applications beyond digital currencies led to the advent of what is now known as blockchain 3.0 (Khan MA et al., 2018). In this chapter, blockchain technology transcended its initial financial use case and found applications in diverse domains, including but not limited to industry, healthcare, and business logistics management. The versatility of self-tuned contracts enabled their integration into a wide variety of sectors, fundamentally reshaping how transactions, data, and agreements are managed in the digital realm. Blockchain 3.0 represents a paradigm shift where the technology's potential is harnessed beyond cryptocurrencies. It signifies a new era of decentralized applications (DApps) and innovative solutions that leverage blockchain's inherent security, transparency, and immutability. As a result, industries are exploring novel ways to optimize processes, enhance security, and improve efficiency, all made possible by the integration of blockchain.

1.3 Objectives of the Review

This remarkable progress has been driven by advancements in both computer science and economic principles. Key innovations, such as computer-to-computer networks, public key encryption, proof of work and proof of stake, decentralized storage, decentralized databases, automatic contracts, and impetus schemes, have played pivotal roles in shaping the evolution of blockchain technology. Blockchain is playing crucial change in traditional technique for managing the data. In conventional approach, the information is maintained and handled with single server along with central administrator. In contract, blockchain has been used for managing the data in a digital register that can be dispersed around the computer – to - computer network along with no centralised administrator for managing the data is described in the Figure 1.1. Peer-to-peer networks (computer-to-computer networks) laid the foundation for decentralized communication and data exchange, allowing nodes in a network to interact directly without the need for a central authority. Asymmetric cryptography provided the means for secure data transmission and user authentication, ensuring privacy and integrity in digital transactions. Consensus protocols enabled decentralized decision-making, confirming all type of network customers approve upon the expiry of the relations and state of the system.

Decentralized storage solutions revolutionized data management by distributing information across a network of nodes, enhancing data resilience and accessibility. Decentralized computing, coupled with smart contracts, introduced the concept of self-executing code, enabling automated and trustless transactions. Smart contracts,

Figure 1. Traditional vs. peer-to-peer network
Source: HIMSS Blockchain Networks Overview (HIMSS 2019)

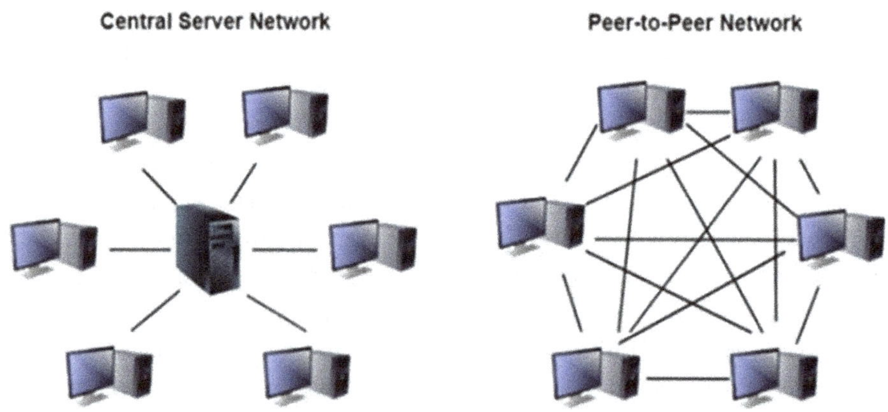

powered by decentralized computing, facilitate agreements between parties without the need for intermediaries, streamlining processes and reducing costs. Additionally, incentive systems, often implemented through cryptocurrencies and tokens, motivate participants to contribute resources and maintain the network's integrity. These economic principles ensure that individuals and entities are rewarded for their participation, fostering a self-sustaining ecosystem of collaborative efforts. Together, these technological and economic advancements have propelled the blockchain industry forward, enabling the development of innovative applications beyond traditional financial use cases. The synergistic integration of these principles continues to fuel the growth of blockchain technology, driving its adoption across various sectors and paving the way for a decentralized and more efficient digital future.

Security is the mainly considered for technological factor of blockchain technology that will projects the medical and IoT applications. A certain consideration encompasses different titles such as, information safety, devices and nodes. Data/information are the major factor in data management. So the management of data is projected by this chapter for covering the data gathering, computation, and outputting, storing, recovery and data safety. Here, necessary to protect or toughen all the activities of data in medical industry and IoT. In medical industry, several challenges hinder the seamless exchange of information. One significant obstacle is to identify the exclusive patient absence that will make it difficult to accurately match patient records across different healthcare providers. Additionally, there is message delay protocols that can support both lexical and connotation interoperability among various devices, leading to communication gaps and data inconsistencies. Furthermore, the absence of standardized data encoding methods exacerbates these issues, making it challenging to establish a cohesive and standardized approach to managing healthcare data. Addressing these impediments is crucial for enhancing the efficiency and effectiveness of healthcare information exchange and ensuring high-quality patient care (Taylor PJ et al., 2019). Huge volume of data are generated in both offline as well as online for confounding the management of data in Web of Things (WoT) framework. At an outcome, many researchers have suggested to elevate to blockchain-based implemented systems are considered as a primary solution for managing data. So the challenges and future prospects of blockchain in medical industry and the web of things are reviewed in this chapter.

1.4 Contributions

In order to attaining the previously outlined objectives, this chapter significantly put up to the existing survey with addressing notable difference in current research. These differences encompass the scarcity of consistent reviews concerning repudiation and protection in blockchain-based systems. Furthermore, there is delay thorough reviews exploring the integration of distributed ledger and web of things technologies. Additionally, this review enhances the understanding of various other pertinent problems, like confidential techniques employed in distributed ledger-based technologies. The following key contributions could be highlighted:

1. Comprehensive Exploration of Access Control and Data Integrity: By delving into integrity mechanisms and data confidentiality within distributed ledger-based systems, this review offers an in-depth analysis of these critical aspects. It fills a void in the literature by providing a comprehensive overview of existing strategies, highlighting their strengths, limitations, and potential areas of improvement.
2. Thorough Examination of Blockchain and IoT Integration: This review bridges the gap in research by thoroughly investigating the integration of blockchain and IoT technologies. By synthesizing existing knowledge and exploring real-world implementations, it sheds light on the synergies between these two transformative technologies. This analysis offers valuable insights into the challenges faced and the opportunities presented by their convergence in various applications, particularly in the healthcare sector.
3. Insightful Analysis of Privacy-Preserving Techniques: Privacy concerns are paramount in blockchain-based systems. This review critically assesses the privacy-preserving techniques employed in these systems, evaluating their effectiveness and suitability for different contexts. By addressing the nuances of privacy preservation within blockchain technology, this review informs future research efforts and practical implementations, ensuring that privacy remains a central focus in blockchain applications.

These contributions not only enrich the existing body of knowledge but also provide valuable guidance for researchers, practitioners, and policymakers. By filling these gaps and offering comprehensive insights, this review advances the understanding of blockchain technology's intricate facets, promoting its effective and responsible integration into various domains, including healthcare, industry, and beyond.

2. RELATED WORK

2.1 Overview of Web of Things in Healthcare

The medical industry data is transfigured by enhancing the tireless amalgamation of different systems, sensors and device to gather, transfer and modify the data in real time in Web of Things technology. This interconnected node of physical systems, often combined with sensors and software, facilitates the monitoring & management of healthcare processes, outputting to patient data improvement and extended efficiency in healthcare delivery.

2.1.1 Internet of Things

The devices used in internet of things can computed from day to day life objects to complex business machinery, and these will communicate with other devices by using central server systems to share information & perform various tasks without human intervention.

Key aspects of IoT include:

1. Sensors and Connectivity: IoT systems are furnished with sensors that can able to gather data such as temperature, humidity, motion, and more. These devices use various communication technologies to transmit data to centralized systems for processing.
2. Data pre-processing and Analysis: The data gathered by IoT systems has been send to cloud servers for pre-processing and analysis. Advanced algorithms and machine learning models are often applied to develop meaningful information from data.
3. Automation and Control: IoT system empowers automation by allowing devices to respond to specific conditions or triggers automatically. For example, a smart thermostat can adjust the temperature based on occupancy or weather conditions without manual intervention.
4. Remote Monitoring and Management: IoT technology empowers real-time monitoring systems from remote locations. This is particularly valuable in applications like healthcare, where patient vitals can be monitored remotely, or in industrial settings, where machinery performance can be tracked.

2.1.2 Applications

- Smart Home: IoT devices in homes include smart thermostats, security cameras, smart appliances, and voice assistants that enhance convenience and energy efficiency.
- Healthcare: IoT devices monitor patients' health, track medications, and assist in remote patient monitoring, improving healthcare outcomes.
- Industrial IoT (IIoT): IoT is extensively used in industries for predictive maintenance, supply chain optimization, and monitoring equipment performance, enhancing operational efficiency.

- Smart Cities: IoT technologies are deployed in urban areas for traffic management, waste management, smart street lighting, and environmental monitoring to create sustainable and efficient cities.
- Agriculture: IoT devices help farmers monitor crop conditions, soil moisture, and weather patterns, leading to precision farming and increased crop yield.

2.1.3 Challenges

- Security: IoT devices are susceptible to cybersecurity threats. Ensuring safety measures, including confidential and authentication, is essential to safeguard data & privacy.
- Interoperability: The lack of standardized protocols can hinder communication among IoT systems, requiring efforts to ensure seamless interoperability.
- Scalability: The scalability is a very big challenges while facing the growth of the data.
- Privacy: Collecting and processing confidential data from IoT systems improve privacy. Implementing privacy policies and practices is crucial to address these issues.

Overall, IoT technology continues to transform various sectors, offering new opportunities for efficiency, automation, and improved decision-making. As the IoT ecosystem evolves, addressing security, interoperability, and privacy challenges will be pivotal in harnessing the full potential of this transformative technology.

2.1.2 Healthcare IT

The key components and aspects of Health Information Technology:

1. Electronic Health Records (EHRs): EHRs are digital versions of patients' data charts. This will provide the patients' medical data, analyses, medicines, management plans, vaccination details, antipathies, radiology, and results of the test, allowing healthcare providers to access and update patient information electronically. EHRs improve accuracy, reduce paperwork, and support better coordination of care among healthcare professionals.
2. Health Information Exchange (HIE): HIE empowers the electronic transferring of patient data among various medical industry. It allows medical persons to analyse and access the patient medical data that leads to care improvement, faster decision-making, and reduced duplicate tests or procedures.

3. Telemedicine and Telehealth: Health IT enables remote consultations and monitoring of patients through telemedicine and telehealth technologies. Patients can connect with doctors through skype calls, messaging apps and wearable devices, allowing for virtual consultations, remote monitoring of vital signs, and managing chronic conditions from the comfort of home.
4. Clinical Decision Support Systems (CDSS): These systems provide evidence-based recommendations, alert healthcare professionals about potential drug interactions, suggest diagnostic tests, and help in the interpretation of test results, enhancing the quality and safety of patient care.
5. Mobile Health (mHealth) Applications: Mobile health apps run on smartphones and other mobile devices, allowing users to track their health, access medical information, schedule appointments, and communicate with healthcare providers. mHealth apps support patient engagement, self-management, and facilitate remote monitoring of health conditions.

Health Information Technology continues to evolve, playing a pivotal role in improving healthcare quality, enhancing patient experiences, reducing costs, and supporting more efficient and effective healthcare delivery systems. As technology advances, the integration of Health IT solutions is expected to further transform the healthcare landscape, driving innovation and improving patient outcomes.

The primary objective of Health Information Technology (HIT) is to attain various advantages, including minimizing medical errors, enhancing patient outcomes, improving the quality of patient care, boosting physician efficiency, increasing the overall value of hospitals, and optimizing the operational and financial performance of healthcare institutions. Generally, research studies have shown that Health Information Technology (HIT) is most effective when utilized collectively as a unified system (Karahanna E et al., 2019). Despite this, there has been a longstanding issue of fragmentation in its implementation. Recognizing this challenge, government initiatives aimed at enhancing health information exchange among healthcare providers have been implemented (Vest JR 2010).

2.2 Blockchain Technology in Healthcare

2.2.1. Blockchain

A universally accepted definition of blockchain technology remains elusive. Different authors have put forward diverse interpretations, leading to varying perspectives on the topic. Some, like (Ducas E et al.,2017, Hammi MT et al., 2018), define blockchain as a distributed digital ledger. In contrast, others, such as (Dagher GG et al., 2018, Danzi P et al., 2018, Qiu T et al., 2019), view this in terms of a specific data structure. Additionally, certain authors, like (Kleinaki A-S et al., 2018, S. Kamble 2009), conceptualize blockchain as a transaction management technology. These divergent viewpoints reflect the multifaceted nature of blockchain technology.

The discrepancies in defining blockchain technology stem from the diverse viewpoints of authors and the technology's continuous evolution, making it a dynamic and evolving concept. As discussed earlier, Blockchain has been progressed through its initial stages (BlockChain Version 1.0) to more advanced iterations (BlockChain Version 3.0). This evolution based on the technique of several foundational elements outlined in references (Dinh TTA et al., 2018, Croman K, et al. 2016). These fundamentals encompass computer-to-computer networks, distributed ledger, consensus protocols, automated contracts, and application domains. Despite the variation in interpretations, these components are universally recognized as critical aspects of blockchain technology.

2.2.2. Distributed Ledger

In a distributed ledger system, blocks are formed by grouping transactions together. To provide a detailed understanding of blocks and transactions, the contents of each are outlined in Table 1.

In the context described, each block contains the transactions hash value and the hash point of previous block in its header part. Here inclusion empowers a durability and safety of both blocks and transactions. The generation of a block hinges on providing solution for computational problems, the level of difficulty can be mentioned in the block header part. This type of process, known as mining, requires substantial timeline and computational energy.

2.2.3. Smart Contract

A smart contract can be conceptualized as an autonomously triggered process that activates while the transaction gets activated. When all of the distributed ledger technology systems support smart contracts, there are variations to programming languages used for writing them and the environments in which they operate. Commonly used smart contract languages include Solidity, Golang, Serpent, Java, Python, and LLL.

2.2.4. Blockchain Use and Applications

As discussed earlier, the progress of blockchain technology is evident in its expanding application areas and diverse purposes. The specific domain of application and the intended purpose significantly impact the distributed ledger technology problems.

Table 1. Blocks content

Block (Bl) Header	
Name of the Block	**Description**
Version of the block	Block version number
Hash value block	Block hash value
Timestamp	Block time
Root	Transactions Root
Nonce	Random value for Consensus protocols
Bl Body: Transactions	
Transactions 1, Transactions 2……Transactions n	
Transaction header	
Hash point	Hash value of transactions
Block number	Block number of transactions
Order number	Transactions number
Timestamp	Transactions timeline
Sender / Receiver	Sender Id / Receiver Id
Signature	Transactions hash value

Payload
data 1, data 2……data n

A mandatory field such as medical industry, economical systems, digital management, and benefits of computer-to-computer blockchain is necessary. In this setup, a central server hosts a single ledger, while peers maintain metadata. Additionally, decentralized technology adopted topology can be suggested in banking applications, as highlighted in Reference (Peters GW et al., 2016). Here, a Distributed Hash Table (DHT) can be used for maintaining the reviews through blockchain. The information could be placed in either centralised store or cloud-based store like randomly selected nodes, with DHT enhancing data accessibility (Zyskind G et al., 2015). Decentralized server based unstructured protocol is a common approach in designing blockchain architectures, especially in cryptocurrency & certain IoT sector involving numerous networks. Similar clustering methods, as mentioned earlier, are also be applied in blockchain systems (Huang B et al.,2017). The communication techniques previously described are similarly relevant in the scenarios involving blockchain technology. For instance, Bitcoin placed as the best example of a decentralized unstructured computer-to-computer network where relations are disseminated among customers. Likewise, Hyperledger Fabric utilizes gossip protocols for similar purposes. The below figure depicts the blockchain components.

Figure 2. Blockchain components

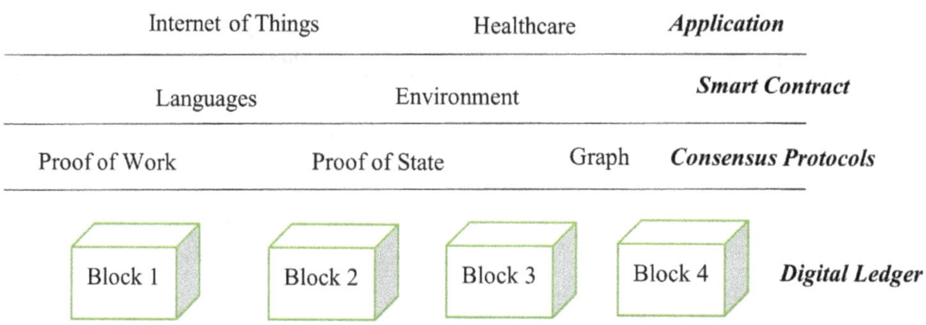

2.4 IoT-Based EHRs and Blockchain Integration

When authors explore the integration of blockchain technology within an IoT context, their approach is often guided by various factors, including the specific application domain they are targeting, the desired levels of latency and throughput, the regulatory landscape of the chosen sector, and the feasibility of managing participants within the blockchain network.

In light of these considerations, some scholarly articles have proposed classification frameworks for integrating blockchain and IoT technologies, aiming to categorize these integrations into distinct types. One approach, outlined in (Danzi P et al., 2018), involves categorizing integration solutions based on the volume of input that can traverses the blockchain through the interchange of information among IoT systems. Meanwhile, another study (Gai K et al., 2018) compares the use of blockchain with traditional cloud services for providing IoT-related services.

Certainly, the integration approaches between blockchain and IoT devices vary based on the emphasis placed on their relationship. In one approach (A. Reyna et al., 2018), the focus is primarily on the interaction between blockchain and IoT devices. In this scenario, blockchain acts as a storage medium, holding certain data or metadata from the IoT devices, a concept often referred to as offline chain usage. Expanding this integration towards cloud, another technique (Gai K et al., 2018) termed as Cloud over Blockchain (CoB) is incorporated. Blockchain acts as a supportive technology enhancing cloud operations.

In the second architecture, a more substantial role is assigned to blockchain. All type of data generated over relations between IoT devices are channelled through blockchain, making it the central service provider. However, it finds analytical and virtualization services from the cloud. This approach, known as Blockchain over Cloud (BoC) (Gai K et al., 2018), emphasizes the pivotal role of blockchain in service provision while leveraging cloud capabilities for specific functions. The third integration setting involves a balanced exchange of data between blockchain and IoT devices. This allows for the simultaneous and direct utilization of the unique qualities of both technologies. From the perspective of cloud versus blockchain dominance, this method is termed Mixed Blockchain-Cloud (MBC) in (Gai K et al., 2018). This approach ensures a harmonious synergy between blockchain and IoT devices, leveraging their strengths for enhanced functionality and efficiency.

3. METHODOLOGY

The pervasive nature of blockchain has been highlighted by huge number of authors (Efanov D et al., 2018), and also many of the publications projects different prospective applications. This can improve the research publications.

3.1 Search Strategy

Search strategy relevant reviews are described in (Webster J et al., 2002, Bandara W et al., 2015). Subsequently, reviews relevant with the term "blockchain", which leads to huge set of documents. At first sight, collects the publications, area of application, languages h-index, impact factor etc. The initial evaluation involved screening the gathered publications based on factors such as application sector, program, and impact factor. Titles and abstracts are then examined to sort the remaining publications into specific application areas, including cryptography, IoT, medical industry, self-tuned contracts, business management, banking and economic industry and others. A detailed analysis was conducted to identify the application areas that required further review. While the majority of publications focused on cryptocurrency, this review specifically concentrates on those generally termed as blockchain version 3.0. Within the category, the primary focus is on the prominent uses of blockchain technology in healthcare, particularly in conjunction with IoT devices. Following the sorting of documents and the selection of application sectors within blockchain version 3.0, a 2nd searching initiated in the year of December 2019. The search queries used were "blockchain in IoT" & "blockchain in healthcare." This particular search complemented by front and back searches as needed. The purpose of performing this searching by one-year difference was used to gain insights into the evolving notion & trends in utilization of blockchain technology in these specific sectors.

Among the above mentioned searches, a comprehensive systematic reading carried out to enhance the understanding of subject then to establish clear standards for including / excluding documents (Boell SK et al., 2014). Whenever disparities were identified between existing information and recent publications on blockchain, further literature was examined to bridge the gap, ensuring a thorough evaluation and establishing connections among predefined knowledge and the latest trends in blockchain process.

3.2 Inclusion and Exclusion Standards

The primary publications were selected based on specific inclusion criteria. Publications falling within the designated sectors / applications and journal publications with an impact factor not less than 1.0, as per the standard publication source database, as well as books/book chapters, were eligible for future consideration. Conference presented/published papers were approached by care (Efanov D et al., 2018). However, papers presented at conferences conducted by reputable professional bodies like AIS, ACM, IEEE, ICIS, INFORM, etc., were recommended in Reference [Levy Y et al., 2006], were also considered for future phase of processing. Additionally, these conference papers were evaluated in contradiction of the Google h-index, with these scoring ten or higher being included in review. Implementing stringent quality requirements has implications, notably the unintentional exception of quality publications from the data bases with lesser rankings. Unlike the impact factor 1.0 standards mentioned in Reference (Levy Y et al., 2006), there isn't a fixed cut-off level indicating a journal's quality, as this metric fluctuates over time. Additionally, the h-5 index is not frequently utilized, leading to potential oversights. Consequently, some papers might be excluded even though if it is high qualified papers, although this doesn't impact the replicability of the review.

Nevertheless, for publications meeting the specified standards, a tough assessment. This critical assessment, as detailed in (Boell SK et al., 2014), involves comprehensive analysis aimed at broadening the understanding of existing knowledge acquisition, types of knowledge produced, and the utility of different knowledge types in explaining the pertinent issues. It also helps in identifying the separation and flaws of the previous data.

The purpose of this critical analysis of literature was twofold: first, to gain insight into the knowledge generated from the application of blockchain in specific areas; and second, to understand the extent to which blockchain has revolutionized these domains. Additionally, it aimed to understand the development of artifacts, comprising hypotheses models, techniques, and instantiations (implemented and prototype systems), as outlined in (Hevner AR et al.,2004).

By conducting the critical assessment, author was able to perform a second evaluation, which facilitated the screening out of publications lacking relevance and deepness in their demonstration. Few publications, such as those cited in (Hoy MB et al., 2017, Zhang P, et al., 2017, Engelhardt MA et al., 2017), were excluded based on this critical analysis. The preparation steps involved in articles are illustrated in the below Figure No. 3.1

4. RESULTS AND DISCUSSION

4.1 The Publications Reviewed

Publications in this domain encompass a broad spectrum of topics, including the incorporation of blockchain with the Internet of Things (IoT), IoT data management, IoT protection, and challenges related to smart cities. Another significant domain where blockchain technology holds transformative potential is healthcare, primarily for data management purposes. The table 2 displays a compilation of paper publications discussing the availability of blockchain technology.

Internet of Things (IoT)

Noteworthy IoT topics enclosed in the literature comprise comprehensive discussions on the advantages of employing blockchain for IoT, the design of systems enhancing IoT data security, and demonstrations of blockchain integration with IoT. Additionally, several papers delve into smart city applications within this context, offering detailed insights into these areas.

Healthcare

In the healthcare sector, authors explore the probable usage of utilizing blockchain technology. These benefits covers the creation of a consistent, safe, undisputable, strong, distributed, and user-managed data background system. Blockchain can be acknowledged for its role in improving drug supply chains, serving as a data store for healthcare research, medical trials, and harmony management, as well as facilitating health payment systems, insurance coverage processing, secure sharing and storage of health records. Furthermore, blockchain enriches data accessibility and facilitates patient identity with ensuring data durability through instantaneous access to medical/clinical data (Gordon WJ et al., 2018).

Figure 3. Review process steps

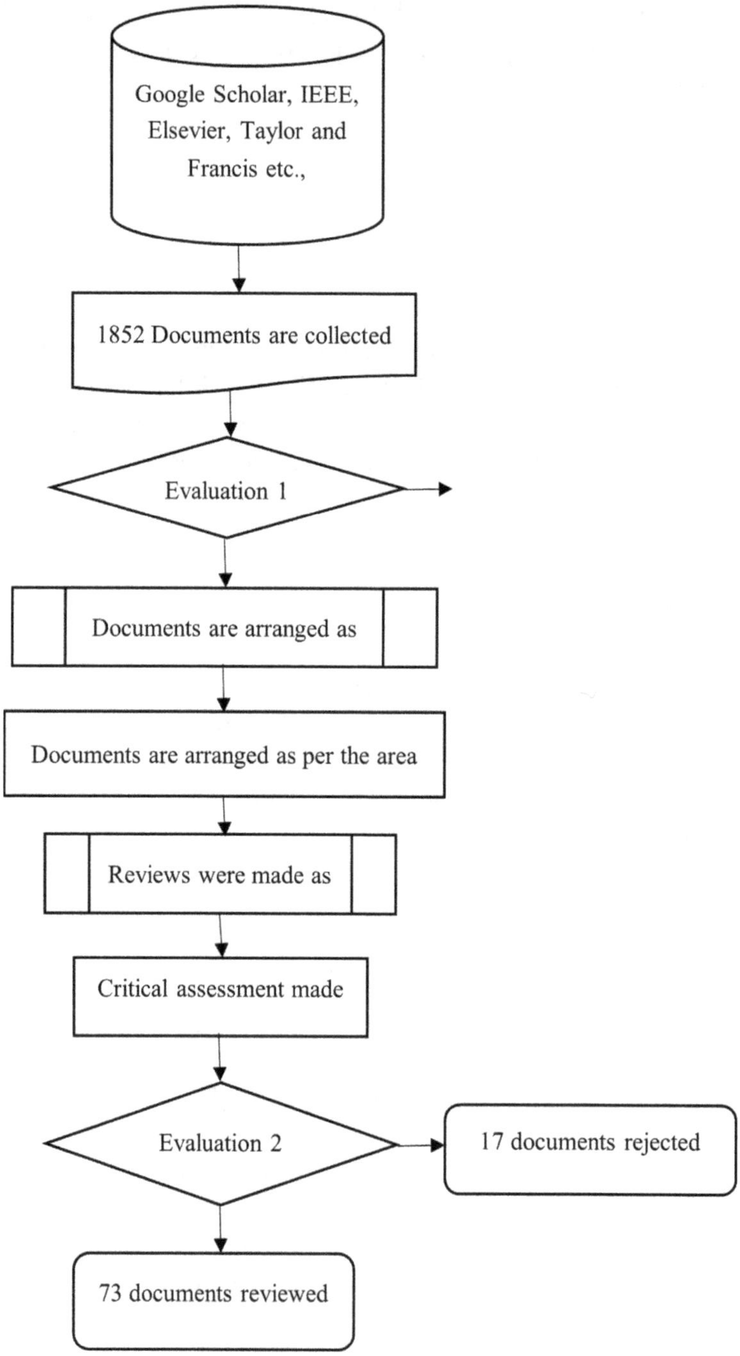

Table 2. Mandatory survey list: Compilation of paper publications along with blockchain technology

Journal Focus on		Procedure
WoT	Healthcare	
Pahl C et.al.,	Angraal S et.al., T.-T. Kuo et.al.,	Framework
Novo et.al., I. Makhdoom et.al., Atlam HF et.al.,	Dwivedi A et.al., Brunese L et.al.,	Amalgamation of blockchain with WoT
Sun J et.al., Yuan Y et.al.,	Mackey TK et.al.,	Smart City
Miller D et.al., J. J. Sikorski et.al.,	Mackey TK et.al.,	Drug supply chain

4.2 Knowledge Management: Medical Industry and IoT Devices

This review underscores knowledge management as a pivotal aspect encompassing various responsibilities all over the information life cycle, with acquisition, handling, safety, distribution, recovery, and storing. Blockchain technology is identified in the literature as instrumental in facilitating these data management processes, with a primary focus on enhancing data security. Within the realm of data safety, blockchain is most widely used to confirm data veracity, access mechanism & confidential technique. These security measures offer numerous advantages across various application domains, particularly in contexts that integrate both blockchain and IoT. Given the diverse and numerous devices in an IoT network generating substantial data, systems addressing data management tasks must consider the network's dynamic nature, operating in both physical and logical modes. Knowledge management is frequently motivated with the objective to address the flaws of IoT in specific functions by adopting the blockchain technology. The authors highlight various authentication methods beyond the conventional use of public keys and pseudonyms, such as voice recognition. Architectural strategies, such as entity assignment for unique IDs, are also noted. Regarding data processing, the literature points to the use of smart contracts and data-processing-friendly architecture.

Data integrity assurance commonly involves encrypting data before or after hashing, with 3rd-party systems like IPFS, Argon2 and Chainpoint used for generating exceptional identifiers, forming digital signatures & creating data structures. Access control and privacy preservation lack a singular, widely adopted strategy. Architectural strategies, like segmenting the nodes into "sidechains" or establishing a hierarchy of blockchains at native and worldwide levels, are employed to protect privacy. Clustering techniques are applied to minimize identification and transaction exposure risks. Overall, no discernible pattern has emerged in these privacy-centric architectural solutions.

4.3 Opportunities and Challenges of IoT-Based EHRs

Blockchain is most effective in scenarios involving relations by a lightweight numerical footprint, where the advantages of clarity and durability is crucial. It finds optimal application in situations characterized by a lack of trust among network participants and where the data block sizes are relatively small. In healthcare, blockchain holds particular promise for patient identity verification, suppliers, or contractors, business chain management, data usage. Blockchain faces challenges when it comes to handling high-volume data due to computational and capacity constraints associated with replicating the blockchain across every network participant (node). Storing extensive records like full electronic medical records or genetic data on the blockchain is inefficient and costly. IoT-based Electronic Health Records (EHRs) offer several benefits but also pose certain challenges. Here's an overview of both aspects:

Benefits of IoT-Based EHRs

Real-Time Monitoring

Advantage: IoT empowers continuous, real-time monitoring of patient health metrics. This constant data flow contributes to a more accurate representation of a patient's health status.

Remote Patient Management

Advantage: IoT-based EHRs allow healthcare providers to remotely monitor patients. This is especially valuable for those with chronic conditions, promoting proactive interference and decreasing the essentials for hospital visits.

Data Accuracy and Completeness

Advantage: Automated data collection through IoT devices improves the accuracy and completeness of patient records. This reduces the chances of errors associated with manual data entry.

Patient Engagement

Advantage: Patients can actively participate in their healthcare by using wearable devices and sensors. This engagement often leads to better adherence to treatment plans and healthier lifestyle choices.

Efficient Data Sharing

Advantage: IoT-based EHRs facilitate seamless and secure sharing of patient data among healthcare providers. This can enhance collaboration and provide a consistent aspects of medical data of the patient's.

Predictive Analytics

Advantage: The continuous data streams created with IoT devices can be influenced for predictive analytics. This allows healthcare providers to anticipate health issues and intervene before they escalate.

Challenges of IoT-Based EHRs

Data Security and Privacy Concerns

Challenge: Massive amount of complex health data collected with IoT devices raises concerns about data safety and protection breaches. Safeguarding this information becomes crucial to maintain patient trust.

Interoperability Issues

Challenge: Ensuring seamless interoperability among various IoT devices and EHR systems from different vendors can be challenging. Standardization efforts are ongoing but are not yet universally adopted.

Data Overload

Challenge: The constant stream of data from IoT devices may lead to information overload.

Integration With Existing Systems

Challenge: Integrating IoT-based EHRs with existing healthcare systems can be complex. Legacy systems may not easily adapt to new technologies, leading to implementation challenges.

Cost and Resource Implications

Challenge: The initial investment in IoT infrastructure and ongoing maintenance costs can be significant. Healthcare organizations need to assess the financial implications and resource requirements carefully.

In end, while IoT-based EHRs offer promising advantages in terms of real-time monitoring, improved patient engagement, and data accuracy, addressing challenges related to security, interoperability, and ethical considerations is crucial for their successful implementation and widespread adoption in the healthcare industry.

5. INTEGRATION OF IOT-BASED EHRS WITH BLOCKCHAIN

When applying blockchain in an IoT context, the authors aim to leverage the uses arising from simultaneous benefits of both engineering and technologies. This outcome has been influenced with factors such as specific technology factor for instantiation, the mandatory potential and quantity, the governing situation of technology area, & maintainability of customers in blockchain.

Two articles contribute to the understanding of amalgamation approaches for distributed ledger and WoT, categorizing them into 3 different approaches. In any classification (A. Reyna et al., 2018), amalgamation elucidations are categorized based on the volume of data flowing through the distributed ledger through information exchange among WoT systems. In another classification (Gai K, 2018), a comparison is made between blockchain and cloud computing services. These methods were not inconsistent but relatively supplement with each other. For instance, [A. Reyna et al., 2018] focuses on an association among blockchain and WoT devices, (Gai K, 2018) extends this relationship from WoT systems to cloud services.

General computation has been carried out among WoT systems in the first amalgamation technique, and blockchain does not play a role in data exchange between WoT devices. Instead, it assists the storage model for few metadata, known as off-chain practice (A. Reyna et al., 2018). Expanding the integration to the cloud services, blockchain is not considered primary service but promotes the cloud, known as Cloud over Blockchain (CoB) according to (Gai K, 2018). In final setup, a substantial portion of information exchanges occurs in the blockchain and WoT systems, enabling the concurrent & direct use of the technologies. Through the perspective of the cloud over blockchain, technique is known as Mixed Blockchain-Cloud (MBC) (Gai K, 2018).

5.1 Ensuring Data Security and Privacy

Data security encompasses a range of issues, with blockchain-based systems primarily focused on addressing three key areas: data veracity, access security, and protection. It's important to note that these security concerns are interconnected rather than distinct from one another. Despite this interconnected nature, journals have been predominantly focused on these specific things are discussed below.

5.2 Data Integrity and Immutability

"Data integrity" denotes the progress of confirming the performance and duration of the information in the lifecycle (Liu B et al., 2017). Previous journals, including (Sivathanu G et al., 2005, Menezes AJ et al., 1997), elaborate the fact that data integrity approaches focus on evading, classifying, modifying data integrity problems. Techniques like publications and constructing cryptographic file devices aim to prevent data integrity problems. In addition, techniques like hash-sum, simulation, Polynomial code checksum (PCC), and equality are employed to perceive data integrity threats. Then, corrective measures for data integrity concerns involve techniques like majority vote and RAID equality.

5.3 Retrieval and Data Sharing

The information is stored as an encrypted file form in the blockchain systems, necessitating the use of documents recovery methods like Searchable Symmetric Encryption (SSE), initially presented by Song et al. (Dawn Xiaoding Songet al., 2000) as a Boolean search scheme. Numerous authors have further advanced SSE, with notable contributions in (Swaminathan A, et al., 2007), who has been introducing the systematic search for coded files. These methods assist as foundational methods for increasing effectiveness of information recovery results. When it comes to encrypted image data, (Lu W et al., 2009) proposed a technique for recovery image over encoded images, with subsequent enhancements incorporating features like protection. (Ferreira B et al., 2015) Introduced a method for protection encoded image recovery.

Few research concentrates the treatment of data retrieval from blockchain varies, with some researchers considering it a relations, whereas others exclude it because of accuracy. For instance, (Gai K, 2018, Zhang P et al., 2017) treat it as a transaction, whereas (Novo O et al., 2018) does not provide the critical control systems. Moreover, there will be many difference in the survey related to the access of the right to recover and learn about information among distributed ledger participants. For example, derives the results of an input query that are encoded with entity known as leader that will explains the gateway server re-encryption.

5.4 Smart Contracts and Automating Processes

To commence, the various instantiations given here aim to enrich the model's power over further analogous results perceived as relevant to addressing the identified problem. However, in conducting this review, the author noted inconsistencies among these instantiations. Consequently, there is a need for a survey to concentrate on systematically associating the accuracy of these diverse instantiations. A smart contract can be conceptualized as spontaneously triggered technique activated upon the execution of a transaction. While all blockchain systems support smart contracts, variations exist in the languages for writing smart contracts and the environments for their execution. The most commonly utilized smart contract languages include Solidity, Golang, Serpent, Java, Python, and LLL.

Secondly, data processing, previously categorized as a data management operation, gains enhanced autonomous processing capacity in blockchain-based systems through smart contracts. However, smart contracts number embedded in systems that varies. As this usage might impact accuracy, due to the exploration of optima number of smart contracts.

6. CONCLUSION AND FUTURE PROSPECTS

To conclude, this chapter investigates how the journals influence blockchain technology to restructure the activities of data management and incorporate blockchain by the Internet of Things (IoT). Additionally, it explores trends in developing instantiations and displays the usage of adopting blockchain in few specific areas, namely smart cities and drug supply chains.

Blockchain in smart cities, including the management of data of consumption energy, employment with smart usage, real time data discussion, and increased traffic related accuracy with final instantiations. So the technology provides the reward based system to stimulate the positive behaviour. Blockchain in Drug Supply Chains play a major role in combating counterfeiting, sub-standardization, and diversion in drug supply chains by increasing transparency throughout the entire supply chain.

Integration approaches for blockchain and IoT are intricately linked to data management. Three diverse integration approaches are identified, with IoT-IoT (BoC) and hybrid approaches being preferred when facing challenges related to file size, strict regulations, a huge amount of participants, subtle information sensitivity, and huge throughput and latency requirements. This systematic survey aims to provide a comprehensive understanding of the integration of IoT-based EHRs with blockchain technology in the medical industry. By analyzing with the current state, challenges, and future prospects, this review pays to the previous knowledge and guides future research and implementation efforts in this domain.

LIMITATIONS

Like any research endeavor, this review has inherent limitations. Firstly, here susceptible to journal publication bias because of the limited availability of literature outputting negative reports relations with usage of blockchain. While some publications, such as (Cheng EC et al., 2018), reject the use of blockchain for certain purposes, and (Pahl C et al., 2018) raises doubts about its scalability, many advocate for its benefits. This imbalance may lead to a lack of comprehensive reporting, with potential exaggeration of positive outcomes and uncertainties about the future of instantiated solutions.

Secondly, irrespective of the reputation of the journals or conferences, this survey allocates identical weight to all the literature with primary requirements. However, a significant portion of valuable blockchain-based journal publications exists in the form of papers, which are considered as disqualified. This unintentional exclusion may result in overlooking valuable contributions to the field.

REFERENCES

Adere, E. M. (2022). Blockchain in healthcare and IoT: A systematic literature review. *Array (New York, N.Y.)*, *14*, 100139. doi:10.1016/j.array.2022.100139

Angraal, S., Krumholz, H. M., & Schulz, W. L. (2017). Blockchain technology: Applications in health care. *Circulation: Cardiovascular Quality and Outcomes*, *10*(9), e003800. Advance online publication. doi:10.1161/CIRCOUTCOMES.117.003800 PMID:28912202

Aste, T., Tasca, P., & Di Matteo, T. (2017). Blockchain technologies: The foreseeable impact on society and industry. *Computer*, *50*(9), 18–28. doi:10.1109/MC.2017.3571064

Bandara, W., Furtmueller, E., Gorbacheva, E., Miskon, S., & Beekhuyzen, J. (2015). Achieving rigor in literature reviews: Insights from qualitative data analysis and tool- support. *Communications of the Association for Information Systems*, *37*. Advance online publication. doi:10.17705/1CAIS.03708

Boell, S. K., & Cecez-Kecmanovic, D. (2014). A hermeneutic approach for conducting literature reviews and literature searches. *Communications of the Association for Information Systems*, *34*. Advance online publication. doi:10.17705/1CAIS.03412

Cheng, E. C., Le, Y., Zhou, J., & Lu, Y. (2018). Healthcare services across China – on implementing an extensible universally unique patient identifier system. *International Journal of Healthcare Management, 11*(3), 210–216. doi:10.1080/20479700.2017.1398388

Croman, K. (2016). On scaling decentralized blockchains: (A position paper). In J. Clark, S. Meiklejohn, P. Y. A. Ryan, D. Wallach, M. Brenner, & K. Rohloff (Eds.), *Financial Cryptography and Data Security* (Vol. 9604, pp. 106–125). Springer Berlin Heidelberg. doi:10.1007/978-3-662-53357-4_8

Dagher, G. G., Mohler, J., Milojkovic, M., & Marella, P. B. (2018). Ancile: Privacy-preserving framework for access control and interoperability of electronic health records using blockchain technology. *Sustainable Cities and Society, 39*, 283–297. doi:10.1016/j.scs.2018.02.014

Danzi, P., Kalor, A. E., Stefanovic, C., & Popovski, P. (2018). Analysis of the communication traffic for blockchain synchronization of IoT devices. *2018 IEEE International Conference on Communications (ICC)*, 1–7. 10.1109/ICC.2018.8422485

De Filippi, P., Mannan, M., & Reijers, W. (2020, August). Blockchain as a confidence machine: The problem of trust & challenges of governance. *Technology in Society, 62*, 101284. doi:10.1016/j.techsoc.2020.101284

Dinh, T. T. A., Liu, R., Zhang, M., Chen, G., Ooi, B. C., & Wang, J. (2018). Untangling blockchain: A data processing view of blockchain systems. *IEEE Transactions on Knowledge and Data Engineering, 30*(7), 1366–1385. doi:10.1109/TKDE.2017.2781227

Dinh, T. T. A., Wang, J., Chen, G., Liu, R., Ooi, B. C., & Tan, K.-L. (2017). BLOCKBENCH: a framework for analyzing private blockchains. *Proceedings of the 2017 ACM International Conference on Management of Data*, 1085–100. 10.1145/3035918.3064033

Ducas, E., & Wilner, A. (2017). The security and financial implications of blockchain technologies: Regulating emerging technologies in Canada. *International Journal (Toronto, Ont.), 72*(4), 538–562. doi:10.1177/0020702017741909

Eberhardt, J., & Tai, S. (2017). On or off the blockchain? Insights on off-chaining computation and data. In F. De Paoli, S. Schulte, & E. Broch Johnsen (Eds.), *Service-Oriented and Cloud Computing* (Vol. 10465). Springer International Publishing. doi:10.1007/978-3-319-67262-5_1

Efanov, D., & Roschin, P. (2018). The all-pervasiveness of the blockchain technology. *Procedia Comput Sci, 123*, 116–21. https://doi.org/.procs.2018.01.019 doi:10.1016/j

Engelhardt, M. A. (2017). Hitching healthcare to the chain: An introduction to blockchain technology in the healthcare sector. *Technology Innovation Management Review*, *7*(10), 22–34. doi:10.22215/timreview/1111

Ferreira, B., Rodrigues, J., Leitao, J., & Domingos, H. (2015). Privacy-preserving content-based image retrieval in the cloud. *2015 IEEE 34th Symposium on Reliable Distributed Systems (SRDS),* 11–20. 10.1109/SRDS.2015.27

Gai, K., Choo, K.-K. R., & Zhu, L. (2018). Blockchain-enabled reengineering of cloud datacenters. *IEEE Cloud Comput*, *5*(6), 21–25. doi:10.1109/MCC.2018.064181116

Geetha, S. K., Kanakaprabha, S., Devipriya, A., Brindha, D., & Vetrimani, E. (2023). Implementation of a Blockchain Based Attendance Tracking System. *2023 International Conference on Computer Communication and Informatics (ICCCI)*, 1-5. 10.1109/ICCCI56745.2023.10128438

Gordon, W. J., & Catalini, C. (2018). Blockchain technology for healthcare: Facilitating the transition to patient-driven interoperability. *Computational and Structural Biotechnology Journal*, *16*, 224–230. doi:10.1016/j.csbj.2018.06.003 PMID:30069284

Hammi, M. T., Hammi, B., Bellot, P., & Serhrouchni, A. (2018). Bubbles of Trust: A decentralized blockchain-based authentication system for IoT. *Computers & Security*, *78*, 126–142. doi:10.1016/j.cose.2018.06.004

Hevner, A. R., March, S. T., Park, J., & Ram, S. (2004). Design science in information systems research. *MIS Q, 28*(1), 75–105. http://misq.org/design-science-in-information-systems-research.html?SID=shpier0675mhpes3hkfagcqee1

Hoy, M. B. (2017). An introduction to the blockchain and its implications for libraries and medicine. *Medical Reference Services Quarterly*, *36*(3), 273–279. doi:10.1080/02763869.2017.1332261 PMID:28714815

Huang, B., Liu, Z., Chen, J., Liu, A., Liu, Q., & He, Q. (2017). Behavior pattern clustering in blockchain networks. *Multimedia Tools and Applications*, *76*(19), 20099–20110. doi:10.1007/s11042-017-4396-4

Kamble, S., Gunasekaran, A., & Arha, H. (2019, April). Understanding the Blockchain technology adoption in supply chains-Indian context. *International Journal of Production Research*, *57*(7), 2009–2033. doi:10.1080/00207543.2018.1518610

Karahanna, E., Adela, C., Liu, Q. B., & Serrano, C. (2019). Capitalizing on health information technology to enable advantage in U.S. Hospitals. *Management Information Systems Quarterly*, *43*(1), 113–140. doi:10.25300/MISQ/2019/12743

Khan, M. A., & Salah, K. (2018). IoT security: Review, blockchain solutions, and open challenges. *Future Generation Computer Systems*, *82*, 395–411. doi:10.1016/j.future.2017.11.022

Kleinaki, A.-S., Mytis-Gkometh, P., Drosatos, G., Efraimidis, P. S., & Kaldoudi, E. (2018). A blockchain-based notarization service for biomedical knowledge retrieval. *Computational and Structural Biotechnology Journal*, *16*, 288–297. doi:10.1016/j.csbj.2018.08.002 PMID:30181840

Kohli, R., & Tan, S. S.-L. (2016). Electronic health records: How can IS researchers contribute to transforming healthcare? [Mar.]. *Management Information Systems Quarterly*, *40*(3), 553–573. doi:10.25300/MISQ/2016/40.3.02

Kuo, T.-T., Kim, H.-E., & Ohno-Machado, L. (2017, November). Blockchain distributed ledger technologies for biomedical and health care applications. *Journal of the American Medical Informatics Association : JAMIA*, *24*(6), 1211–1220. doi:10.1093/jamia/ocx068 PMID:29016974

Levy, Y., & Ellis, T. J. (2006). A systems approach to conduct an effective literature review in support of information systems research. *Info Sci Int J Emerg Transdiscipl*, *9*, 181–212. doi:10.28945/479

Liu, B., Yu, X. L., Chen, S., Xu, X., & Zhu, L. (2017). Blockchain based data integrity service framework for IoT data. *2017 IEEE International Conference on Web Services*, 468–75. 10.1109/ICWS.2017.54

Lu, W., Swaminathan, A., Varna, A. L., & Wu, M. (2009). *Enabling search over encrypted multimedia databases*. doi:10.1117/12.806980

Menezes, A. J., Van Oorschot, P. C., & Vanstone, S. A. (1997). *Handbook of applied cryptography*. CRC Press.

Novo, O. (2018). Blockchain meets IoT: An architecture for scalable access management in IoT. *IEEE Internet of Things Journal*, *5*(2), 1184–1195. doi:10.1109/JIOT.2018.2812239

Pahl, C., El Ioini, N., & Helmer, S. (2018). A decision framework for blockchain platforms for IoT and edge computing. *Proceedings of the 3rd International Conference on Internet of Things, Big Data and Security*, 105–13. 10.5220/0006688601050113

Peters, G. W., & Panayi, E. (2016). Understanding modern banking ledgers through blockchain technologies: future of transaction processing and smart contracts on the internet of money. In P. Tasca, T. Aste, L. Pelizzon, & N. Perony (Eds.), *Banking Beyond Banks and Money* (pp. 239–278). Springer International Publishing. doi:10.1007/978-3-319-42448-4_13

Qiu, T., Zhang, R., & Gao, Y. (2019). Ripple vs. SWIFT: Transforming cross border remittance using blockchain technology. *Procedia Computer Science*, *147*, 428–434. doi:10.1016/j.procs.2019.01.260

Reyna, A., Martín, C., Chen, J., Soler, E., & Díaz, M. (2018, November). On blockchain and its integration with IoT. Challenges and opportunities. *Future Generation Computer Systems*, *88*, 173–190. doi:10.1016/j.future.2018.05.046

Roman-Belmonte, J. M., De la Corte-Rodriguez, H., & Rodriguez-Merchan, E. C. (2018). How blockchain technology can change medicine. *Postgraduate Medicine*, *130*(4), 420–427. doi:10.1080/00325481.2018.1472996 PMID:29727247

Sivathanu, G., Wright, C. P., & Zadok, E. (2005). Ensuring data integrity in storage: techniques and applications. *Proceedings of the 2005 ACM workshop on Storage security and survivability - StorageSS '05*, 26. . Fairfax, VA, USA.10.1145/1103780.1103784

Swaminathan, A. (2007). Confidentiality-preserving rank-ordered search. *Proceedings of the 2007 ACM workshop on Storage security and survivability - StorageSS '07*, 7. 10.1145/1314313.1314316

Swan, M. (2015). Blockchain: blueprint for a new economy. O'Reilly.

Taylor, P. J., Dargahi, T., Dehghantanha, A., Parizi, R. M., & Choo, K.-K. R. (2019). A systematic literature review of blockchain cyber security. *Digital Communications and Networks*. Advance online publication. doi:10.1016/j.dcan.2019.01.005

Vest, J. R., & Gamm, L. D. (2010). Health information exchange: persistent challenges and new strategies: table. *Journal of the American Medical Informatics Association : JAMIA*, *17*(3), 288–294. doi:10.1136/jamia.2010.003673 PMID:20442146

Webster, J., & Watson, R. T. (2002). Analyzing the past to prepare for the future: Writing a literature review. *Management Information Systems Quarterly*, *26*(2), xiii–xxii.

Zhang, P., Walker, M. A., White, J., Schmidt, D. C., & Lenz, G. (2017). Metrics for assessing blockchain-based healthcare decentralized apps. *2017 IEEE 19th International Conference on e-Health Networking, Applications and Services (Healthcom),* 1–4. 10.1109/HealthCom.2017.8210842

Zyskind, G., & Nathan, O. A. (2015). Decentralizing privacy: using blockchain to protect personal data. 2015 IEEE Security and Privacy Workshops, 180–4. doi:10.1109/SPW.2015.27

Chapter 6
Human-Centric AI Applications for Remote Patient Monitoring

Sunil Kadyan
Manav Rachna University, Faridabad, India

Yogita Sharma
Manav Rachna University, Faridabad, India

Atul Kumar Agnihotri
https://orcid.org/0009-0001-6770-8316
University Institute of Engineering and Technology, Kanpur, India

Veer Bhadra Pratap Singh
Symbiosis Skills and Professional University, India

Rakshit Kothari
https://orcid.org/0000-0003-2893-1504
College of Technology and Engineering, Maharana Pratap University of Agriculture and Technology, India

Fateh Bahadur Kunwar
https://orcid.org/0009-0007-5749-9892
Geetanjali Institute of Technical Studies, India

ABSTRACT

This research analyses the deployment of a human-centric IoT gadget for remote impacted person monitoring, employing sophisticated technology to beautify healthcare operations. The suggested approach incorporates a community of sensors, together with temperature, stress, coronary heart charge, and oxygen sensors, strategically situated at the afflicted person's frame. These sensors capture actual-time physiological information, which is processed via a signal converter, delivered to character controllers, and consolidated within the cloud for complete analysis. Subsequently, machine studying styles, including artificial neural network (ANN),

DOI: 10.4018/979-8-3693-1662-7.ch006

decision tree (DT), random forest (RF), and naive bayes (NB), are used to anticipate impacted person fitness outcomes based at the accumulated dataset. The analysis assesses each version's performance using a dataset of 3233 items, of which 70% are designated for learning and 30% for experimentation. Results suggest that the proposed ANN model achieves an outstanding accuracy of 97.5%, outperforming DT, RF, and NB. Decision tree and random forest comply closely with accuracies of 92.33% and 91.22%, correspondingly, while naive bayes demonstrates a superb accuracy of 86.5%. These outcomes underline the potential of sophisticated machine learning models, notably ANN, within the field of remote affected person monitoring, giving a transformational method to healthcare. The merger of human-centric layout ideas, IoT technologies, and device learning contributes to the continuous dialogue on improving affected person care, opening the way for extra proactive, customized, and successful healthcare treatments. This investigation suggests a leap forward in utilising generation to alter healthcare practices, highlighting the crucial significance of facts-driven decision-making in making sure best patient impacts.

INTRODUCTION

In the evolving landscape of healthcare, the integration of innovative technologies has remarkable potential for improving impacted person care. The introduction of the Internet of Things (IoT) has brought in a new technology of potential, especially within the realm of far-flung patient monitoring (Adeosun & Asiri, 2020; Aggarwal, 2022). This study objectives to develop a system for monitoring the health of the patient from the remote location. Several research are done in developing a remote health monitoring of the patients (Bilal & Sajid, 2022). This is accomplished using the set of various sensor and wireless data communication and cloud storage (Rani et al., 2022). In the setting of far-flung patient monitoring, human-centric design becomes vital, guaranteeing that the age is user-friendly, less intrusive, and comprises the varied wants of sufferers. Research emphasizes the good influence of human-centric layout in increasing impacted person engagement and adherence to remote monitoring techniques (Pathak & Kulkarni, 2015).

The Internet of Things has seen exponential expansion, providing remarkable potential for redesigning healthcare services. In afar patient monitoring, IoT programs play a vital role through supporting the smooth collection and transfer of physiological facts (Raza & Sajid, 2022). Wearable devices geared up with sensors, together with temperature, pressure, heart price, and oxygen sensors, offer continuous surveillance of sufferers in actual-time. Research underlines the potential of IoT in increasing the efficiency and accuracy of healthcare statistics collecting, establishing the muse for our research of a sophisticated IoT-based affected person monitoring gadget (Shaik et al., 2023).

The Internet of Things (IoT) has experienced unprecedented growth, presenting substantial opportunities for the transformation of healthcare services. In the realm of remote patient monitoring, IoT applications play a pivotal role by facilitating the seamless collection and transmission of physiological data (Singh, 2020; Sharan, 2015). Wearable devices equipped with an array of sensors, including those for temperature, pressure, heart rate, and oxygen levels, contribute to continuous real-time surveillance of patients. This integration of IoT technology holds great promise for enhancing the efficiency and accuracy of healthcare data collection.

Research underscores the immense potential of IoT in advancing the capabilities of patient monitoring systems. The continuous, real-time monitoring enabled by wearable IoT devices allows for a more comprehensive and dynamic understanding of patients' health status. The ability to collect diverse physiological data points in real-time offers a nuanced and holistic view, contributing to a more accurate assessment of patients' well-being (Sellamuthu et al., 2023).

Our research focuses on the development of an advanced IoT-based patient monitoring system, leveraging the capabilities of wearable devices and IoT applications. By harnessing the potential of IoT, we aim to enhance the precision and efficiency of healthcare data collection, ultimately leading to improved patient care and outcomes. The integration of IoT in patient monitoring not only streamlines the process of data collection but also opens avenues for proactive healthcare interventions based on real-time insights.

The expansion of IoT in healthcare, particularly in remote patient monitoring, represents a transformative shift in how we gather and utilize health-related data. As we delve into the possibilities offered by IoT, our research endeavors to contribute to the evolution of patient monitoring systems, ensuring that technological advancements are effectively translated into tangible benefits for both healthcare providers and patients (Vellappally et al., 2019).

Artificial Intelligence, primarily machine learning models, has evolved as a significant tool in healthcare analytics. These styles, together with Artificial Neural Networks (ANN), Decision Trees (DT), Random Forest (RF), and Naive Bayes (NB), exhibit the power to examine difficult datasets and anticipate fitness outcomes. While the capacity advantages of far-flung patient monitoring are extensive challenging scenarios continue in its enormous adoption. Issues related with records security, privateness issues, and the interoperability of distinct IoT devices offer major difficulties (Sharan, 2016; Shaik et al., 2023). Research explores into these difficult conditions, offering insights into the complications connected with integrating IoT technology into healthcare organizations. Addressing such problems is crucial for a success deployment and reputation of remote impacted person monitoring structures.

Artificial Intelligence, particularly machine learning models, has emerged as a pivotal tool in healthcare analytics, contributing to the advancement of predictive and personalized medicine. Key models, such as Artificial Neural Networks (ANN), Decision Trees (DT), Random Forest (RF), and Naive Bayes (NB), showcase the ability to analyze complex datasets and predict health outcomes. While the potential benefits of remote patient monitoring are extensive, there are significant challenges hindering its widespread adoption (Sajid & Gupta, 2022).

One major hurdle lies in issues related to data security and privacy concerns. The sensitive nature of health data requires robust security measures to safeguard patient information and maintain confidentiality. Additionally, ensuring the interoperability of various Internet of Things (IoT) devices poses a substantial challenge. The integration of diverse devices and technologies into a cohesive and seamless remote monitoring system demands careful consideration and standardized protocols (Prasad et al., 2015).

Research is actively delving into these intricate challenges, providing valuable insights into the complications associated with the integration of IoT technology into healthcare frameworks. Understanding and addressing these issues are imperative for the successful deployment and widespread acceptance of remote patient monitoring systems. A comprehensive exploration of data security protocols, privacy frameworks, and strategies for achieving interoperability is crucial to establish trust among healthcare providers, patients, and stakeholders.

The evolving landscape of AI in healthcare, especially in the context of remote patient monitoring, holds immense promise. However, a concerted effort is required to overcome the existing challenges and ensure the seamless integration of these technologies into healthcare organizations, ultimately contributing to improved patient care and outcomes.

Despite advances in character domains, there existing a research gap that needs an integrated investigation of human centric IoT structures with device mastering styles for remote patient monitoring. While research exist at the individual components, their aggregate usability and assessment in a real-international healthcare context remain underexplored. This research objectives to bridge this hole by offering a holistic technique, thinking about the human aspects, IoT technologies, and machine learning algorithms in concert, and analyzing their cumulative effect on the success of far-flung patient monitoring (Sharma et al., 2021; Singh, 2020).

As we engage in this investigation, the merger of human-centric design, IoT packages, and device learning styles heralds a new technology in healthcare. The complicated interplay of these additives is expected to now not best increase the accuracy of fitness forecasts but also transform the administration of affected person-centric treatment. By addressing existing gaps in the literature and harnessing the capacity synergies between those technologies, our investigations intend to contribute substantively to the continuing conversation on the integration of better technology in healthcare practices. The following sections will discuss the method, outcomes, and consequences of our research, culminating in an in-depth understanding of the suggested remote patient monitoring.

RELATED WORK

The integration of Artificial Intelligence (AI) applications in healthcare, particularly in the domain of remote patient monitoring, represents a significant paradigm shift in healthcare delivery. Human-centric AI applications have the potential to revolutionize patient care by providing personalized and proactive monitoring, enabling early detection of health issues, and fostering a more patient-centric approach. This section reviews the existing body of literature and research related to Human-Centric AI Applications for Remote Patient Monitoring.

A. Evolution of Remote Patient Monitoring

Remote Patient Monitoring (RPM) has evolved over the years, spurred by advancements in technology and the need for more efficient and patient-friendly healthcare solutions. Early forms of RPM primarily involved basic data collection, such as vital signs, through telecommunication channels. With the integration of AI, RPM has entered a new era where sophisticated algorithms can analyze complex datasets, enabling more comprehensive monitoring of patients' health status (Verma, 2024).

The landscape of healthcare has undergone a transformative shift with the evolution of Remote Patient Monitoring (RPM), a dynamic field shaped by technological advancements and the imperative for more effective and patient-centric healthcare solutions. The early stages of RPM were characterized by rudimentary data collection, focusing on essential metrics like vital signs, facilitated through telecommunication channels. However, the integration of Artificial Intelligence (AI) has propelled RPM into a new era marked by sophisticated algorithms and enhanced capabilities (Singh & Srivastva, 2022).

Traditionally, RPM involved the remote collection of basic health data, enabling healthcare providers to monitor vital signs and other fundamental parameters from a distance. This approach facilitated a degree of patient care beyond the confines of traditional healthcare settings. The introduction of telecommunication channels allowed for the transmission of data between patients and healthcare professionals, laying the groundwork for remote monitoring systems.

The advent of AI has catalyzed a paradigm shift in RPM, introducing advanced analytical capabilities that transcend the limitations of basic data collection. The integration of sophisticated algorithms empowers RPM systems to navigate and interpret complex datasets, facilitating a more nuanced and comprehensive monitoring of patients' health statuses (Sajid et al., 2022). AI's analytical prowess enables the identification of subtle patterns, trends, and anomalies within patient data, offering a more holistic understanding of individuals' health conditions.

This integration not only enhances the accuracy of diagnostics but also opens avenues for proactive healthcare interventions. AI-driven RPM systems can now detect early signs of health deterioration, predict potential issues, and provide timely alerts to healthcare providers. The result is a more proactive and personalized approach to patient care, aligning with the broader goals of achieving efficiency and patient-centricity in modern healthcare practices (Gupta et al., 2023).

B. AI in Healthcare

The use of AI in healthcare has gained traction across various applications, including diagnostics, treatment planning, and patient management. AI technologies such as Machine Learning (ML), Natural Language Processing (NLP), and computer vision have demonstrated capabilities in analyzing medical data, predicting health outcomes, and optimizing treatment strategies. This body of research provides a foundation for exploring the potential applications of AI in the specific context of remote patient monitoring.

The integration of Artificial Intelligence (AI) into healthcare has become increasingly prevalent, finding applications in diverse areas such as diagnostics, treatment planning, and patient management. AI technologies, including Machine Learning (ML), Natural Language Processing (NLP), and computer vision, have showcased their efficacy in parsing and analyzing vast sets of medical data. From discerning intricate patterns within data to predicting health outcomes and optimizing treatment strategies, AI has emerged as a powerful ally in the realm of healthcare innovation (Mall, 2023).

This robust foundation of research underscores the transformative potential of AI in shaping the landscape of healthcare delivery. As the applications of AI continue to expand, there is a growing interest in exploring its nuanced role in remote patient monitoring. The capabilities demonstrated by AI in analyzing medical data and predicting outcomes position it as a valuable asset in the evolution of remote patient monitoring systems, promising more effective, personalized, and proactive healthcare solutions.

C. Wearable Devices and IoT Integration

Wearable devices equipped with sensors have become integral components of remote patient monitoring systems. These devices continuously collect a diverse range of physiological data, including heart rate, temperature, activity levels, and more. The seamless integration of wearable devices with the Internet of Things (IoT) allows for real-time transmission of this data to centralized systems. The literature reveals insights into the challenges and opportunities associated with wearable devices and IoT integration in healthcare (Babu & Anirudh, 2016).

D. Human-Centric AI Applications

The concept of human-centric AI emphasizes the integration of AI technologies that prioritize human needs, values, and experiences. In the context of remote patient monitoring, human-centric AI applications aim to enhance patient engagement, satisfaction, and overall well-being. Research in this domain explores user-centered design principles, usability studies, and the impact of AI on the patient experience.

In the realm of remote patient monitoring, wearable devices have emerged as indispensable tools, equipped with an array of sensors that enable the continuous collection of diverse physiological data. These wearables, capable of monitoring parameters such as heart rate, temperature, and activity levels, play a pivotal role in providing a comprehensive understanding of a patient's health status. The seamless integration of these wearable devices with the Internet of Things (IoT) facilitates the real-time transmission of the collected data to centralized healthcare systems (Bahat, 2021).

The literature surrounding remote patient monitoring delves into the nuanced landscape of wearable devices and IoT integration in healthcare, shedding light on both the challenges and opportunities inherent in this technological convergence. As wearables continue to evolve and their integration with IoT matures, the potential for more effective and responsive remote patient monitoring systems becomes increasingly promising, paving the way for enhanced patient care and improved health outcomes.

E. Privacy and Security Concerns

The deployment of AI applications in healthcare, especially in remote patient monitoring, raises concerns about privacy and data security. Existing literature addresses the ethical considerations, regulatory frameworks, and security measures required to ensure the confidentiality and integrity of patient data.

F. Patient Empowerment and Engagement

Human-centric AI applications have the potential to empower patients by providing them with personalized insights into their health status. Research explores the impact of AI-driven monitoring on patient engagement, adherence to treatment plans, and self-management of chronic conditions (Mall, 2023).

G. Challenges and Future Directions

While the literature acknowledges the transformative potential of Human-Centric AI Applications for Remote Patient Monitoring, it also highlights challenges. These include issues related to interoperability, standardization, and the need for a collaborative healthcare ecosystem. Future directions in research involve addressing these challenges, refining AI algorithms, and exploring novel applications that enhance the overall patient experience (Shaik et al., 2023).

In summary, the related work provides a comprehensive understanding of the evolution of remote patient monitoring, the integration of AI in healthcare, the role of wearable devices and IoT, human-centric AI applications, privacy concerns, patient empowerment, and the challenges and future directions in this dynamic field. This synthesis of existing knowledge serves as a valuable foundation for advancing research in Human-Centric AI Applications for Remote Patient Monitoring.

METHODOLOGY

Remote patient monitoring, using a variety of sensors, is becoming increasingly important, particularly in the context of the ongoing epidemic. Remote monitoring of patients' vital signs enables prompt action and alleviates the burden on healthcare facilities. This study presents a complete methodology for remote patient monitoring using temperature sensors, pressure sensors, heart rate sensors, and oxygen sensors as shown in figure 1. These sensors acquire crucial information, that is subsequently communicated via a chain of linked components, sooner or later reaching the cloud storage.

The basic premise of our technology is the deployment of a pair of sensors strategically positioned on the patient's body. These sensors characteristic as statistics creditors, continually accumulating and recording crucial physiological information. By together with a temperature sensor, it will become practical to show the patient's body temperature in actual-time. This is crucial to appraising their health repute, particularly in the course of intervals of infectious disease outbreaks. At the identical time, a stress sensor measures changes in strain, offering data on elements associated to breathing characteristic. Heart fee and oxygen sensors perform a critical part in figuring out essential data concerning cardiovascular health, bearing in mind a full knowledge of the patient's normal properly-being.

The Several sensor facts are subsequently fed into a signal converter, that is an essential detail in our approach. The sign converter translates the raw information, converting them into a layout appropriate for similarly transmission. This stage assures that the facts acquired from the different sensors is standardized and can be successfully transmitted in the course of the tracking system. Following the signal conversion, the processed information is transferred to an individual controller. This controller acts as a local hub, integrating the information from a handful of sensors attached to a single patient. The main controller now not finest gathers the information but also plays preliminary analysis, keeping in mind quick evaluations of the afflicted person's wellness condition. This localized processing lowers the requirement for non-stop excessive-bandwidth communication, making the device and more responsive.

The second phase in our approach entails the discussion of data from induvial controllers to the chief controller. This centralized unit operates as a storehouse for patient statistics from numerous sources. By integrating details from distinct persons, the main controller supplies a full overview of the fitness repute of more people. This stage is crucial for healthcare firms and directors to make informed decisions, spend resources appropriately, and respond right promptly to developing fitness qualities. The last connection in our method is the transfer of data from the essential controller to the cloud. Cloud-primarily based garage gives scalability, accessibility, and safety

Figure 1. Architecture of the proposed research

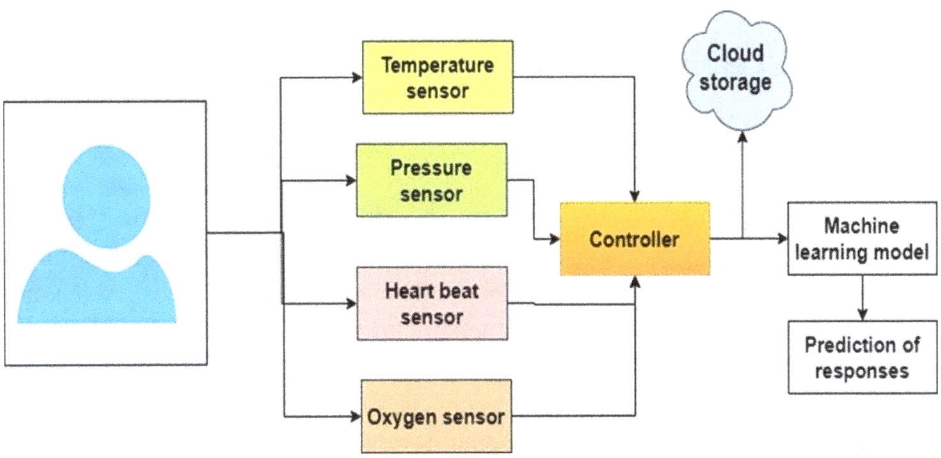

for the huge volumes of information created by far flung affected person monitoring structures. The cloud acts as a centralized database, keeping past impacted person information and enables enhanced analytics. This recorded data may be valuable for lengthy-time period trend analysis, research, and retrospective investigations, adding to the larger field of healthcare information science.

A. Need for Machine Learning

Beyond actual-time monitoring, the capacity to forecast future fitness states is essential for proactive and well-timed action. In our research, we incorporate better machine learning models to anticipate fitness patterns mainly based on the actual-time facts collected from the sensor network. Specifically, we designate Artificial Neural Networks (ANN), Random Forest (RF), Decision Trees (DT), and Naive Bayes (NB) as our preferred models. The training method incorporates each model to a carefully picked dataset, comprising a varied range of impacted person features and medical conditions.

Following training, extensive testing is performed to examine every version ability to foretell fitness repercussions. The use of ANN lets in for the finding of state-of-the-art patterns and correlations within the facts, delivering detailed forecasts. Random Forest excels in dealing with big sized datasets and gives high performance, whereas Decision Trees supply interpretable insights into the selection-making approach. Naive Bayes, praised for its simplicity and efficacy, offers a probabilistic scale to our predictive analytics.

By the utilization of those several system studying tactics, our research targets to place up a comprehensive and proper forecasting framework. This approach now provides healthcare organizations with useful information to enable informed decision-making and prompt action, in addition to enhancing the accuracy of fitness forecasts.

B. Machine Learning Models

(i) Artificial Neural Network

A key component of our research methods, artificial neural networks (ANN) are essential for identifying complex patterns and associations from the large, dynamic information created by remote patient monitoring devices. ANNs are computational designs influenced by the structure and functioning like the brain of humans, including linked nodes or neurons constructed in layers. In the context of our investigations, the entry layer obtains the standardized sensor data, and the community analyses these facts via hidden layers to offer an output layer, which depicts the predicted health implications. What makes ANNs in particular useful is their power to parent complicated, non-linear connections within the information. In healthcare programs, this relates to the capacity to comprehend small patterns which could overcome standard analytical tools. The adaptive nature of ANNs enables them to continually learn from the data they are subjected to, modifying their inner parameters to increase forecast accuracy over time. This capability is particularly cherished in the context of afar patient monitoring, where health problems might display various and developing patterns.

The training phase of the ANN comprises exposing the community to a diverse and properly curated dataset, inclusive of a spectrum of afflicted person profiles and fitness circumstances. This training technique helps the network to analyze the underlying styles and institutions among exceptional variables. Once trained, the ANN will become excellent at creating predictions relying completely on fresh, unseen facts, so supplying a beneficial method for anticipating future health circumstances within the area of distant patient surveillance. In our study, the usefulness of ANN increases the predictive abilities of our remote affected person monitoring system, adding to a larger complete understanding of patients' fitness patterns. Our objective is to not only improve the accuracy of health forecasts but also open the door for more proactive and customized healthcare treatments by using the computational capacity of ANNs.

(ii) Random Forest

Random Forest (RF) stands as a major aspect in our study technique for remote patient monitoring, giving a strong and diverse approach to predictive analytics. This machine learning model helps to know technique works by utilizing generating a multiplicity of decision trees at some time of the training section. The energy of RF comes in its capacity to manage huge and difficult information, making it especially properly-proper for the diverse and dynamic fitness statistics created in distant impacted person monitoring situations.

The core building blocks of RF are selection trees, each of which acts independently, creating predictions largely based on a subset of the input capabilities. The randomization in RF is twofold – first, in the course of the advent of every selection tree, a random subset of capabilities is examined at each split, adding variability many of the wood. Second, the learning dataset for every tree is produced by utilizing sampling with replace, from the original dataset. This randomization mitigates overfitting and adds to the version's generalizability (Shaik et al., 2023). The predictive energy of RF is obtained from the variety of predictions produced with the use of multiple choice questions. Each tree might do well in taking photos certain styles inside the data, and by means of pooling their outputs, RF generates a more powerful and accurate forecast. This machine learning now not only increases prediction accuracy but also supplies insights into feature importance, highlighting the factors that contribute considerably to the predictive ultimate results.

(iii) Decision Tree

Decision Trees (DT) offer a vital feature inside our study framework for far off influenced character monitoring, supplying an interpretable and useful way to predictive modeling. A Decision Tree is a hierarchical structure made from nodes, in which every internal node represents an option based fully on a specific function, and each leaf node relates to an ultimate results or prediction. This tree-like model depicts a sequence of alternatives built dependent solely on access abilities, providing it a clear and straightforward instrument for knowing the choice-making mechanism. The operational core of a Decision Tree requires recursively separating the dataset significantly principally depending on skills, with the purpose of putting up homogeneous subsets at every level of the tree. The approach endures until a preventing condition is satisfied, mixed with a predetermined depth or a minimal variety of samples in a node. This hierarchical choice-making should permit the version to store complex correlations within the facts even though keeping transparency in terms of feature significance.

One amazing benefit of Decision Trees is in its capacity to manage both numerical and explicit statistics, accommodating the distinct types of information frequently seen in healthcare datasets. Additionally, Decision Trees are less delicate to outliers, since the hierarchical structure permits them to form judgements in large part based solely on the bulk of samples inside every node. In our work, Decision Trees add to the interpretability of the prediction version and assist in discovering essential features affecting health impacts in remote affected person monitoring. The honest and perceptive man or woman of Decision Trees helps the extraction of crucial insights into the factors fundamental to distinctive fitness forecasts.

(iv) Navie Bayes

Naive Bayes (NB) is a vital part in our research approach for remote affected person monitoring, supplying a probabilistic technique to predictive modeling. NB, or naïve Bayes, is a probabilistic classifier that depends on the belief of independence of capacities given the elegant label. Despite its simplicity, NB constantly works astoundingly adequately, especially in instances wherever interpretability and computational economy are vital. The essential premise of

NB rests in Bayes' theorem, which predicts the likelihood of a specific prevalence given the preponderance of every other event. In the context of our investigations, NB assesses the opportunity of a favorable health outcome given the observed sensor data. The naïve assumption of function independence simplifies the calculation, making it computationally green and primarily suitable for datasets with multiple features.

NB is well-ideal for managing both explicit and non-forestall facts, making it flexible to the one of a kind types of facts observed in healthcare datasets. The training strategy comprises computing the likelihood of different repercussions based upon the diagnostic features. This recognized probabilistic version is then employed for producing predictions on modern-day, unknown information. In our take a look at, NB performs as a crucial instrument for its simplicity, quickness, and efficiency in categorizing health outcomes primarily based solely on far off impacted person monitoring information. Its charge fits with situations wherever real-time choice-making is crucial, which includes in healthcare settings. Additionally, NB gives a clear information regarding the likelihood of distinct fitness states given the provided sensor data, contributing to the interpretability of our prediction model.

RESULT AND DISCUSSION

Table 1 displays a simulated dataset exhibiting sensor readings gathered at half-hour intervals from 9:00 AM to 5:00 PM for a patient inside the proposed IoT system for remote patient monitoring. The following parameters are recorded: heart rate (beats per minute), blood pressure (systolic/diastolic mmHg), temperature (°C), and oxygen saturation (%). Starting at 9:00 AM with a baseline temperature of 37.2°C, the table depicts changes in vital signs throughout the day.

For instance, blood pressure displays usual changes, heart rate rises steadily, and oxygen levels indicate a declining trend. These numbers, albeit hypothetical, show the possible variety of sensor data provided by the IoT system. Such extensive databases allow healthcare practitioners to monitor patients remotely, discover abnormalities, and make educated choices for early therapies based on real-time physiological information.

In the evaluation segment of our investigations, each machine learning models—Artificial Neural Network (ANN), Decision Tree (DT), Random Forest (RF), and Naive Bayes (NB)—became submitted to checking out the utilization of the dataset obtained by the IoT machine. The dataset, which comprises a total of 3233 items, was partitioned, designating 70% for instructional purposes and reserving the final

Table 1. Sensor reading of each model

Timestamp	Temperature (°C)	Pressure (mmHg)	Heart Rate (bpm)	Oxygen Level (%)
9:00 AM	37.2	120/80	75	98
9:30 AM	37.1	121/81	76	97
10:00 AM	37.0	119/79	78	96
10:30 AM	37.3	122/82	80	95
11:00 AM	37.2	120/80	82	94
11:30 AM	37.1	121/81	85	93
12:00 PM	37.0	119/79	88	92
12:30 PM	37.2	120/80	90	91
1:00 PM	37.1	121/81	92	90
1:30 PM	37.0	119/79	94	89
2:00 PM	37.3	122/82	96	88
2:30 PM	37.2	120/80	98	87
3:00 PM	37.1	121/81	100	86
3:30 PM	37.0	119/79	102	85
4:00 PM	37.2	120/80	104	84
4:30 PM	37.1	121/81	106	83
5:00 PM	37.0	119/79	108	82

30% for testing. After thorough trying out, the findings demonstrated the efficiency of the machine learning in forecasting impacted person fitness.

The Artificial Neural Network displayed an exceptional accuracy score of 97.5%, displaying its skill ability in capturing the health troublesome patterns within the data. Decision Tree and Random Forest watched closely with accuracies of 92.33% and 91.22%, respectively, underlining their solid overall performance in fitness prediction. Naive Bayes revealed a respectable accuracy of 86.5%, reaffirming its trustworthiness in probabilistic modeling. Figure 2 graphically summarizes those data, displaying the comparative performance of each model. The excessive accuracy obtained by the presented ANN version stresses its capacity for precise fitness forecasts, strengthening its usefulness for implementation in remote patient monitoring systems.

The overall performance rankings offered in figure 3 show off the effectiveness of every machine learning model. Accuracy, showing the total validity of predictions, is substantially high for ANN at 97.5%, highlighting its competence in identifying intricate patterns within the data. Precision, representing the ratio of successfully anticipated pleasant observations to the whole projected positives, is consistently high

Figure 2. Accuracy of each model

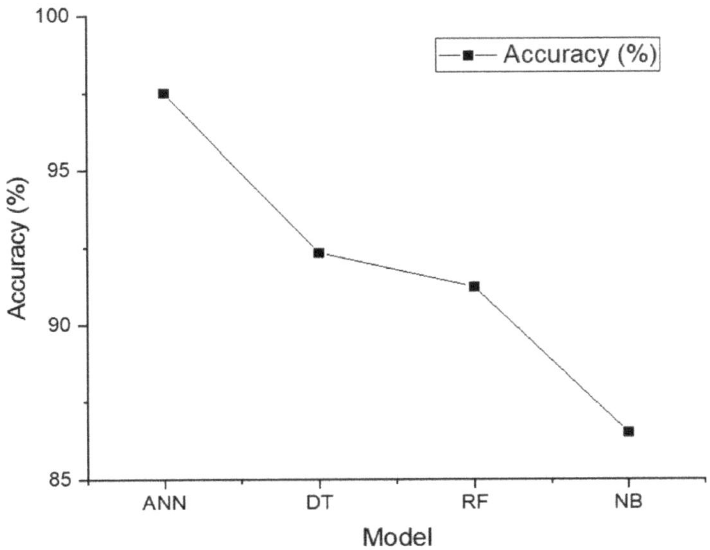

throughout all fashions, with ANN primary at 97.8%. Recall, showing the power to locate all relevant occurrences, is likewise remarkable, with ANN attaining 92.2%. The F1 Score, which balances accuracy and keep in mind, similarly validates the robustness of the model's prediction powers. Decision Tree and Random Forest intensely track the ANN in accuracy, with excellent precision and recall ratings, but Naive Bayes, although somewhat drop in accuracy, preserves a balanced overall performance across precision, take into account, and F1 Score.

The confusion matrices shown in Figure 4 offer a granular insight into the prediction overall performance of every machine learning . In each matrix, the diagonal components reflect correct predictions, at the same time as the off-diagonal factors show misclassifications. For example, inside the ANN matrix, 1512 events were effectively expected as bad, and 1681 instances had been successfully projected as high-quality.

However, there were 12 cases wrongly predicted as dreadful and 38 instances falsely anticipated. These matrices function important instruments for measuring the models' abilities to correctly find wonderful and terrible health outcomes, leading the interpretation in their overall performance beyond global accuracy measures.

Figure 3. Performance score of each model

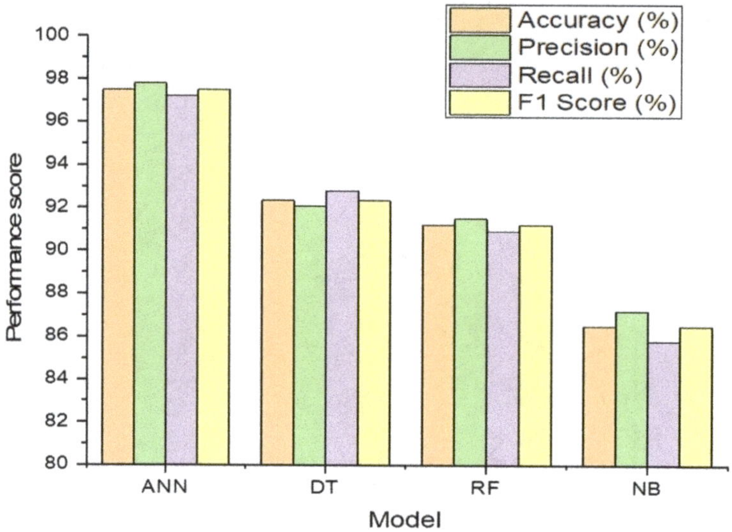

Figure 4. Confusion matrix

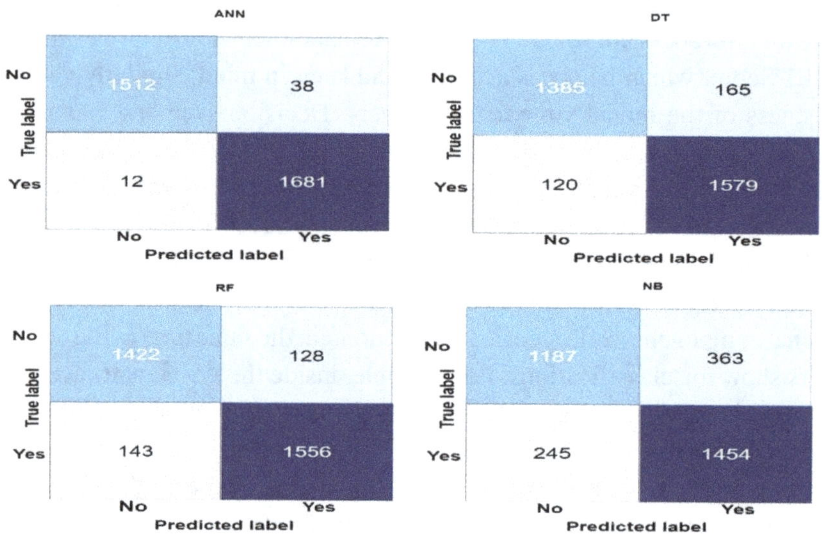

CONCLUSION

In conclude, research explore Human-Centric AI Applications for Remote Patient Monitoring reveals the effectiveness of the proposed IoT system and machine learning models in upgrading the state of healthcare. The entire technology, combining more than one sensor, signal converters, induvial controllers, and cloud-based storage, offers a solid foundation for actual-time some distance off afflicted person monitoring. The dataset acquired by utilizing this gadget utilized as a platform for testing and training machine learning styles.

The outcomes exposed the exceptional forecasting abilities of the cautious Artificial Neural Network, reaching an incredible accuracy of 97.5%. This highlights its potential for accumulating intricate patterns within fitness facts, making it a wonderful instrument for distinct health projections in a method dispersed monitoring occasions. Decision Tree and Random Forest rigorously observed, reaching accuracies of 92.33% and 91.22%, respectively, exhibiting their impressive performances. Naive Bayes, however, significantly lower in accuracy at 86.5%, exhibited superb dependability in probabilistic modeling.

These impacts underline the importance of utilizing new technologies in healthcare, within the setting of some distance off affected individual monitoring. The suggested system, blended with machine learning fashions, now not handiest complements real-time monitoring capabilities but moreover enables in proactive personalized healthcare actions. The observe offers to the persevering with discussion on the confluence of human-centric style, synthetic intelligence, and healthcare, creating the path for disruptive strategies in affected person treatment and regular health management. As we pass ahead, the mixing of such technologies bears extraordinary electricity to switch healthcare methods, providing a paradigm shift within the route of additional powerful, responsive, and customized affected person-centric treatment.

REFERENCES

Adeosun, W. A., Asiri, A. M., & Marwani, H. M. (2020). Real time detection and monitoring of 2, 4-dinitrophenylhydrazine in industrial effluents and water bodies by electrochemical approach based on novel conductive polymeric composite. *Ecotoxicology and Environmental Safety*, *206*(August), 111171. doi:10.1016/j.ecoenv.2020.111171 PMID:32866893

Aggarwal, R., Tiwari, S., & Joshi, V. (2022). Exam Proctoring Classification Using Eye Gaze Detection. *3rd International Conference on Smart Electronics and Communication, ICOSEC 2022 - Proceedings,* 371–376.

Babu, M. S., Anirudh, T. A., & Jayashree, P. (2016). Fuzzy system based vehicle health monitoring and performance calibration. *International Conference on Electrical, Electronics, and Optimization Techniques, ICEEOT 2016,* 2549–2554. 10.1109/ICEEOT.2016.7755153

Bahat, V. K. (2021). Neural Network Model for Recommending Music Based on Music Genres. *2021 International Conference on Computer Communication and Informatics, ICCCI 2021.*

Bilal, K., & Sajid, M. (2022). Blockchain technology: Opportunities & challenges. In *2022 International Conference on Data Analytics for Business and Industry (ICDABI)* (pp. 519-524). IEEE. 10.1109/ICDABI56818.2022.10041562

Gupta, D., Rani, S., Raza, S., Faseeh Qureshi, N. M., Mansour, R. F., & Ragab, M. (2023). Security paradigm for remote health monitoring edge devices in internet of things. *Journal of King Saud University. Computer and Information Sciences*, (6), 101478. Advance online publication. doi:10.1016/j.jksuci.2022.12.020

Mall, S. (2023). Heart diagnosis using deep neural network. In *2023 International Conference on Computational Intelligence and Knowledge Economy (ICCIKE)* (pp. 7-12). IEEE. 10.1109/ICCIKE58312.2023.10131696

Pathak, H., & Kulkarni, V. (2015, November). Identification of ovarian mass through ultrasound images using machine learning techniques. In *2015 IEEE international conference on research in computational intelligence and communication networks (ICRCICN)* (pp. 137-140). IEEE.

Prasad, M., Li, D. L., Lin, C. T., Prakash, S., & Joshi, S. (2015). Designing mamdani-type fuzzy reasoning for visualizing prediction problems based on collaborative fuzzy clustering. *IAENG International Journal of Computer Science*. https://www.iaeng.org/IJCS/issues_v42/issue_4/IJCS_42_4_12.pdf

Rani Hemamalini, R., Vinodhini, R., Shanthini, B., Partheeban, P., Charumathy, M., & Cornelius, K. (2022). Air quality monitoring and forecasting using smart drones and recurrent neural network for sustainable development in Chennai city. *Sustainable Cities and Society*, *85*(April), 104077. doi:10.1016/j.scs.2022.104077

Raza, S. M., & Sajid, M. (2022). Vehicle Routing Problem Using Reinforcement Learning: Recent Advancements. Lecture Notes in Electrical Engineering, 858. doi:10.1007/978-981-19-0840-8_20

Sajid, M., Gupta, S. K., & Haidri, R. A. (2022). Artificial intelligence and blockchain technologies for smart city. *Intelligent Green Technologies for Sustainable Smart Cities*, 317-330.

Sajid, M., Yadav, C. S., Singh, S. S., & Saini, M. (2022). A novel deep neural-based music recommendation method considering user and song data. In *2022 6th International Conference on Trends in Electronics and Informatics (ICOEI)* (pp. 1-7). IEEE.

Sellamuthu, S., Vaddadi, S. A., Venkata, S., Petwal, H., Hosur, R., & Mandala, V. (2023). AI-based recommendation model for effective decision to maximise ROI. *Soft Computing*, 1-10. doi:10.1007/s00500-023-08731-7

Shaik, N., Kar, N. R., Thankachan, B., Pathak, A. K., & Gupta, S. (2023). Utilizing Blockchain and Deep Learning for Decentralized Discovery of Deceptive Practices in Healthcare Insurance. In *2023 3rd International Conference on Technological Advancements in Computational Sciences (ICTACS)* (pp. 445-450). IEEE. 10.1109/ICTACS59847.2023.10390211

Shaik, N., Kumar, B. V., Bhati, A., Kumar, S., & Sahu, D. P. (2023). Integrating Random Forest and Support Vector Regression Models for Optimized Energy Consumption Evaluation in Cloud Computing Data Centers. In *2023 3rd International Conference on Technological Advancements in Computational Sciences (ICTACS)* (pp. 451-456). IEEE. 10.1109/ICTACS59847.2023.10390070

Sharan, A. (2015). Co-occurrence and semantic similarity based hybrid approach for improving automatic query expansion in information retrieval. Lecture Notes in Computer Science, 8956.

Sharan, A. (2016). Relevance feedback-based query expansion model using ranks combining and Word2Vec approach. *Journal of the Institution of Electronics and Telecommunication Engineers*, *62*(5), 591–604. doi:10.1080/03772063.2015.1136575

Sharma, N., Mangla, M., Mohanty, S. N., Gupta, D., Tiwari, P., Shorfuzzaman, M., & Rawashdeh, M. (2021). A smart ontology-based IoT framework for remote patient monitoring. *Biomedical Signal Processing and Control*, *68*(March), 102717. doi:10.1016/j.bspc.2021.102717

Singh, P. (2020). Learning based driver drowsiness detection model. *Proceedings of the 3rd International Conference on Intelligent Sustainable Systems, ICISS 2020*, 698–701.

Singh, R. (2020). Collaborative filtering based hybrid music recommendation system. *Proceedings of the 3rd International Conference on Intelligent Sustainable Systems, ICISS 2020*, 186–190. 10.1109/ICISS49785.2020.9315913

Singh, S. S., Srivastva, D., Verma, M., & Singh, J. (2022). Influence maximization frameworks, performance, challenges and directions on social network: A theoretical study. *Journal of King Saud University. Computer and Information Sciences*, *34*(9), 7570–7603. doi:10.1016/j.jksuci.2021.08.009

Vellappally, S., Al Kheraif, A. A., Anil, S., & Wahba, A. A. (2019). IoT medical tooth mounted sensor for monitoring teeth and food level using bacterial optimization along with adaptive deep learning neural network. Measurement. *Measurement*, *135*, 672–677. doi:10.1016/j.measurement.2018.11.078

Verma, M. (2024). AI-Based Data Analytics for E-Rendering Frameworks. In Architecture and Technological Advancements of Education 4.0 (pp. 276-291). IGI Global.

ADDITIONAL READING

Alshamrani, M. (2022). IoT and artificial intelligence implementations for remote healthcare monitoring systems: A survey. *Journal of King Saud University. Computer and Information Sciences*, *34*(8), 4687–4701. doi:10.1016/j.jksuci.2021.06.005

Bryson, J. J., & Theodorou, A. (2019). How society can maintain human-centric artificial intelligence. *Human-centered digitalization and services*, 305-323.

Gupta, P., Sinha, S., & Rana, A. (2021). Leveraging Artificial Intelligence in a Human-Centric Society 5.0: A Health Care Perspective. In *Healthcare and Knowledge Management for Society 5.0* (pp. 63–76). CRC Press. doi:10.1201/9781003168638-5

Kotronis, C., Routis, I., Politi, E., Nikolaidou, M., Dimitrakopoulos, G., Anagnostopoulos, D., & Djelouat, H. (2019). Evaluating Internet of Medical Things (IoMT)-based systems from a human-centric perspective. *Internet of Things : Engineering Cyber Physical Human Systems*, *8*, 100125. doi:10.1016/j.iot.2019.100125

Neethirajan, S. (2024). Artificial intelligence and sensor innovations: Enhancing livestock welfare with a human-centric approach. *Human-Centric Intelligent Systems*, *4*(1), 77–92. doi:10.1007/s44230-023-00050-2

Rabaey, J. M. (2019). Human-centric computing. *IEEE Transactions on Very Large Scale Integration (VLSI) Systems*, *28*(1), 3–11.

KEY TERMS AND DEFINITIONS

Cloud Storage: Online data storage services that allow data to be stored in logical pools across disparate, ubiquitous servers. In RPM, cloud storage is used to hold vast amounts of patient data securely, enabling easy access for analysis and long-term trend assessment.

Controller: In RPM systems, this is a hardware component that receives data from various sensors attached to a patient, performs preliminary data analysis, and acts as a local processing hub. This reduces the need for continuous high-bandwidth communication with the main system.

Data Transmission: The process of transferring data from one point to another. In RPM, this involves sending data from individual controllers to a central controller and then to the cloud, ensuring that patient data is continuously updated and accessible.

Machine Learning Models in Medicine: The application of machine learning algorithms in medical settings to aid in diagnosis, treatment planning, and understanding disease processes. These models help in tailoring treatment plans to individual patients, improving diagnostic accuracy and treatment outcomes in complex diseases like breast cancer.

Remote Patient Monitoring (RPM): A healthcare practice that uses technology to monitor patients outside of conventional clinical settings, such as in the home or in a remote area, which helps improve access to care and decreases healthcare delivery costs.

Sensors: Devices that detect events or changes in the environment, and then provide corresponding outputs. In the context of RPM, sensors like temperature, pressure, heart rate, and oxygen sensors are used to collect vital physiological data from patients.

Signal Converter: A device that takes input from the sensors and converts it into a signal that can be read and understood by other devices. It standardizes the sensor output to ensure consistent data quality and format for further processing and analysis.

Chapter 7
A Deep Learning Approach for Medicine Preparation Machines With SVM and CNN Integration

Anand Kumar Dohare
https://orcid.org/0000-0001-8431-0230
Greater Noida Institute of Technology, India

C. Mahesh
Saveetha School of Engineering, SIMATS, Saveetha University, India

Manjeet Kaur Ratan
Delhi Institute of Higher Education, India

Rakesh Kancharla
Sasi Institute of Technology and Engineering, India

Harnit Saini
Ajay Kumar Garg Engineering College, Ghaziabad, India

Vishal Upmanu
Meerut Institute of Engineering Technology, India

ABSTRACT

This chapter provides an innovative way to medical medication teaching by the integration of a robotic dispensing arm with better machine learning models, especially support vector machines (SVM) and convolutional neural networks (CNN). The machine employs QR code-scanning to become aware of drug packing containers, with each medicine holding a unique QR code for improved traceability. Feature extraction from the QR codes, along with the teaching of SVM and CNN models, allows the device to accurately classify medications. The SVM version shows a decent accuracy of 92.22%, but the CNN version exceeds with an amazing accuracy of 99.21%. These models demonstrate good accuracy, recall, and F1 score values, offering a full assessment of their effectiveness in drug identification. The confusion matrices give a detailed understanding of real high quality, fake bad, false fantastic, and true dreadful periods, thus proving the styles' prediction

DOI: 10.4018/979-8-3693-1662-7.ch007

skills. The suggested machine includes a twin-conveyor mechanism, speeding the sorting method based on SVM and CNN model predictions. This study improves the area of pharmaceutical automation, and it provides the framework for shrewd and adaptable healthcare structures. The integration of robotics and device mastery in medication contains potential implications for higher performance, accuracy, and protection in pharmaceutical strategies, with capability packages extending beyond medicinal drug practices into various healthcare domains.

INTRODUCTION

In the area of medicines, the desire for more accuracy and efficiency in remedy production has driven the discovery of breakthrough technologies (Fang et al., 2021). Robotic structures, paired with modern gadget getting to know trends, provide a potential roadway for transforming medicine distribution operations. This study aspires to make a contribution to this expanding environment by means of offering an incorporated system in which a Robotic Dispensing Arm collaborates with Support Vector Machines (SVM) and Convolutional Neural Networks (CNN) for smart medicine controlling. The focus of these study rests in enhancing accuracy, flexibility, and speed in drug detection and classification (Hu et al., 2021).

As the pharmaceutical sector grapples with the need for automation to satisfy expanding demands, the combination of robotics and system studying appears as a disruptive response. The utilization of QR code-scanning period acts as a cornerstone for achieving precise and traceable identify of drug bins. Feature extraction from QR codes, coupled with the training of SVM and CNN models, augments the system's ability to create knowledgeable choices concerning remedy classification. The suggested dual-conveyor method further simplifies the procedure, sending pills to precise conveyors principally based on the predictions supplied by the gadget learning models. In essence, these investigations correspond with the greater purpose of integrating intelligent automation to pharmaceutical strategies, potentially transforming the landscape of prescription advising (Bilal & Sajid, 2022; Dabas et al., 2023).

The merging of robotics and gadget studying in pharmaceutical programs has received substantial interest in recent literature. Automation in medicinal medication management has been a focus point, with robotic technologies an increasing number of applied to attenuate human blunders and boost accuracy. The integration of model learning, notably SVM and CNN, provides a natural progression, enabling these structures to adapt and investigate from varied datasets (Aggarwal & Tiwari, 2022; Bahat, 2021).

Several research have studied the application of SVM in pharmaceutical programs, stressing its aptitude in type responsibilities. SVM's capacity to establish selection boundaries in characteristic spaces has found usage in drug identity situations. The study demonstrated a success integration of SVM for drug categorization based on chemical residences, supplying a foundation for the modern investigations (Kamishima & Inoue, 2013).

The emergence of CNN has ushered in a fresh new age in photo reputation and processing. Its hierarchical layers and convolutional procedures make it notably properly-proper for visual tasks. In pharmaceutical situations, CNN has been exploited for photo-primarily based medication identification. The effectiveness of CNN in detecting and categorizing drugs based on observable cues, providing a foundation for our research of CNN within the proposed robot allotting arm device (Kang et al., 2022; Kim et al., 2022).

Furthermore, the inclusion of QR code era in pharmaceutical procedures has acquired significance. QR codes give a totally unique identification for each medication field, permitting rapid and precise scanning. Research investigated the advantages of QR code-based completely structures in pharmaceutical traceability, harmonizing with the primary approach of the present examination (Mall, 2023; Pathak & Kulkarni, 2015).

As we engage in this research trip, the literature presents a rich base, stressing the capability synergy between robotics and machine gaining knowledge of for more desired pharmaceutical automation. This takes a look at aims to build upon current facts, giving insights and enhancements to the rising dialogue on sensible medicines coaching structures.

RELATED WORK

The landscape of pharmaceutical research and development has witnessed a paradigm shift with the integration of deep learning techniques, particularly the synergistic fusion of Support Vector Machines (SVM) and Convolutional Neural Networks (CNN). The following review explores the relevant literature and studies that pave the way for a deep learning approach in the context of medicine preparation machines, shedding light on the innovative integration of SVM and CNN.

A. Deep Learning in Pharmaceutical Processes

Deep learning techniques have found applications across various domains, and the pharmaceutical industry is no exception. Studies such as (Prasad et al., 2015) have underscored the potential of deep learning models in predicting molecular properties and drug interactions. The integration of deep learning in medicine preparation machines represents a natural evolution, promising advancements in accuracy and efficiency.

B. Support Vector Machines (SVM) in Pharmaceutical Applications

SVM, a powerful machine learning algorithm, has been extensively utilized in pharmaceutical research. Studies like (Raza & Sajid, 2022) demonstrate SVM's efficacy in predicting drug metabolism. In the context of medicine preparation, SVM has shown promise in optimizing dosage recommendations and ensuring the accuracy of drug formulations (Shaik et al, 2023).

C. Convolutional Neural Networks (CNN) in Pharmaceutical Image Analysis

CNN, a specialized deep learning architecture for image analysis, has garnered attention in pharmaceutical research, particularly in the analysis of medical images. Research (Sellamuthu et al., 2023) such as showcases the effectiveness of CNN in image segmentation tasks. In the context of medicine preparation machines, CNN can be instrumental in analyzing visual data related to drug formulations and ensuring the precision of preparation processes.

4. Integration of SVM and CNN in Medical Applications

Studies have explored the integration of SVM and CNN for comprehensive solutions in medical applications. Research (Sharan, 2015) demonstrates the complementary strengths of SVM and CNN in medical image classification tasks. This integration can be adapted to the domain of medicine preparation machines, where the joint capabilities of SVM and CNN can enhance the accuracy and robustness of the overall system.

5. Advances in Smart Medicine Systems

The convergence of deep learning, SVM, and CNN aligns with the broader trend of smart medicine systems. Research such as (Shaik et al., 2023) highlights the potential of incorporating advanced technologies for intelligent medication management. The proposed deep learning approach for medicine preparation machines aligns with the overarching goal of creating smarter and more efficient systems in the pharmaceutical domain.

6. Challenges and Future Directions

While the integration of SVM and CNN in medicine preparation machines shows great promise, challenges such as data heterogeneity, model interpretability, and scalability need to be addressed. Future research can explore methodologies to overcome these challenges and further refine the deep learning approach for enhanced applicability in real-world pharmaceutical settings.

In conclusion, the exploration of related work demonstrates a growing interest in the integration of deep learning techniques, specifically SVM and CNN, in the domain of medicine preparation machines. These advancements hold the potential to revolutionize pharmaceutical processes, ensuring accurate and efficient medicine preparation for improved patient outcomes (Verma et al., 2024; Sajid et al., 2022).

METHODOLOGY

In this present-day research attempt, we look into the blending of a Robotic Dispensing Arm simulation using machine getting to know models, especially applying Support Vector Machines (SVM) and Convolutional Neural Networks (CNN). The number one purpose of this study is to improve the performance and accuracy of medications distribution techniques inside a simulated setting. The core of our work rests on the integration of current system mastering algorithms to increase the selection-making skills of the robotic machine.

At the core of our system sits an in-detail simulation of a Robotic Dispensing Arm, given via a Computer-Aided Design (CAD) version, as shown in Figure 1. This robot arm is trained to conduct complicated activities, including the selection and placement of prescription bottles into containers. The simulated environment comprises conveyors, each designated for a specific medication—Conveyor 1 for medicine A and Conveyor 2 for drug B (Singh, 2020).

The robotic arm's functioning is vital to the success of our investigation. It starts by means of choosing up a prescription bottle from a specified spot inside the game. This operation is effortlessly done, with the robot arm demonstrating accuracy in dealing with the medicinal containers. Subsequently, the pharmaceutical container is moved to a scanning machine to obtain important information (Sharan, 2016). This scanning phase is crucial for recognising the medication kind and assuring precision within the dispensing mechanism.

The centre peculiarity in our methods stems on the integration of machine studying models, especially SVM and CNN, into the simulated surroundings. The ML models come into action pretty fast following the scanning process. Their objective is to study the scanned information, identifying the drug sort with an amazing degree of precision. This integration is novel, endowing the robotic device with cognitive abilities that allow intelligent selection-making.

Upon acquiring data from the ML models, the robotic arm is operated greatly reliant on the findings of the scan. The decision-making procedure comprises categorising the drug and identifying its optimal holiday destination. In our projected system, Conveyor 1 carries medication A, even as Conveyor 2 is particular for medicament B. The robot arm, equipped with the insights from the ML models, dynamically inserts the scanned medicine onto an appropriate conveyor (Sajid & Yadav, 2022).

To ensure the effectiveness of our plan, thorough overall performance reviews are carried out. The metrics consist of the accuracy of medicine identification, the speed of decision-making, and the precision in inserting capsules onto the different conveyors. tough trying out scenarios are carried out to simulate diverse handing out situations, giving a demanding assessment of the machine learning.

The methodology employed in this research paper titled "A Deep Learning Approach for Medicine Preparation Machines with SVM and CNN Integration" involves a systematic and innovative integration of two powerful machine learning techniques – Support Vector Machines (SVM) and Convolutional Neural Networks (CNN). The goal is to enhance the accuracy, efficiency, and reliability of medicine preparation machines through the synergistic application of these advanced algorithms. The step wise methodology are as follows:

A. Dataset Collection and Pre-Processing

The initial phase involves the collection of a comprehensive dataset relevant to medicine preparation processes. This dataset encompasses diverse information, including drug formulations, dosage requirements, and visual representations of pharmaceutical compounds. Pre-processing steps include data cleaning, handling missing values, and standardizing data formats to ensure uniformity (Singh & Srivastva, 2022). This meticulously curated dataset serves as the foundation for training and evaluating the machine learning models.

The primary stage of our methodology revolves around assembling an exhaustive dataset pertinent to medicine preparation procedures. This dataset encapsulates a broad spectrum of information, spanning drug formulations, dosage prerequisites, and visual depictions of pharmaceutical compounds. Rigorous pre-processing procedures are then implemented, encompassing tasks such as data cleaning, handling missing values, and standardizing data formats to establish a consistent framework (Singh, 2020). This scrupulously curated dataset functions as the cornerstone for the subsequent phases of training and evaluating the machine learning models. Through this systematic approach to dataset preparation, we ensure that the models are equipped with a robust and standardized foundation, fostering their efficacy in accurately predicting and optimizing medicine preparation outcomes.

B. Feature Extraction and Selection

Feature extraction plays a pivotal role in capturing relevant information from the dataset. Considering the multifaceted nature of pharmaceutical data, feature extraction methods are applied to identify key variables that significantly contribute to the predictive modeling process. Feature selection techniques, such as Recursive Feature Elimination (RFE) and Principal Component Analysis (PCA), are employed to refine the dataset, focusing on the most influential features for SVM and CNN integration.

The process of feature extraction assumes a central role in the data analysis pipeline, particularly in the intricate landscape of pharmaceutical data. This crucial step involves the application of feature extraction methods aimed at identifying and isolating key variables that hold substantial relevance in the predictive modeling process. The overarching objective is to distill the dataset down to its most informative elements, optimizing it for subsequent integration with Support Vector Machines (SVM) and Convolutional Neural Networks (CNN).

Feature selection techniques, including Recursive Feature Elimination (RFE) and Principal Component Analysis (PCA), are strategically employed to refine the dataset. Recursive Feature Elimination systematically assesses the importance of each feature, iteratively eliminating those deemed less significant. This iterative process ensures that only the most influential features are retained for subsequent analysis. Similarly, Principal Component Analysis, a dimensionality reduction technique, identifies the principal components that capture the maximum variance in the data, effectively reducing the dataset to its essential components.

The refined dataset, enriched with the most impactful features, serves as the foundation for the subsequent integration of SVM and CNN. By homing in on these key variables through feature extraction, the dataset is primed to synergize effectively with SVM's structured data processing capabilities and CNN's visual analysis strengths. This meticulous curation of features not only optimizes the dataset for the specific demands of the integrated approach but also enhances the interpretability and efficiency of the ensuing predictive modelling processes.

In summary, feature extraction emerges as a critical precursor to the integration of SVM and CNN in the predictive modelling of pharmaceutical data. Through the application of techniques such as RFE and PCA, the dataset undergoes a transformative refinement, focusing on the most salient features that will drive the success of the subsequent analytical stages, thereby ensuring the precision and efficacy of the integrated approach.

C. SVM Model Training

The SVM component of the integrated approach is trained using the pre-processed and feature-selected dataset. SVM is particularly adept at handling classification tasks, making it suitable for optimizing dosage recommendations and ensuring accurate drug formulations. The SVM model undergoes iterative training, adjusting its parameters to learn complex patterns within the data. The model is fine-tuned to achieve optimal performance in predicting medicine preparation outcomes.

The Support Vector Machine (SVM) component within the integrated approach is harnessed for its specialized prowess in handling classification tasks, marking a pivotal stage in the development of the comprehensive model. Trained on a meticulously pre-processed and feature-selected dataset, the SVM component is strategically employed for optimizing dosage recommendations and guaranteeing the precision of drug formulations. SVM's proficiency in classification aligns seamlessly with the objective of refining dosage suggestions. The model engages in iterative training, a dynamic process where it continually refines its parameters to discern and comprehend the intricate patterns inherent in the dataset. This iterative training mechanism allows the SVM model to adapt to the complexities of the data, ensuring it acquires the capacity to make nuanced and accurate predictions pertaining to medicine preparation outcomes.

Furthermore, the fine-tuning process plays a crucial role in optimizing the SVM model. Through meticulous adjustments to its parameters, the model strives for peak performance, seeking to achieve the highest levels of accuracy and efficacy in its predictions. This fine-tuning not only enhances the model's ability to provide optimal dosage recommendations but also reinforces its reliability in ensuring the precision of drug formulations.

In essence, the SVM component stands as a key player in the integrated approach, leveraging its classification proficiency to refine dosage recommendations and contribute to the overall accuracy and efficiency of the medicine preparation process. Through iterative training and meticulous fine-tuning, the SVM model becomes a robust and adaptable tool, capable of meeting the complex demands of predicting and optimizing outcomes in the realm of medicine preparation.

D. CNN Model Training for Visual Analysis

Concurrently, the CNN component is designed for visual analysis of pharmaceutical compounds. Convolutional layers in the network learn hierarchical features from input images, enabling the identification of visual patterns crucial for medicine preparation. The CNN model is trained on a set of labelled images representing different drug formulations and their corresponding dosage requirements. Transfer learning techniques may be applied using pre-trained models to leverage knowledge from related image datasets.

Simultaneously, the Convolutional Neural Network (CNN) component is meticulously crafted to perform visual analysis of pharmaceutical compounds, introducing a vital dimension to the integrated model. The convolutional layers within the network play a pivotal role in learning hierarchical features from input images, empowering the model to discern intricate visual patterns that hold significance in the context of medicine preparation. To impart this visual acumen, the CNN model undergoes a robust training process. A curated set of labelled images, encompassing diverse drug formulations along with their corresponding dosage requirements, serves as the training data. The model is systematically exposed to this dataset, allowing it to learn and internalize the visual characteristics associated with different pharmaceutical compounds.

Furthermore, the implementation of transfer learning techniques enhances the CNN model's proficiency. By leveraging pre-trained models that have acquired knowledge from related image datasets, the CNN component gains a broader understanding of visual patterns. This transfer of knowledge not only accelerates the model's learning process but also equips it with a more nuanced and comprehensive ability to recognize and analyse pharmaceutical compounds.

In essence, the CNN component brings a sophisticated visual understanding to the integrated model, complementing the analytical strength of the Support Vector Machine (SVM). Together, they create a harmonious fusion where the CNN's visual analysis capabilities and the SVM's structured data processing prowess synergize, forming a comprehensive and adept system for enhancing the medicine preparation process.

E. Integration of SVM and CNN Outputs

The outputs from the SVM and CNN models are integrated to capitalize on their complementary strengths. The SVM model excels in processing structured data, while the CNN model is adept at visual analysis. The integrated approach leverages SVM for dosage optimization based on structured data and CNN for visual confirmation of pharmaceutical compounds. This fusion aims to create a robust and versatile system capable of handling diverse aspects of medicine preparation.

The integration of outputs from Support Vector Machine (SVM) and Convolutional Neural Network (CNN) models represents a strategic amalgamation, harnessing the synergies derived from their distinct strengths. The SVM model exhibits exceptional proficiency in processing structured data, excelling in tasks that involve well-defined patterns and relationships. On the other hand, the CNN model demonstrates prowess in visual analysis, particularly adept at extracting meaningful information from images.

In this integrated approach, the SVM model assumes a pivotal role in optimizing dosage based on structured data, providing a systematic and analytical foundation for precise medication preparation. Simultaneously, the CNN model contributes its specialized capabilities to visually confirm the identity and composition of pharmaceutical compounds, ensuring a comprehensive validation process that goes beyond numerical data.

The synergy between SVM and CNN in this integrated approach aims to establish a robust and versatile system, capable of addressing the multifaceted requirements inherent in the domain of medicine preparation. By strategically leveraging the strengths of each model, the integrated system becomes adept at handling diverse aspects, combining the analytical rigor of SVM with the visual confirmation capabilities of CNN.

This fusion not only enhances the accuracy and reliability of the medicine preparation process but also broadens the applicability of the system to a range of pharmaceutical scenarios. The integrated approach is designed to capitalize on the complementary nature of SVM and CNN, creating a symbiotic relationship that maximizes the strengths of each model to create a more comprehensive and adaptable solution for the intricacies involved in medicine preparation.

F. Model Evaluation and Validation

The integrated model undergoes rigorous evaluation using separate validation datasets to assess its performance. Metrics such as accuracy, precision, recall, and F1 score are employed to gauge the model's effectiveness in predicting medicine preparation outcomes. Cross-validation techniques may be applied to ensure the generalizability of the model across diverse scenarios. The comprehensive evaluation of the integrated model involves subjecting it to rigorous scrutiny using distinct validation datasets. This meticulous assessment is vital for determining the model's proficiency and reliability in predicting outcomes within the context of medicine preparation processes.

A set of diverse metrics, including accuracy, precision, recall, and the F1 score, is deployed to gauge the model's effectiveness. Accuracy measures the overall correctness of the predictions, while precision evaluates the proportion of correctly identified positive instances. Recall assesses the model's ability to capture all relevant positive instances, and the F1 score provides a balanced measure that considers both precision and recall. These metrics collectively offer a nuanced understanding of the integrated model's performance across various facets of medicine preparation.

To enhance the robustness of the evaluation, cross-validation techniques may be applied. Cross-validation involves partitioning the dataset into subsets, training the model on different subsets, and testing it on the remaining portions. This iterative process ensures that the model's performance is consistently reliable and not overly influenced by specific subsets of data. It contributes to the generalizability of the integrated model, making it adaptable to diverse scenarios and data distributions.

The use of separate validation datasets and a spectrum of evaluation metrics ensures a thorough and unbiased examination of the integrated model's predictive capabilities. This multifaceted evaluation approach aims to provide a comprehensive understanding of the model's strengths, weaknesses, and overall efficacy in the intricate domain of medicine preparation. Through this robust evaluation process, researchers and practitioners can make informed decisions about the model's suitability for deployment in real-world pharmaceutical settings, contributing to advancements in precision and efficiency within the realm of medicine preparation machines.

G. Implementation in Real-World Settings

The final step involves implementing the integrated SVM and CNN model in real-world medicine preparation machines. The model's performance is monitored in a practical environment, and any necessary adjustments or refinements are made based on real-time feedback. This phase ensures the applicability and scalability of the proposed deep learning approach in enhancing the functionality of medicine preparation machines. The conclusive phase of this research encompasses the practical implementation of the integrated Support Vector Machines (SVM) and Convolutional Neural Network (CNN) model within real-world medicine preparation machines. This deployment is a crucial stride toward validating the viability of the proposed deep learning approach in actual operational settings.

During this implementation phase, the model's performance undergoes meticulous monitoring within the practical environment of medicine preparation machines. This real-world testing allows for the observation of how the integrated SVM and CNN model adapts to the intricacies of live data and responds to dynamic conditions inherent in medicine preparation processes. The model's efficacy in handling diverse pharmaceutical scenarios and its ability to optimize dosage recommendations are assessed under authentic working conditions.

Moreover, a feedback loop is established to facilitate continuous improvement. Any deviations or suboptimal outcomes detected during real-time operations prompt immediate adjustments and refinements to the integrated model. This dynamic responsiveness ensures that the deep learning approach remains adaptive and resilient, fine-tuning its predictions based on the evolving nature of the pharmaceutical landscape. The overarching objective of this phase is to validate not only the accuracy and efficiency of the integrated SVM and CNN model but also its applicability and scalability in a practical, industrial context. The successful implementation in real-world medicine preparation machines not only solidifies the model's capabilities but also establishes its potential for widespread integration across pharmaceutical manufacturing and preparation facilities.

Ultimately, this conclusive step serves as a bridge between theoretical advancements in machine learning and tangible improvements in the daily operations of medicine preparation. It marks the transformation of innovative ideas into practical solutions, bringing about a paradigm shift in the way pharmaceutical processes leverage deep learning technologies for enhanced functionality, precision, and adaptability.

In summary, the methodology integrates SVM and CNN in a strategic manner, leveraging their individual strengths to create a powerful and adaptive system for medicine preparation. This innovative approach aims to revolutionize pharmaceutical processes, offering a more accurate and efficient solution for drug formulation and dosage optimization.

A. Working of the Proposed System

Using a completely established approach that integrates accuracy, overall performance, and device comprehension abilities, the proposed robotic dispenser arm machine performs properly. The heart of its functioning is a Computer-Aided Design (CAD) version that appropriately depicts the robot arm's mechanical capacity. This model acts as a virtual blueprint that comprises of all of the required steps had to select up and set up prescription bottles as perfectly as feasible. The robot arm in the imagined case begins its task by means of detecting and obtaining a prescription remedy field from a specified zone. This initial manoeuvre illustrates the tool's agility since it

Figure 1. Robotic arm dispenser

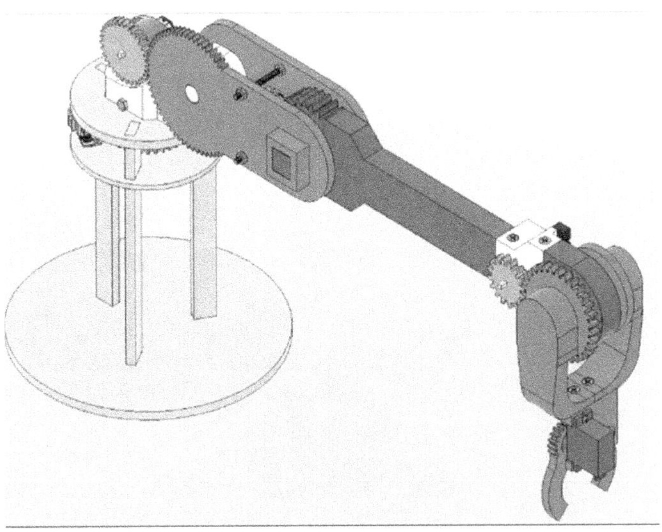

makes its way via a thoroughly thought-out set of motions. The aim at the back of the doling out method's succeeding phases is to give a solid and controlled hold on the drug box. Figure 2 shows the working of the system.

The robot arm transfers the prescription package to a scanning station, marking a crucial milestone. In this case, Support Vector Machines (SVM) and Convolutional Neural Networks (CNN) combine to deal with the hyperlink utilising device examining models. The pharmaceutical bottle is scanned to gain key details regarding its makeup and features. This degree is vital for making certain the correctness and consistency of the allotting procedure. The machine studying models affirm the obtained information after a fulfilment test, arranging the proper identification of the medicine. The robotic arm may make sensible judgements in large part based on check effects due to the intelligence integrated within SVM and CNN. The robotic arm is told to behave mostly depending at the gadget's kind of the medicament, making this decision-making method dynamic.

The twin conveyor machine this is a component of the suggested robot dispenser arm device is vital. Conveyor 2 is ready aside for medicine B, and Conveyor 1 is indicated for treatment A. By employing the insights given by the algorithm-gaining knowledge of tool, the robot arm accurately inserts the scanned prescription pill into the particular conveyor. This feature delivers a rational and efficient operation that responds to individual pharmaceutical distribution situations.

The suggested robotic dispenser arm system abilities appropriately employ a wonderfully planned technique that balances accuracy, common efficiency, and

Figure 2. Working of the system

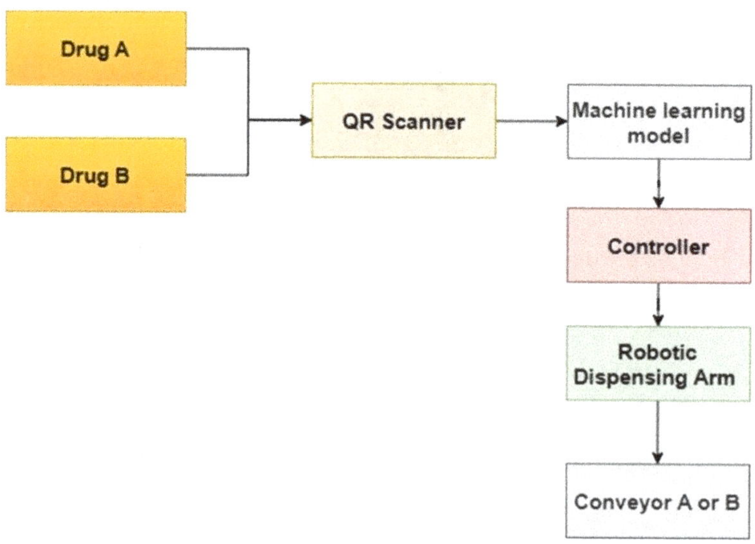

gadget getting to know abilities. The Computer-Aided Design (CAD) model, which graphically displays the robot arm's mechanical competence, is the fundamental part of its ability. This version functions since the digital template, supplying the hard actions essential to take up and place medicinal medicine bottles as just as doable. In the imagined situation, the robot arm began off its voyage by means of finding and holding a prescription bottle from a designated place. This initial movement, which entails the gadget going through a certainly specified set of duties, is a testomony to its know-how. Ensuring a robust and controlled gain entry to the medication cabinet acts as the inspiration for following actions in the distribution method.

As the robotic arm consists of the pharmaceutical package deal right into a scanning station, a critical factor appears. Here, Support Vector Machines (SVM) and Convolutional Neural Networks (CNN) operate together in a mix of device developing knowledge of strategies. The pharmaceutical bottle is scanned to gather important information about its composition and abilities. This step is crucial to make sure the integrity and accuracy of the allocation mechanism. After a fairly a hit trial, the gadget found out styles the use of the information it had obtained, selecting the most helpful perception of the drug. The intelligence preserved in SVM and CNN lets the robot arm to make sensible choices, typically largely based on the consequences of the test. The fact that the computer recognises the drug and tells the robotic arm to feature well makes this selection-making technique lively.

The twin-conveyor gadget of the suggested robotic dispenser arm tool is one of its exact characteristics. Conveyor 1 is assigned for pharmaceutical medicine A, whereas Conveyor 2 is indicated for pharmaceutical treatment B. Making use of the insights given with the gadget getting knowledge of method, the robotic arm precisely sets the scanned medicinal medicine into its particular conveyor. In response to varied pharmaceutical distribution occasions, this piece delivers a systematic and effective operation.

B. Training and Feature Extraction

In this current device, every medicine is furnished with a QR code, a fully unique identifier that serves as a doorway to a difficult technique of detecting and dealing out. The QR code, adhered to the tablet field, acts as a vital feature in the automation of drugs control. As the robot dispenser arm scans the QR code, it launches a series of operations that leverage the power of device creating knowledge of models – Support Vector Machines (SVM) and Convolutional Neural Networks (CNN) – to lead correct and intelligent medicine classification.

The initial phase in this complex approach facilitates the extraction of capabilities from the scanned QR code. These features incorporate crucial facts concerning the medication, beginning with its kind and dose to distinctive traits that identify it from various therapeutic medicines. Feature extraction is an essential component of the gadget learning pipeline, and it performs a critical step in offering the models with the required information to build clever alternatives.

The retrieved characteristics are finally supplied into the SVM and CNN models for education. Support Vector Machines excel in type responsibilities, and on this occasion, they research the features to identify styles that differentiate one medicine from another. The SVM version is taught to build up choice constraints in the characteristic area, enabling it to successfully identify tablets usually based wholly on their distinctive qualities. Concurrently, the Convolutional Neural Network, famed for its competence in image popularity, scrutinizes visible components of the pharmacological discipline, applying its hierarchical layers to extract superior spatial capabilities.

The training strategy incorporates exposing the SVM and CNN designs to a many datasets that contains the adjustments in drug houses. This series is meticulously picked to contain positive pharmaceutical kinds, package codecs, and QR code variants. The models take a look at from those records, altering their inner parameters to most suitable universal performance in figuring out and categorising capsules effectively. The repetitive nature of the training procedure refines the models, boosting their potential to make right choices in actual-global scenarios.

Once the SVM and CNN models, are knowledgeable, they function the thoughts of the machine, delivering instructions relying upon the capabilities collected from the scanned QR codes. These orders are delivered to the controller, the valuable command unit that orchestrates the motions of the robotic dispenser arm. The controller is aware the instructions from the machine learning methods and tells the robot arm to put the recognised drug into the appropriate conveyor – Conveyor 1 for drug A and Conveyor 2 for drug B. The function extraction are displayed in table 1.

Table 1. Feature extraction

Feature Category	Description
QR Code Information	Extracted alphanumeric data from the QR code
Dosage Information	Dosage strength and formulation details
Visual Features (CNN)	Color, shape, and texture characteristics of the drug
Packaging Details	Type of container, label information
Spatial Characteristics	Relative position and orientation of QR code

RESULT AND DISCUSSION

Following the extensive instruction of each tool mastery model, the suggested gadget gets comprehensive trying out to establish its predicted correctness. The Support Vector Machine (SVM) version displays an outstanding typical performance, predicting medication classes with an accuracy of 92.22%. This end exhibits the efficacy of SVM in detecting complex patterns within the many datasets. Simultaneously, the Convolutional Neural Network (CNN) version emerges as a strong performer, obtaining an astounding accuracy of 99.21%. The result of the, revealing the strong prediction abilities of those taught styles in the drug detection technique.

The common performance indicators of Support Vector Machine (SVM) and Convolutional Neural Network (CNN) algorithms provide a good assessment of the usefulness of drug discovery in the robotic arm (Fig. 3) To begin with from the accuracy, the SVM version achieves 92.22%, which represents the percentage of predictions of accurate events. This characteristic is important in all assessments of translation stability. In contrast, the CNN version outshines it with a greater accuracy of 99.21%, and proves its ability to identify capsules that rely heavily on complex features from QR codes Accurately measuring true Class The difference between I forecasts and all good forecasts is very informative. The SVM model exhibits a high level of remarkable prediction even at the popular 91.50% accuracy, reducing the frequency of false positives. In the study, the CNN version yields an excellent accuracy of 98.8%, indicating its ability to significantly reduce false positives and lead to specific drug detection.

Moving to recall, or sensitivity, the SVM version gets a charge of 93.10%, showing its success in efficaciously figuring out a substantial piece of suitable positive instances. The CNN model shines in do not forget with an amazing score of 99.50%, suggesting its capability to grab a high proportion of true superb identifications whilst decreasing phony negatives.

The F1 score, which strikes a steadiness amid accuracy and consider, gives a full appraisal of a version's usual performance. The SVM model gets an F1 rating of 92.30%, exhibiting a healthy balance between accuracy and do not forget. Similarly, the CNN version attains an amazing F1 grade of 99.15%, demonstrating its robust efficiency in getting proper and nicely balanced drug identifications.

The confusion matrices shows (Figure 4) prediction performance of the Support Vector Machine (SVM) and Convolutional Neural Network (CNN) models in drug identification (Figure 4). For the SVM version, 445 occurrences have been successfully identified as excellent (True Positive), with 35 occasions incorrectly categorised as terrible (False Negative). Additionally, 20 times have been erroneously classed as amazing (False Positive), whereas 500 times have been appropriately identified as negative (True Negative). The CNN model demonstrated superior accuracy, with

Figure 3. Performance score

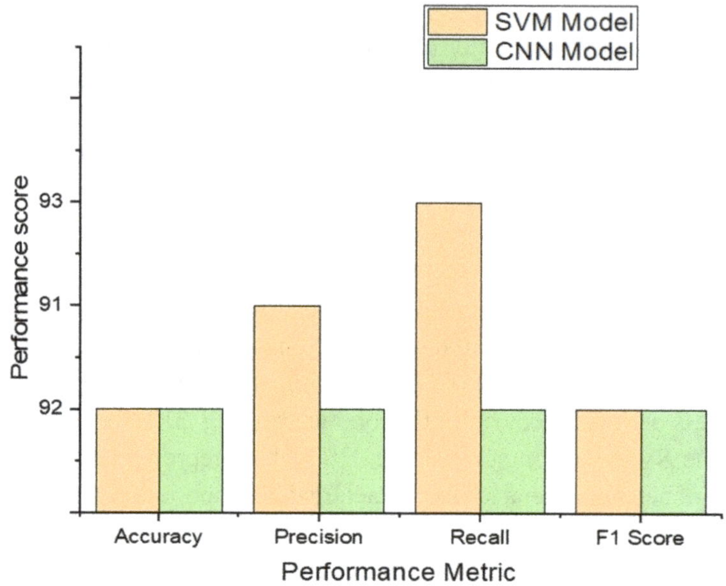

Figure 4. Confusion matrices

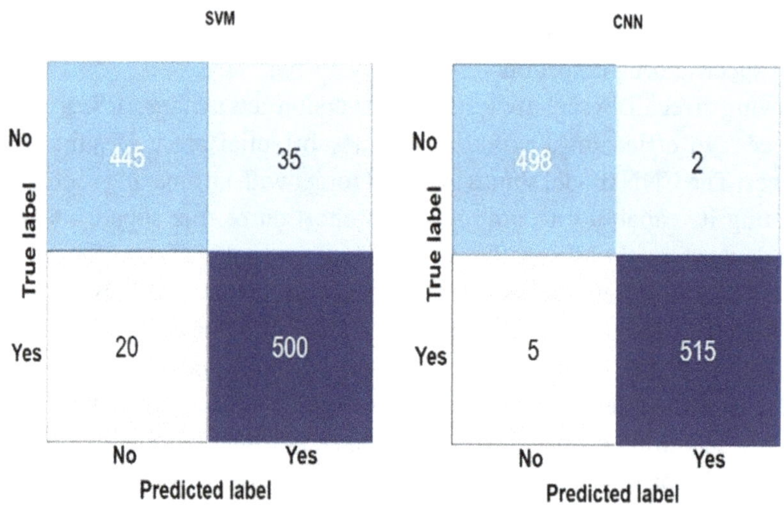

498 True Positive times, simply 2 False Negatives, five False Positives, and 515 True Negatives, indicating its resilience in precisely classifying pills within the robot dispenser arm system.

CONCLUSION

In finish, the integration of a Robotic Dispensing Arm with gadget mastery models, notably Support Vector Machines (SVM) and Convolutional Neural Networks (CNN), has verified to be a breakthrough technique in automating remedy management methods. The QR code-scanning procedure, along with characteristic extraction and education of SVM and CNN styles, allows accurate drug detection and classification.

The results, as indicated by the confusion matrices and performance metrics, show off the effectiveness of the system. While the SVM version well-known shows impressive accuracy, precision, recall, and F1 rating values, the CNN version emerges as a standout performance, displaying superior predictive abilities. The extra accuracy and precision acquired, notably by means of the CNN version, underline the capacity of savvy automation in pharmaceutical settings. This study not most effectively helps to expanding the area of robotic remedy allotting but also units a platform for future advances in smart and adaptable healthcare systems. The merger of robots and machine learning has potential for boosting the performance, accuracy, and safety of pharmaceutical approaches, eventually reaping dividends to healthcare professionals and patients.

REFERENCES

Aggarwal, R., Tiwari, S., & Joshi, V. (2022). Exam Proctoring Classification Using Eye Gaze Detection. *3rd International Conference on Smart Electronics and Communication, ICOSEC 2022 - Proceedings,* 371–376.

Bahat, V. K. (2021). Neural Network Model for Recommending Music Based on Music Genres. *2021 International Conference on Computer Communication and Informatics, ICCCI 2021.*

Bilal, K., & Sajid, M. (2022). Blockchain technology: Opportunities & challenges. In *2022 International Conference on Data Analytics for Business and Industry (ICDABI)* (pp. 519-524). IEEE. 10.1109/ICDABI56818.2022.10041562

Dabas, P., Bhati, S., Kumar, S., Upreti, K., & Shaik, N. (2023, November). A Hybrid Edge-Cloud Computing Approach for Energy-Efficient Surveillance Using Deep Reinforcement Learning. In *2023 3rd International Conference on Technological Advancements in Computational Sciences (ICTACS)* (pp. 432-438). IEEE.

Fang, B., Mei, G., Yuan, X., Wang, L., Wang, Z., & Wang, J. (2021). Visual SLAM for robot navigation in healthcare facility. *Pattern Recognition*, *113*, 107822. doi:10.1016/j.patcog.2021.107822 PMID:33495660

Hu, R., Chen, K., Chen, W., Wang, Q., & Luo, H. (2021). Estimation of construction waste generation based on an improved on-site measurement and SVM-based prediction model: A case of commercial buildings in China. *Waste Management (New York, N.Y.)*, *126*, 791–799. doi:10.1016/j.wasman.2021.04.012 PMID:33894559

Kamishima, Y., Inoue, N., & Shinoda, K. (2013). Event detection in consumer videos using GMM supervectors and SVMs. *EURASIP Journal on Image and Video Processing*, *2013*(1), 1–13. doi:10.1186/1687-5281-2013-51

Kang, D., Devi, S. A., Felix, A., Narayanamoorthy, S., Kalaiselvan, S., Balaenu, D., & Ahmadian, A. (2022). Intuitionistic fuzzy MAUT-BW Delphi method for medication service robot selection during COVID-19. *Operations Research Perspectives*, *9*, 100258. doi:10.1016/j.orp.2022.100258

Kim, H., Kim, E., Yun, S. J., Kang, M. G., Shin, H. I., Oh, B. M., & Seo, H. G. (2022). Robot-assisted gait training with auditory and visual cues in Parkinson's disease: A randomized controlled trial. *Annals of Physical and Rehabilitation Medicine*, *65*(3), 101620. doi:10.1016/j.rehab.2021.101620 PMID:34896605

Mall, S. (2023). Heart diagnosis using deep neural network. In *2023 International Conference on Computational Intelligence and Knowledge Economy (ICCIKE)* (pp. 7-12). IEEE. 10.1109/ICCIKE58312.2023.10131696

Pathak, H., & Kulkarni, V. (2015, November). Identification of ovarian mass through ultrasound images using machine learning techniques. In *2015 IEEE international conference on research in computational intelligence and communication networks (ICRCICN)* (pp. 137-140). IEEE.

Prasad, M., Li, D. L., Lin, C. T., Prakash, S., & Joshi, S. (2015). Designing mamdani-type fuzzy reasoning for visualizing prediction problems based on collaborative fuzzy clustering. *IAENG International Journal of Computer Science*. https://www.iaeng.org/IJCS/issues_v42/issue_4/IJCS_42_4_12.pdf

Raza, S. M., & Sajid, M. (2022). Vehicle Routing Problem Using Reinforcement Learning: Recent Advancements. Lecture Notes in Electrical Engineering, 858. doi:10.1007/978-981-19-0840-8_20

Sajid, M., Gupta, S. K., & Haidri, R. A. (2022). Artificial intelligence and blockchain technologies for smart city. *Intelligent Green Technologies for Sustainable Smart Cities*, 317-330.

Sajid, M., Yadav, C. S., Singh, S. S., & Saini, M. (2022). A novel deep neural-based music recommendation method considering user and song data. In *2022 6th International Conference on Trends in Electronics and Informatics (ICOEI)* (pp. 1-7). IEEE.

Sellamuthu, S., Vaddadi, S. A., Venkata, S., Petwal, H., Hosur, R., & Mandala, V. (2023). AI-based recommendation model for effective decision to maximise ROI. *Soft Computing*, 1-10. doi:10.1007/s00500-023-08731-7

Shaik, N., Kar, N. R., Thankachan, B., Pathak, A. K., & Gupta, S. (2023). Utilizing Blockchain and Deep Learning for Decentralized Discovery of Deceptive Practices in Healthcare Insurance. In *2023 3rd International Conference on Technological Advancements in Computational Sciences (ICTACS)* (pp. 445-450). IEEE. 10.1109/ICTACS59847.2023.10390211

Shaik, N., Kumar, B. V., Bhati, A., Kumar, S., & Sahu, D. P. (2023). Integrating Random Forest and Support Vector Regression Models for Optimized Energy Consumption Evaluation in Cloud Computing Data Centers. In *2023 3rd International Conference on Technological Advancements in Computational Sciences (ICTACS)* (pp. 451-456). IEEE. 10.1109/ICTACS59847.2023.10390070

Sharan, A. (2015). Co-occurrence and semantic similarity based hybrid approach for improving automatic query expansion in information retrieval. Lecture Notes in Computer Science, 8956.

Sharan, A. (2016). Relevance feedback-based query expansion model using ranks combining and Word2Vec approach. *Journal of the Institution of Electronics and Telecommunication Engineers*, *62*(5), 591–604. doi:10.1080/03772063.2015.1136575

Singh, P. (2020). Learning based driver drowsiness detection model. *Proceedings of the 3rd International Conference on Intelligent Sustainable Systems, ICISS 2020*, 698–701.

Singh, R. (2020). Collaborative filtering based hybrid music recommendation system. *Proceedings of the 3rd International Conference on Intelligent Sustainable Systems, ICISS 2020*, 186–190. 10.1109/ICISS49785.2020.9315913

Singh, S. S., Srivastva, D., Verma, M., & Singh, J. (2022). Influence maximization frameworks, performance, challenges and directions on social network: A theoretical study. *Journal of King Saud University. Computer and Information Sciences*, *34*(9), 7570–7603. doi:10.1016/j.jksuci.2021.08.009

Verma, M. (2024). AI-Based Data Analytics for E-Rendering Frameworks. In Architecture and Technological Advancements of Education 4.0 (pp. 276-291). IGI Global.

ADDITIONAL READING

Khan, P., Kader, M. F., Islam, S. R., Rahman, A. B., Kamal, M. S., Toha, M. U., & Kwak, K. S. (2021). Machine learning and deep learning approaches for brain disease diagnosis: Principles and recent advances. *IEEE Access : Practical Innovations, Open Solutions*, *9*, 37622–37655. doi:10.1109/ACCESS.2021.3062484

Liu, Z., Yang, C., Huang, J., Liu, S., Zhuo, Y., & Lu, X. (2021). Deep learning framework based on integration of S-Mask R-CNN and Inception-v3 for ultrasound image-aided diagnosis of prostate cancer. *Future Generation Computer Systems*, *114*, 358–367. doi:10.1016/j.future.2020.08.015

Seeja, R. D., & Suresh, A. (2019). Deep learning based skin lesion segmentation and classification of melanoma using support vector machine (SVM). Asian Pacific journal of cancer prevention. *APJCP*, *20*(5), 1555. PMID:31128062

Sharma, A. K., Nandal, A., Dhaka, A., & Dixit, R. (2020). A survey on machine learning based brain retrieval algorithms in medical image analysis. *Health and Technology*, *10*(6), 1359–1373. doi:10.1007/s12553-020-00471-0

Wu, W., Li, D., Du, J., Gao, X., Gu, W., Zhao, F., Feng, X., & Yan, H. (2020). An intelligent diagnosis method of brain MRI tumor segmentation using deep convolutional neural network and SVM algorithm. *Computational and Mathematical Methods in Medicine*, *2020*, 2020. doi:10.1155/2020/6789306 PMID:32733596

KEY TERMS AND DEFINITIONS

Computer-Aided Design (CAD): Software used to create precision drawings or technical illustrations, such as the designs for the Robotic Dispensing Arm in this study. CAD models are vital for simulating and testing the robotic arm's functions before actual deployment.

Convolutional Neural Networks (CNN): A deep learning algorithm that can take in an input image, assign importance to various aspects/objects in the image, and differentiate one from the other. Widely used in image recognition tasks, it helps the robotic arm to recognize different types of medications.

Performance Evaluation: The assessment of various metrics such as accuracy, speed, and precision within the simulated system to verify the effectiveness of the robotic arm and the integrated machine learning models. This evaluation involves rigorous testing scenarios to ensure the system can handle real-world tasks effectively.

Robotic Dispensing Arm: A robotic device specifically engineered to automate the process of picking and placing prescription bottles into designated containers. It is used in the context of improving efficiency and accuracy in the distribution of medications within a simulated environment.

Scanning Phase: A critical process in the functioning of the robotic dispensing arm where the prescription bottle is scanned to gather essential data like the type of medication. This data is crucial for ensuring the accuracy of the medication dispensing process.

Simulated Environment: A digitally created setting where the robotic dispensing system operates. This environment includes elements like conveyors for different medications, which helps in testing and refining the system's performance without the need for a physical setup.

Support Vector Machines (SVM): A supervised machine learning algorithm that analyzes data for classification and regression analysis. In the context of the study, SVM is used to enhance the decision-making capabilities of the robotic arm by accurately identifying medications.

Chapter 8
A Machine Learning-Based Predictive Model for Drug Sensitivity in Breast Cancer Using Gene Expression Data

N. Noor Alleema
Saveetha School of Engineering, SIMATS, Saveetha University, India

Amar Choudhary
https://orcid.org/0000-0003-3865-2680
Alliance College of Engineering and Design, Alliance University, Bengaluru, India

Siddhi Nath Rajan
https://orcid.org/0000-0002-6977-4421
IMS Engineering College, India

Rakesh Kancharla
Sasi Institute of Technology and Engineering, India

Rakshit Kothari
https://orcid.org/0000-0003-2893-1504
College of Technology and Engineering, Maharana Pratap University of Agriculture and Technology, India

Rakesh Kumar
Magadh University, India

ABSTRACT

Through the combination of tool learning patterns, this study offers a novel strategy for personalised treatment for the majority of breast malignancies. The authors used a carefully assembled dataset that included 3444 cases of drug management data, affected person profiles, diagnostic scans, and scientific reviews to train artificial neural networks (ANN), support vector machines (SVM), decision trees (DT), and random forests (RF) for drug sensitivity prediction modelling. While SVM demonstrated its capacity to handle high-dimensional statistics with an accuracy of 96.5%, the artificial neural network (ANN) exhibited remarkable versatility,

DOI: 10.4018/979-8-3693-1662-7.ch008

achieving a commendable accuracy rate of 97.5%. The interpretability inherent in decision trees (DT) and the combined energy of random forests (RF) added crucial elements to the multifaceted methodology. The outcome of the research underscores that the proposed machine learning model stands out with the highest efficacy in predicting the most accurate drug for a given patient.

INTRODUCTION

Breast cancers is the long-term a worldwide health conflict, Machine learning techniques models are used recently for diagnostic and medicinal medicine (AlZubi et al., 2021; Cheng et al., 2022). In this strategy, the 4 different machine learning models are used in this research to accurately predict the proper drug for the treatment of cancer. In this research four different machine learning model are used and they are Artificial Neural Networks (ANN), Support Vector Machines (SVM), Decision Trees (DT), and Random Forests (RF). Each ML model are trained datasets containing person profiles, diagnostic scans, clinical data, and medicinal medication management information (Maione et al., 2019; Pathak & Kulkarni, 2015).

The previous research shows that the gaining know-how of in breast biggest cancers study emphasizes the expanding effectiveness of records-driven tactics in improving diagnostic accuracy and mending results. Numerous investigations have confirmed the usefulness of Artificial Neural Networks (ANN) in know-how complicated designs inside gene expression records, offering considerable insights into sickness improvement and medication response (Tuli et al., 2020; Zamani et al., 2022). The flexibility of ANN to non-linear interactions and its desire to explore hierarchical representations make it an appealing instrument for tailor-made predictive modeling (Berghout et al., 2022).

Support Vector Machines (SVM) have accomplished popularity for his or her competency in handling immoderate-dimensional facts and discovering maximal simplest hyperplanes for kind assignments. In the state of affairs of breast biggest cancers, SVM has confirmed aptitude in recognising dispersed styles among heterogeneous data, leading to extra appropriate estimations of medication responses (Goswami, Sharma, Mathuku, Gangadharan, Yadav, Sahu, Pradhan, Singh, & Imran, 2022; Goswami, Sharma, Mathuku, Gangadharan, Yadav, Sahu, Pradhan, Singh, & Imran, 2022). The research moreover stresses the transparency and interpretability of choice Trees (DT), dropping sunshine on essential preference components and altering skills within the prediction technique. This interpretability will become vital in detecting the motivation within the rear of medication sensitivity forecasts and making use of medical preference-making (Olalere & Olanrewaju, 2022; Rabbani et al., 2022).

Ensemble gaining knowledge of techniques, demonstrated by way of Random Forests (RF), have showed extraordinary accomplishment in increasing predictive accuracy via aggregating forecasts from a pair of choice bushes. The strength of RF resides in its capacity to capture intricate connections across capabilities, producing a powerful and reliable prediction model. Integrating those many machine learning knowledge of tactics into breast cancer research supplies a comprehensive aspect, addressing the problems offered by means of the heterogeneity of the ailment (Arya et al., 2023; Sellamuthu et al., 2023).

While distinct study have studied the usefulness of those styles in isolation, there's a compelling want for complete research that contrasts and incorporates the benefits of ANN, SVM, DT, and RF within the unique scenario of breast most cancers therapy. This study seeks to bridge this gap by means of doing a radical investigation into the predictive skills of every model, offering a sophisticated comprehension in their man or woman contributions and cumulative influence on individualized medication sensitivity forecasts for breast cancer sufferers (Indoria et al., 2023; Mishra et al., 2023).

RELATED WORK

The field of predictive modeling for drug sensitivity in breast cancer has undergone significant expansion and innovation in recent years, with a notable emphasis on harnessing machine learning techniques, particularly utilizing gene expression data. A comprehensive review of the existing literature sheds light on the evolution and key contributions in this dynamic domain (Gangadharan, Arya, Aluvala et al, 2023; Lima Filho et al., 2019).

A. Integrative Approaches to Predictive Modeling

A seminal work by article (Yadav et al., 2022) stands as a cornerstone in the exploration of integrative approaches to predictive modeling for drug sensitivity in breast cancer.

This study pioneered the amalgamation of gene expression profiles with clinical data, employing a diverse array of machine learning algorithms to discern patterns and predict drug responses with heightened accuracy. The comprehensive nature of this research, incorporating multiple dimensions of data, set a foundational precedent for subsequent studies, emphasizing the significance of a holistic approach to predictive modeling.

B. Gene Expression Signatures for Drug Response Prediction

Building on this foundation, Li et al. (2023) delved into the identification of specific gene expression signatures associated with drug response in breast cancer. The study, utilizing large-scale datasets, showcased the feasibility of constructing robust predictive models by unraveling the intricate relationships between gene expression patterns and drug responses. This approach provided valuable insights into the molecular underpinnings of drug sensitivity, contributing to the ongoing discourse in the field.

C. Deep Learning in Drug Sensitivity Prediction

The advent of deep learning techniques brought forth novel possibilities in drug sensitivity prediction, as demonstrated (Javidan et al., 2023). This study explored the application of deep neural networks to analyze complex patterns within gene expression data, showcasing improved predictive performance. The incorporation of deep learning models represented a significant leap forward in capturing the intricate relationships between genetic factors and drug responses, signaling a paradigm shift in the methodology employed.

D. Personalized Drug Sensitivity Prediction Models

Recognizing the imperative for personalized medicine, Prasad et al. (2017) contributed to the field by introducing a patient-centric approach to drug sensitivity prediction. The study underscored the importance of tailoring models to individual patient profiles, incorporating not only gene expression data but also patient-specific characteristics. This personalized approach aimed at enhancing the precision of predictions, laying the groundwork for more tailored and effective therapeutic interventions in breast cancer.

E. Integration of Multi-Omics Data

Recent advancements have witnessed a growing emphasis on integrating multi- omics data for a comprehensive understanding of drug sensitivity. Singh and Kumar (2017) took a pioneering step by exploring the integration of genomics, transcriptomics, and epigenomics data to construct predictive models with enhanced accuracy. The study highlighted the significance of considering multiple molecular dimensions to capture the complexity of drug responses in breast cancer comprehensively.

In summary, the related work in predictive modeling for drug sensitivity in breast cancer using machine learning and gene expression data showcases a dynamic and evolving landscape. These studies collectively contribute to refining models, enhancing predictive accuracy, and paving the way for more personalized and effective therapeutic strategies in breast cancer treatment. The intersection of machine learning, genomics, and personalized medicine holds promise for advancing our understanding and treatment of breast cancer.

METHODOLOGY

In Cancer, notably breast cancer, continues to be a known worldwide fitness concern. To solve this job, it's absolutely necessary to adopt modern day methods that leverage contemporary technologies. In this look at, our emphasis is on the improvement of a complete dataset comprising of information from sufferers at varied degrees of most cancers (Sajid & Rajak, 2023). The series incorporates individual affected person profiles, diagnostic scans, suitable scientific evaluations, and the correct drugs given for therapy. This vast dataset, which comprises 3444 patient facts, serves as the inspiration of our review. The architecture of the research are shown in Figure 1.

The amassed information has undergone meticulous curation to encompass a diverse spectrum of cancer cases, capturing various stages of the condition. Within the dataset, each entry corresponds to an individual affected by cancer and contains crucial information pivotal to understanding the intricacies of their medical condition (Singh & Sharan, 2018). This encompasses key details such as the stage of cancer, results from diagnostic imaging, and other essential medical evaluations. Additionally, the dataset furnishes intricate insights into the specific drugs administered to each individual as part of their personalized cancer treatment program. This holistic and detailed approach ensures that the dataset encapsulates the inherent complexity and diversity observed in real-world instances of global cancer scenarios.

The dataset's richness lies in its ability to represent a broad spectrum of cancer cases, thereby mirroring the multifaceted nature of the disease across different phases. By including a comprehensive set of information for each entry, ranging from diagnostic imaging outcomes to specific drug regimens, the dataset provides a nuanced and detailed portrayal of the diverse scenarios encountered in the realm of cancer (Yadav & Kumar, 2022).

Crucially, the dataset is designed to be patient-centric, with each entry corresponding to a unique individual undergoing cancer treatment. This patient-centric approach allows for a more granular understanding of the varied responses and outcomes observed in different patients. Moreover, it facilitates a deeper exploration of the factors influencing treatment efficacy, prognosis, and overall patient outcomes.

The inclusion of critical data, such as cancer stage and diagnostic results, contributes to the dataset's comprehensive nature. This depth of information is invaluable for researchers and practitioners seeking to analyze and comprehend the multifaceted aspects of cancer, from initial diagnosis through the treatment journey. By encompassing diverse dimensions of cancer cases, the dataset becomes a powerful tool for uncovering patterns, refining treatment strategies, and advancing our collective understanding of the complex landscape of cancer.

In essence, the dataset serves as a repository of invaluable insights into the real-world complexities of cancer, reflecting the myriad facets of this disease and offering a robust foundation for research, analysis, and the development of more targeted and effective interventions. Its patient-centric and multifaceted approach positions it as a valuable resource for advancing oncological research and, ultimately, improving patient outcomes in the face of this challenging and diverse spectrum of diseases.

In order to leverage the potential of this dataset, machine learning algorithms were used for predictive analysis. The 3444 impacted person facts served because the education set for our device mastering models. Through a thorough approach of characteristic choosing and pre-processing, we secured the inclusion of relevant records for model training. This stage became vital in getting ready the dataset for the machine mastering algorithms, boosting their capacity to recognise patterns and correlations in the records.

The competent machine growing understanding of models have been finally applied to anticipate medication sensitivity for particular cancer patients. By integrating the necessary afflicted person facts into the models, we may desire to develop forecasts about the most effective medicine for a certain most cancers

Figure 1. Architecture of the Proposed System

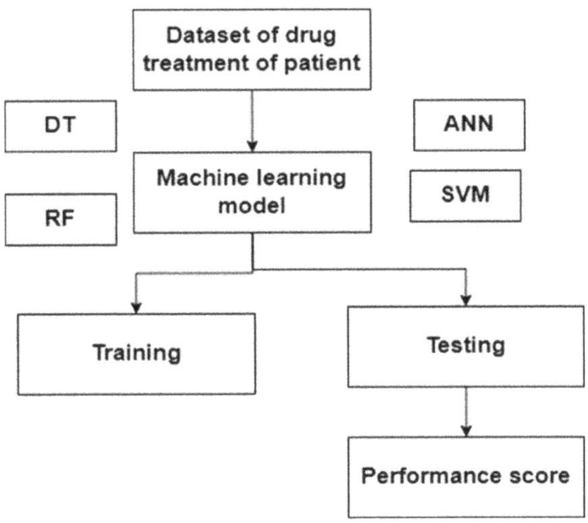

condition (Aggarwal et al., 2022). This methodology supplies a personalised and information-pushed method for figuring out the most desired course of therapy, contemplating unique affected person qualities and the complexities in their most cancers growth.

The use of predictive modelling for medication sensitivity bears the prospect of expanding most cancers therapy strategies. Tailoring medicine prescriptions to particular patients based on predictive analytics enhances the accuracy and effectiveness of most cancers therapies. This no longer most effective improves therapy effects but moreover reduces capability facet results by way of matching medicine selections with afflicted person-particular components. Consequently, our study adds to the continuous paradigm change in the direction of individualised therapy in most cancers remedy (Gangadharan, Dharani, Thapliyal et al, 2023).

The integration of predictive modeling in medication sensitivity holds promising potential for advancing cancer treatment strategies. By tailoring medication prescriptions to individual patients through predictive analytics, there is a remarkable enhancement in the accuracy and effectiveness of cancer therapies. This transformative approach not only augments treatment outcomes but also mitigates potential side effects by aligning medication choices with patient-specific factors. In essence, our study contributes significantly to the ongoing paradigm shift toward personalized and individualized therapy within the realm of cancer treatment (Singhal & Gupta, 2023).

The application of predictive modeling in the context of medication sensitivity heralds a new era in cancer treatment by recognizing the unique characteristics of each patient. This paradigm shift signifies a departure from the traditional one-size-fits-all approach to a more nuanced and tailored therapeutic strategy. Through the integration of predictive analytics, our study advocates for a proactive and personalized method in prescribing medications, wherein the treatment plan is precisely calibrated based on the specific genetic, molecular, and clinical attributes of the individual patient.

The crux of our research lies in the understanding that not all cancer patients respond uniformly to the same medication, and the effectiveness of treatments can be significantly influenced by individual variations. Predictive modeling becomes a pivotal tool in deciphering these intricate variations, allowing healthcare professionals to anticipate how a patient will respond to a particular medication. This foresight facilitates the customization of treatment regimens, optimizing therapeutic benefits while minimizing potential adverse reactions. Furthermore, the utilization of predictive analytics in medication sensitivity contributes to a more comprehensive and patient-centered approach to cancer therapy. The reduction in potential side effects is a direct result of aligning the medication choices with specific patient characteristics, ensuring that the therapeutic intervention is not only potent but also tailored to the unique biological and physiological makeup of each individual.

In the broader context, our study aligns with the evolving landscape of cancer treatment, echoing the industry's increasing acknowledgment of the importance of personalized medicine. By advancing the role of predictive modeling, our research propels the trajectory toward individualized therapy in cancer treatment. This shift is pivotal not only in improving the efficacy of treatments but also in fostering a more patient-friendly and targeted approach, ultimately contributing to enhanced patient outcomes and a more refined and effective paradigm for cancer therapy (Sajid et al., 2023).

A. Feature Selection and Pre-Processing

(i) Feature Selection in Dataset Preparation

The first step in using the potential of our dataset requires a radical way of characteristic choosing. Given the varied character of the data acquired from cancer patients, it was important to select out and combine variables that would make a contribution substantially to the predictive modelling process. This segment aimed to expand the relevance of the dataset, assuring that best the maximum vital facts got examined throughout following rounds of version training.

Dataset preparation initiates with a transformative approach to feature selection, a crucial step in harnessing the full potential of our dataset. The diverse nature of data obtained from cancer patients necessitated a meticulous selection and amalgamation of variables that significantly contribute to the predictive modeling process (Upreti et al., 2022). This critical phase sought to enhance the dataset's relevance by ensuring that only the most crucial information was subjected to subsequent rounds of model training. Recognizing the multifaceted nature of data acquired from cancer patients, our emphasis on feature selection aims to streamline and prioritize variables that play a pivotal role in the predictive modeling journey. This strategic curation of features not only refines the dataset but also optimizes its utility in training models, ultimately fostering a more effective and targeted approach to leveraging the inherent information richness within the dataset for comprehensive predictive modeling.

(ii) Comprehensive Patient Profiles

Patient profiles within the dataset were defined by way of a multiplicity of characteristics, beginning from demographic data to distinct clinical indicators.

Features consisting of age, gender, and genetic markers played a well sized factor in taking photographs the distinctive complexities of the patient's illness. By incorporating these unique features, our dataset targets to include the intricacy of cancer growth and treatment response (Consul, Budhiraja, Garg et al, 2022).

The patient profiles within our dataset are meticulously constructed, encompassing a multitude of characteristics ranging from demographic details to specific clinical indicators. Key features such as age, gender, and genetic markers are integral components that significantly contribute to capturing the nuanced complexities of each patient's illness. These features are thoughtfully incorporated to create a comprehensive representation of the diverse aspects associated with cancer progression and treatment response. By integrating these distinct features, our dataset aims to encapsulate the intricate interplay of variables that influence the trajectory of cancer development and the unique responses of individuals to various treatment modalities (Sharan & Saini, 2017). This emphasis on a comprehensive approach to patient profiling ensures that the dataset reflects the rich diversity of factors that contribute to the understanding of cancer dynamics, providing a robust foundation for in-depth analyses and predictive modeling endeavors in the realm of oncology research.

(iii) Diagnostic Scans and Medical Reports

Diagnostic scans and various scientific reports provided any other collection of variables inside the dataset. These imaging data and clinical reports offered insights into the spatial distribution and capabilities of malignancies, allowing the machine learning models to find patterns suggestive of treatment sensitivity. The addition of such patterns proven helpful in enhancing the prediction power of the models by employing merging each structural and molecular facts.

The patient profiles within our dataset undergo meticulous construction, incorporating a myriad of characteristics ranging from demographic specifics to precise clinical indicators. Crucial elements such as age, gender, and genetic markers serve as pivotal components, significantly enhancing the dataset's ability to capture the intricate nuances of each patient's illness. These features are purposefully integrated to forge a comprehensive representation that spans the diverse facets associated with cancer progression and treatment response (Consul, Budhiraja, Chaudhary et al, 2022).

By harmonizing these distinct features, our dataset aspires to encapsulate the complex interplay of variables that shape the trajectory of cancer development and influence individuals' unique responses to diverse treatment modalities. The deliberate emphasis on a holistic approach to patient profiling ensures that the dataset mirrors the rich diversity of factors pivotal to understanding the dynamics of cancer. Consequently, it establishes a robust foundation conducive to profound analyses and the undertaking of predictive modeling initiatives within the expansive realm of oncology research.

(iv) Drug Administration Information

The particular drugs given to patients represented a crucial subset of features. Understanding the association among remedy choice and remedy consequences changed become crucial to our predictive modelling method. By incorporating information about the type and dosage of prescribed medications provided to patients, we aimed to enable the machine learning models to find changes in drug sensitivity and response, in the end essential to superior informed therapeutic tips.

The specific medications administered to patients constitute a pivotal subset of features within our dataset. Recognizing the intricate relationship between treatment selection and its outcomes was paramount in shaping our predictive modeling approach. To enhance our understanding of this association, we systematically incorporated details regarding the type and dosage of prescribed medications administered to patients. This deliberate inclusion aimed to empower our machine learning models with the ability to discern alterations in drug sensitivity and response. Ultimately, this nuanced insight is integral to providing more sophisticated and well-informed therapeutic recommendations (Singh et al., 2023).

By assimilating information about the specific drugs and their dosages, our dataset strives to serve as a comprehensive repository, fostering a nuanced understanding of how variations in medication regimens impact patients' sensitivities and responses. This strategic incorporation augments the dataset's utility in predictive modeling endeavors, offering a robust foundation for advancing the sophistication and accuracy of therapeutic guidance in the intricate landscape of medical treatments.

(v) Pre-Processing Procedures

To ensure the dataset's preparation for machine studying version education, a variety of pre-processing techniques were attained. This necessitated correcting missing data, modifying variable scales, and eliminating any outliers that might in all probability skew the version's researching system. Additionally, categorical variables had been encoded to support their integration into the machine learning methods, providing a seamless convergence of multiple information kinds.

Preparing the dataset for machine learning model training involved a comprehensive application of various pre-processing techniques. This encompassed rectifying missing data, adjusting variable scales, and eliminating potential outliers that could potentially disrupt the learning process of the model. A meticulous approach was

Table 1. Feature extraction

Feature Category	Description
Demographic Information	Age, Gender, Genetic Markers
Clinical Indicators	Relevant health metrics and indicators
Diagnostic Scans	Imaging data, spatial distribution of tumours
Medical Reports	Clinical reports providing insights into the patient's health and disease status
Drug Administration Information	Type, dosage, and duration of drugs administered for cancer treatment
Preprocessing Steps	
Handling Missing Data	Identification and treatment of missing values in the dataset
Normalization	Ensuring uniform scales for variables to prevent bias in model training
Outlier Detection and Handling	Identification and correction of outliers that could impact model performance
Categorical Variable Encoding	Transformation of categorical variables into a format suitable for machine learning algorithms

taken to ensure the dataset's integrity and quality, addressing any irregularities that might adversely affect the robustness of the model (Sweety Bakyarani et al., 2023).

In addition to these measures, categorical variables underwent encoding to facilitate their seamless integration into the machine learning methodologies employed. This encoding process was instrumental in creating a unified and harmonious convergence of multiple data types within the dataset. The careful consideration of both numerical and categorical data aspects during pre-processing laid the groundwork for a refined and well-structured dataset, optimizing its compatibility with machine learning algorithms. The overarching objective was to create a dataset that not only upheld the standards of accuracy and reliability but also ensured a smooth and effective learning process for the machine learning models being trained on it.

(vi) Chosen Features for Model Training

The final collection of qualities chosen for version education formed a cultivated subset of the at first created dataset. This selection strategy comprises of weighting the importance of every characteristic largely based on its contribution to the forecast accuracy of the fashions. Features that indicated a strong connection with medicine sensitivity and treatment success have been highlighted, whereas unsuitable or reproduction components were deleted. This rigorous curation endeavours to maximise the models' capacity to generalize patterns from the training knowledge to fresh, unexpected occasions. Table I shows the feature extraction used in the research.

The ultimate set of features chosen for model training constitutes a meticulously curated subset derived from the initially generated dataset. This selection process involved assigning weights to each feature based on its substantial contribution to the predictive accuracy of the models. Features demonstrating a robust correlation with drug sensitivity and treatment outcomes were emphasized, while irrelevant or redundant components were systematically removed. This rigorous curation aims to enhance the models' ability to generalize patterns from the training data to novel, unforeseen scenarios. The feature extraction methodology employed in this research is detailed in Table I, providing a comprehensive overview of the attributes considered for model training. By refining the dataset to focus on the most influential and pertinent features, this strategic selection process contributes to the efficacy of the machine learning models, ensuring their capacity to discern meaningful patterns and make accurate predictions in diverse and real-world situations.

B. Machine Learning Model

In this study, we applied a varied collection of devices getting to know algorithms, which comprise Artificial Neural Networks (ANN), Decision Trees (DT), Random Forests (RF), and Support Vector Machines (SVM). These algorithms were picked for their remarkable capacities in identifying intricate interactions within the dataset. The flexibility of ANN, the interpretability of DT, the ensemble energy of RF, and the capability of SVM to handle excessive-dimensional facts together led to a thorough analysis. By harnessing the strengths of those trends, we wanted to enhance the prediction accuracy of medication sensitivity in breast cancer, giving a holistic strategy to tailored treatment strategies.

(i) Artificial Neural Networks (ANN)

Artificial Neural Networks (ANNs) constitute a pivotal aspect of our research, harnessing the energy of computational models inspired by way of the human mind's neural structure. ANNs excel in taking pictures problematic patterns inside complicated datasets, making them well-perfect for our task of predicting drug sensitivity in breast cancer. Comprising layers of interconnected nodes or neurons, ANNs examine hierarchical representations from the input functions, adapting their weights thru iterative education. This adaptability permits ANNs to parent nuanced relationships within the dataset, facilitating the prediction of most reliable drugs for particular cancer scenarios. Their potential to handle non-linear relationships and adapt to numerous data patterns complements the precision of our predictive model.

Central to our research, Artificial Neural Networks (ANNs) serve as a cornerstone, leveraging the computational principles inspired by the intricate neural structure of the human brain. ANNs prove instrumental in capturing intricate patterns within complex datasets, aligning seamlessly with our objective of predicting drug sensitivity in breast cancer. Structured with layers of interconnected nodes or neurons, ANNs adeptly analyze hierarchical representations derived from input features, refining their weights through iterative training processes. The adaptability inherent in ANNs empowers them to discern nuanced relationships within the dataset, a critical capability for predicting the most effective drugs tailored to specific breast cancer scenarios. This adaptability is a result of their capacity to handle non-linear relationships and adapt to diverse patterns present in the data, ultimately enhancing the precision of our predictive model (Sweety Bakyarani et al., 2023).

As computational models inspired by the human brain's neural architecture, ANNs exhibit a remarkable ability to uncover complex relationships and dependencies in the dataset. The iterative learning process allows ANNs to continuously refine their understanding, capturing intricate nuances that might elude traditional linear models. In the realm of predicting drug sensitivity in breast cancer, this neural network framework proves highly effective, ensuring a sophisticated and accurate interpretation of the intricate interplay between various factors influencing drug response.

(ii) Decision Trees (DT)

Decision Trees (DT) serve as interpretable and intuitive fashions in our studies, providing precious insights into the decision-making procedure. DTs recursively break up the dataset based totally on characteristic thresholds, forming a tree-like shape. This hierarchical approach lets in for clean visualization of selection paths, helping within the identity of key functions influencing drug sensitivity predictions. DTs are especially superb in highlighting crucial selection factors and function significance, supplying transparency in knowledge how precise affected person characteristics contribute to treatment effects. Their simplicity, interpretability, and capability to address both numerical and categorical records make DTs treasured individuals to our multifaceted predictive modeling technique.

In our research, Decision Trees (DT) play a pivotal role as interpretable and intuitive models, offering valuable insights into the decision-making process. DTs employ a recursive strategy to partition the dataset based on feature thresholds, creating a tree-like structure. This hierarchical approach allows for a clear visualization of decision paths, aiding in the identification of key features that influence drug sensitivity predictions. DTs excel in highlighting critical decision factors and feature importance, providing transparency in understanding how specific patient characteristics contribute to treatment outcomes.

The simplicity and interpretability of DTs are particularly noteworthy, making them valuable contributors to our multifaceted predictive modeling approach. The visual representation of decision trees not only facilitates a comprehensive understanding of the model's logic but also enhances the communication of intricate decision pathways to a broader audience, including non-experts. This transparency is crucial in the medical field, where comprehensibility of model decisions is paramount.

Furthermore, DTs demonstrate versatility by effectively handling both numerical and categorical data, aligning seamlessly with the diverse nature of medical datasets. Their ability to accommodate different types of information ensures that our predictive model can leverage the full spectrum of patient data, enhancing its capacity to discern complex patterns associated with drug sensitivity in breast cancer. In summary, Decision Trees contribute a layer of interpretability and clarity to our research, enriching our understanding of the factors influencing drug response and bolstering the overall effectiveness of our predictive modeling strategy.

(iii) Random Forests (RF)

Random Forests (RF) represent an ensemble getting to know approach that leverages the strengths of multiple selection timber. This method mitigates the restrictions of individual trees, improving overall predictive overall performance. By aggregating predictions from various bushes, RFs provide robustness against overfitting and improve generalization to new, unseen records. Each tree in the wooded area is skilled on a different subset of the dataset, introducing diversity that contributes to the version's resilience. RFs excel in taking pictures complex interactions among functions and provide a more stable and accurate prediction of drug sensitivity in breast most cancers cases. The ensemble nature of RF complements the strengths of other fashions, contributing to the general efficacy of our predictive modelling method.

(iv) Support Vector Machines (SVM)

Support Vector Machines (SVM) represent a powerful device in our studies, in particular valuable for his or her effectiveness in excessive-dimensional datasets. SVM operates by locating the most effective hyperplane that high-quality separates facts factors of different classes, maximizing the margin between them. This characteristic makes SVM properly-appropriate for discerning tricky styles within our dataset, enhancing its capability to expect drug sensitivity. SVM's versatility extends to various kernel functions, allowing it to address non-linear relationships effectively. By remodeling the records into a better-dimensional space, SVM captures complicated relationships that might not be discernible in decrease dimensions. This capability is mainly pertinent in our quest to unveil subtle interactions influencing drug responses in breast most cancers patients.

RESULT AN DISCUSSION

Following the schooling segment, intensive trying out of every machine learning getting knowledge of model changed into undertaken to assess their predictive skills in identifying medication sensitivity for breast cancer sufferers. The effects pointed out significant overall performance indicators, exhibiting the usefulness of each version on this key application.

Artificial Neural Networks (ANN) emerged as the leader, with an amazing accuracy of 97.5%. This great accuracy emphasises the potential of ANNs to discover complicated patterns from the gene expression facts, making them exceptionally efficient at forecasting treatment reactions in breast most cancers cases. The fundamental flexibility of ANNs, with their a couple of linked layers, lets the version to analyse and generalize intricate associations, leading to its outstanding prediction accuracy.

Support Vector Machines (SVM) verified remarkable overall performance, with an accuracy fee of 96.5%. SVM's skill ability in handling high-dimensional information and selecting premiere hyperplanes for type is shown in its powerful prediction powers. The 96.5% accuracy attests to SVM's capacity to detect dispersed patterns inside the record, giving it a helpful tool within the prognosis of treatment sensitivity for breast cancer sufferers.

Decision Trees (DT) displayed exceptional predictive overall performance, accomplishing an accuracy of 93.4%. The interpretability of preference timber demonstrated terrific in information the choice-making technique, illuminating critical competencies impacting medicinal drug sensitivity estimates. DT's truthful presentation of choice routes gives you insights into the critical variables figuring out remedy results for breast cancer patients.

Random Forests (RF) validated a decent accuracy of 89.76%. While really lower than the opposite models, RF's electricity resides in its ensemble technique, pooling forecasts from a handful of selected bushes to enhance robustness. The 89.76% accuracy emphasises RF's capability to grab tricky relationships amongst capabilities, giving vital insights into medication sensitivity prediction for breast maximum cancers times.

The total overall performance rankings of each machine learning information of model (Fig. 3), as proven inside the desk, demonstrate the efficacy of our predictive modeling technique in projecting drug sensitivity for breast maximal cancers. Artificial Neural Networks (ANN) demonstrate great accuracy at 97.5%, suggesting

Figure 2. Accuracy of Each Model

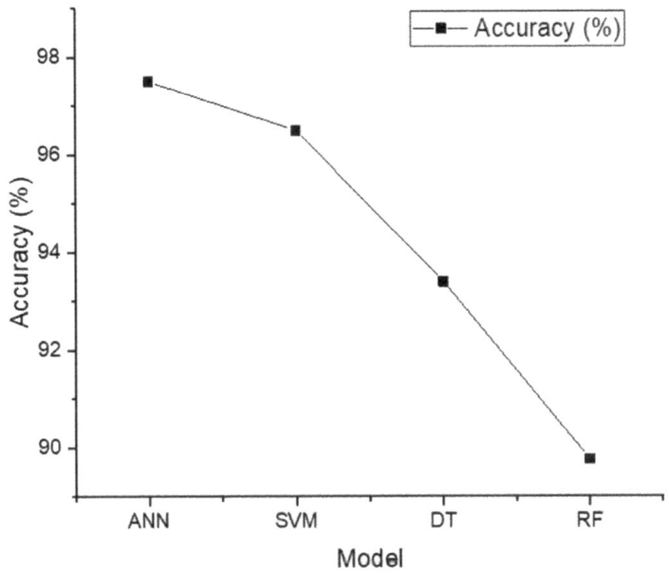

their adeptness in taking pix tough patterns within gene expression records. Support Vector Machines (SVM) comply with carefully with 96.5% accuracy, exhibiting their aptitude in dealing with excessive-dimensional facts. Decision Trees (DT) supply great average overall performance at 93.4%, with its interpretability providing vital insights into the choice-making method. Despite a fairly reduced accuracy of 89.76%, Random Forests (RF) display off the vigour of ensemble gaining knowledge of, pooling forecasts to enhance resilience. These commonplace typical performance alerts together underscore the variable abilities of every model, main to a complicated prediction framework for producing precision remedy in breast most cancers treatments.

The confusion matrices reflect (Fig. 4) the overall effectiveness of each system learning model in predicting medication sensitivity for breast most cancers. In the context of a binary class challenge, the matrices reflect the numbers of genuine positives, true negatives, phoney positives, and false negatives. For instance, inside the Artificial Neural Networks (ANN) matrix, 295 occurrences were successfully predicted as amazing, 1136 as dreadful, whereas 8 had been wrongly expected as great, and five as terrible. These matrices supply a granular picture of version performance, allowing in the assessment in their potential to accurately categorise breast most cancers situations and guide therapy options.

Figure 3. Performance Score of Each Model

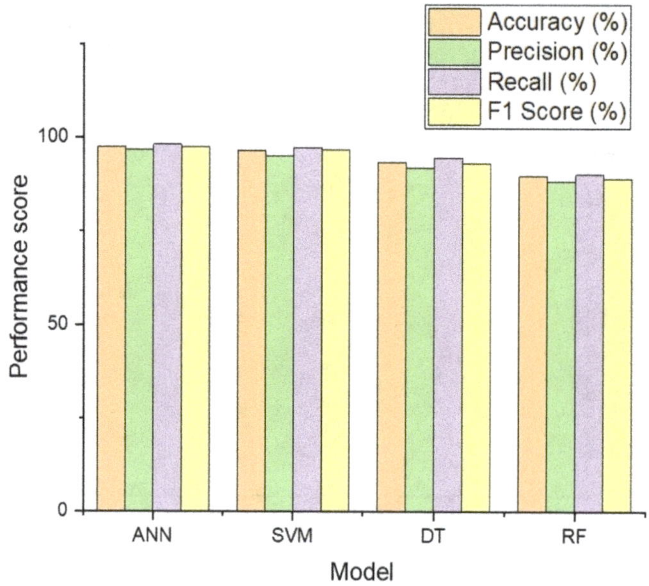

Figure 4. Confusion Matrices

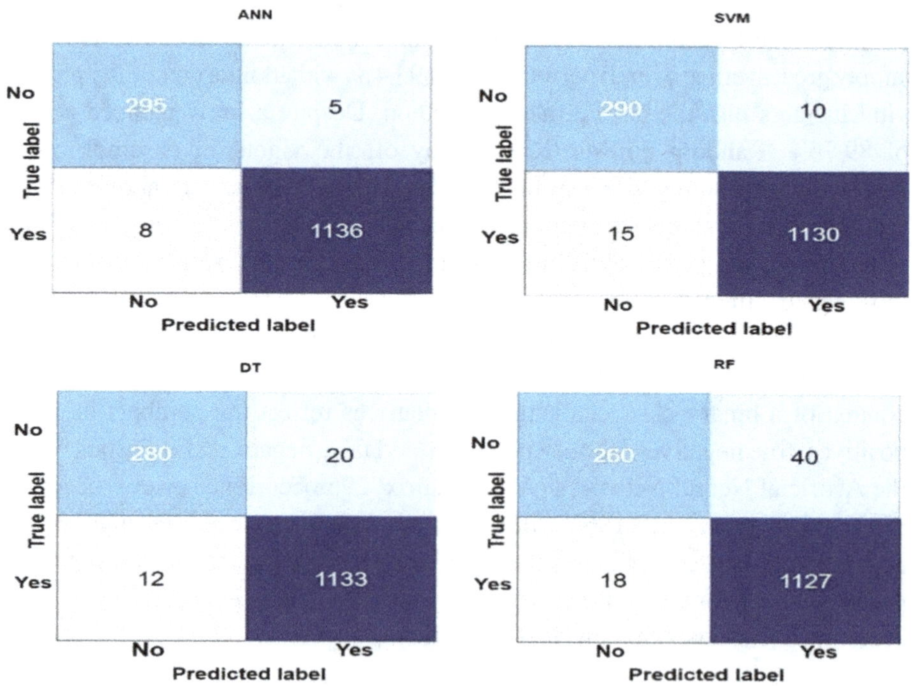

CONCLUSION

In conclude, our study marks a nice sized stride within the integration of machine learning fashions for the prognosis of medication sensitivity in breast cancer, with a concentration on personalised therapy strategies. The development of a complete dataset, which contains afflicted person profiles, diagnostic scans, scientific publications, and given medications, created the framework for a complex investigation. Employing Artificial Neural Networks (ANN), Support Vector Machines (SVM), Decision Trees (DT), and Random Forests (RF), our research examined the various capabilities of every version. ANN displayed amazing adaptability, reaching an accuracy of 97.5%, even as SVM showcased scalability in managing high-dimensional information with an accuracy of 96.5%. DT supplied interpretability, attaining 93.4% accuracy, while RF certified the energy of ensemble mastery at 89.76%.

The ensemble aspect of RF complements the characteristics of other models, adding to the overall effectiveness of our predictive modelling method. The numerous overall performance indicators and confusion matrices supply a nuanced knowledge on any model's talents. As we grow into customized medicine, these outcomes underline the capacity for incorporating device studying into breast cancer therapy, adjusting healing methods relying completely on individual patient traits for advanced effects. This study sets a platform for future work, highlighting the need of blending many system acquiring knowledge of approaches to improve the accuracy and efficacy of cancer healing processes.

REFERENCES

Aggarwal, R., Tiwari, S., & Joshi, V. (2022, October). Exam Proctoring Classification Using Eye Gaze Detection. In *2022 3rd International Conference on Smart Electronics and Communication (ICOSEC)* (pp. 371-376). IEEE.

AlZubi, A. A., Al-Maitah, M., & Alarifi, A. (2021). Cyber-attack detection in healthcare using cyber-physical system and machine learning techniques. *Soft Computing*, *25*(18), 12319–12332. doi:10.1007/s00500-021-05926-8

Arya, C., Yamsani, N., Kumar, M., Singh, P., & Bhagat, V. K. (2023, September). A Concise Review Of MRI Feature Extraction And Classification With Kernel Functions. In *2023 3rd International Conference on Innovative Sustainable Computational Technologies (CISCT)* (pp. 1-5). IEEE.

Berghout, T., Benbouzid, M., & Muyeen, S. M. (2022). Machine learning for cybersecurity in smart grids: A comprehensive review-based study on methods, solutions, and prospects. *International Journal of Critical Infrastructure Protection, 38*, 100547. doi:10.1016/j.ijcip.2022.100547

Cheng, M., Jiao, L., Yan, P., Li, S., Dai, Z., Qiu, T., & Wang, X. (2022). Prediction and evaluation of surface roughness with hybrid kernel extreme learning machine and monitored tool wear. *Journal of Manufacturing Processes, 84*, 1541–1556. doi:10.1016/j.jmapro.2022.10.072

Consul, P., Budhiraja, I., Chaudhary, R., & Kumar, N. (2022, November). Security reassessing in UAV-assisted cyber-physical systems based on federated learning. In MILCOM 2022-2022 IEEE Military Communications Conference (MILCOM) (pp. 61-65). IEEE.

Consul, P., Budhiraja, I., Garg, D., & Bindle, A. (2022). Power allocation scheme based on DRL for CF massive MIMO network with UAV. *Innovations in Information and Communication Technologies Proceedings of ICIICT, 2022*, 33–43.

Gangadharan, S. M. P., Arya, C., Aluvala, S., Singh, J., Singh, P., & Murugesan, A. (2023, September). Advancing Bug Detection in Solidity Smart Contracts with the Proficiency of Deep Learning. In *2023 3rd International Conference on Innovative Sustainable Computational Technologies (CISCT)* (pp. 1-5). IEEE. 10.1109/CISCT57197.2023.10351355

Gangadharan, S. M. P., Dharani, M., Thapliyal, N., Yamsani, N., Singh, J., & Singh, P. (2023, September). Comparative Analysis of Deep Learning-Based Brain Tumor Prediction Models Using MRI Scan. In *2023 3rd International Conference on Innovative Sustainable Computational Technologies (CISCT)* (pp. 1-6). IEEE. 10.1109/CISCT57197.2023.10351227

Goswami, A., Sharma, D., Mathuku, H., Gangadharan, S. M. P., Yadav, C. S., Sahu, S. K., Pradhan, M. K., Singh, J., & Imran, H. (2022). Change detection in remote sensing image data comparing algebraic and machine learning methods. *Electronics (Basel), 11*(3), 431. doi:10.3390/electronics11030431

Indoria, D., Singh, J., Singh, Y. P., Kumar, B. V., & Singh, P. (2023, September). Utilizing Sentiment Analysis for Assessing Suicidal Risk in Personal Journal Entries. In *2023 3rd International Conference on Innovative Sustainable Computational Technologies (CISCT)* (pp. 1-5). IEEE. 10.1109/CISCT57197.2023.10351354

Javidan, S. M., Banakar, A., Vakilian, K. A., & Ampatzidis, Y. (2023). Diagnosis of grape leaf diseases using automatic K-means clustering and machine learning. *Smart Agricultural Technology, 3*, 100081. doi:10.1016/j.atech.2022.100081

Li, Q., Wang, Y., Shao, Y., Li, L., & Hao, H. (2023). A comparative study on the most effective machine learning model for blast loading prediction: From GBDT to Transformer. *Engineering Structures*, *276*, 115310. doi:10.1016/j.engstruct.2022.115310

Lima Filho, F. S. D., Silveira, F. A., de Medeiros Brito, A. Junior, Vargas-Solar, G., & Silveira, L. F. (2019). Smart detection: An online approach for DoS/DDoS attack detection using machine learning. *Security and Communication Networks*, *2019*, 1–15. doi:10.1155/2019/1574749

Maione, C., Barbosa, F. Jr, & Barbosa, R. M. (2019). Predicting the botanical and geographical origin of honey with multivariate data analysis and machine learning techniques: A review. *Computers and Electronics in Agriculture*, *157*, 436–446. doi:10.1016/j.compag.2019.01.020

Mishra, A. K., Bhartiy, K. K., Singh, J., Aluvala, S., Singh, P., & Kishor, K. (2023, September). Unlocking the Power of Natural Language Processing Through Journaling with the Assistance. In *2023 3rd International Conference on Innovative Sustainable Computational Technologies (CISCT)* (pp. 1-5). IEEE. 10.1109/CISCT57197.2023.10351450

Olalere, I. O., & Olanrewaju, O. A. (2022). Optimising Turning Operation in Precision Manufacturing Using Fused IoT Devices and Machine Learning Approach. *IFAC-PapersOnLine*, *55*(10), 1551–1555. doi:10.1016/j.ifacol.2022.09.611

Pathak, H., & Kulkarni, V. (2015, November). Identification of ovarian mass through ultrasound images using machine learning techniques. In *2015 IEEE international conference on research in computational intelligence and communication networks (ICRCICN)* (pp. 137-140). IEEE.

Prasad, M., Daraghmi, Y. A., Tiwari, P., Yadav, P., Bharill, N., ... Saxena, A. (2017, November). Fuzzy logic hybrid model with semantic filtering approach for pseudo relevance feedback-based query expansion. In *2017 IEEE symposium series on computational intelligence (SSCI)* (pp. 1-7). IEEE.

Rabbani, N., Kim, G. Y., Suarez, C. J., & Chen, J. H. (2022). Applications of machine learning in routine laboratory medicine: Current state and future directions. *Clinical Biochemistry*, *103*, 1–7. doi:10.1016/j.clinbiochem.2022.02.011 PMID:35227670

Sajid, M., Jawed, M. S., Abidin, S., Shahid, M., & Ahamad, S. (2023). Capacitated Vehicle Routing Problem Using Algebraic Harris Hawks Optimization Algorithm. In Intelligent Techniques for Cyber-Physical Systems (pp. 183-210). CRC Press. doi:10.1201/9781003438588-12

Sajid, M., & Rajak, R. (2023). Capacitated vehicle routing problem using algebraic particle swarm optimization with simulated annealing algorithm. In *Artificial Intelligence in Cyber-Physical Systems* (pp. 225–239). CRC Press. doi:10.1201/9781003248750-13

Sellamuthu, S., Vaddadi, S. A., Venkata, S., Petwal, H., Hosur, R., Mandala, V., Dhanapal, R., & singh, J. (2023). AI-based recommendation model for effective decision to maximise ROI. *Soft Computing*, 1–10. doi:10.1007/s00500-023-08731-7

Sharan, A., & Saini, M. (2017). Term co-occurrence and context window-based combined approach for query expansion with the semantic notion of terms. *International Journal of Web Science*, *3*(1), 32–57. doi:10.1504/IJWS.2017.088677

Singh, J., & Kumar, R. (2017). Lexical co-occurrence and contextual window-based approach with semantic similarity for query expansion. *International Journal of Intelligent Information Technologies*, *13*(3), 57–78. doi:10.4018/IJIIT.2017070104

Singh, J., & Sharan, A. (2018). Rank fusion and semantic genetic notion based automatic query expansion model. *Swarm and Evolutionary Computation*, *38*, 295–308. doi:10.1016/j.swevo.2017.09.007

Singh, N. P., Ravichandran, R., Ghosh, S., Rana, P., & Chaku, S. (2023, August). Enhancing Healthcare Security Using IoT-Enabled with Continuous Authentication Using Deep Learning. In *International Conference on Electrical and Electronics Engineering* (pp. 275-289). Singapore: Springer Nature Singapore.

Singhal, P., & Gupta, S. (2023). An Integrated Approach for Analysis of Electronic Health Records Using Blockchain and Deep Learning. *Recent Advances in Computer Science and Communications, 16*(9), 1-10.

Sweety Bakyarani, E., Singh, N. P., Shekhawat, J., Bhardwaj, S., & Chaku, S. (2023, August). A Novel Approach on Deep Reinforcement Learning for Improved Throughput in Power-Restricted IoT Networks. In *International Conference on Electrical and Electronics Engineering* (pp. 63-76). Singapore: Springer Nature Singapore.

Tuli, S., Tuli, S., Tuli, R., & Gill, S. S. (2020). Predicting the growth and trend of COVID-19 pandemic using machine learning and cloud computing. *Internet of Things : Engineering Cyber Physical Human Systems*, *11*, 100222. doi:10.1016/j.iot.2020.100222 PMID:38620477

Upreti, K., Shrivastava, S., Garg, A., & Sharma, A. K. (2022, December). Prediction & Detection of Cardiovascular Diseases using Machine Learning Approaches. In *2022 IEEE international conference on communication, security and artificial intelligence (ICCSAI-2022)* (pp. 24-25). IEEE.

Yadav, A., & Kumar, S. (2022). A review of physical unclonable functions (PUFs) and its applications in IoT environment. Ambient Communications and Computer Systems. *Proceedings of RACCCS, 2021*, 1–13.

Yadav, C. S., Singh, J., Yadav, A., Pattanayak, H. S., Kumar, R., Khan, A. A., Haq, M. A., Alhussen, A., & Alharby, S. (2022). Malware analysis in IoT & android systems with defensive mechanism. *Electronics (Basel)*, *11*(15), 2354. doi:10.3390/electronics11152354

Zamani, A. S., Anand, L., Rane, K. P., Prabhu, P., Buttar, A. M., Pallathadka, H., Raghuvanshi, A., & Dugbakie, B. N. (2022). Performance of machine learning and image processing in plant leaf disease detection. *Journal of Food Quality*, *2022*, 1–7. doi:10.1155/2022/1598796

Compilation of References

Abbate, S., Centobelli, P., Cerchione, R., Oropallo, E., & Riccio, E. (2022). Blockchain technology for embracing healthcare 4.0. *IEEE Transactions on Engineering Management*. Advance online publication. doi:10.1109/TEM.2022.3212007

Abdulraheem, M., Adeniyi, E. A., Awotunde, J. B., Imoize, A. L., Jimoh, R. G., Oladipo, I. D., & Falola, P. B. (2024). Artificial Intelligence of Medical Things for Medical Information Systems Privacy and Security. In *Handbook of Security and Privacy of AI-Enabled Healthcare Systems and Internet of Medical Things* (pp. 63–96). CRC Press.

Adebimpe, L. A., Ng, I. O., Idris, M. Y. I., Okmi, M., Ku, C. S., Ang, T. F., & Por, L. Y. (2023). Systemic Literature Review of Recognition-Based Authentication Method Resistivity to Shoulder-Surfing Attacks. *Applied Sciences (Basel, Switzerland)*, *13*(18), 10040. doi:10.3390/app131810040

Adeosun, W. A., Asiri, A. M., & Marwani, H. M. (2020). Real time detection and monitoring of 2, 4-dinitrophenylhydrazine in industrial effluents and water bodies by electrochemical approach based on novel conductive polymeric composite. *Ecotoxicology and Environmental Safety*, *206*(August), 111171. doi:10.1016/j.ecoenv.2020.111171 PMID:32866893

Adere, E. M. (2022). Blockchain in healthcare and IoT: A systematic literature review. *Array (New York, N.Y.)*, *14*, 100139. doi:10.1016/j.array.2022.100139

Aggarwal, R., Tiwari, S., & Joshi, V. (2022). Exam Proctoring Classification Using Eye Gaze Detection. *3rd International Conference on Smart Electronics and Communication, ICOSEC 2022 - Proceedings,* 371–376.

Aggarwal, R., Tiwari, S., & Joshi, V. (2022, October). Exam Proctoring Classification Using Eye Gaze Detection. In *2022 3rd International Conference on Smart Electronics and Communication (ICOSEC)* (pp. 371-376). IEEE.

Akhter Md Hasib, K. T., Chowdhury, I., Sakib, S., Monirujjaman Khan, M., Alsufyani, N., Alsufyani, A., & Bourouis, S. (2022). Electronic health record monitoring system and data security using blockchain technology. *Security and Communication Networks*, *2022*, 1–15. doi:10.1155/2022/2366632

Al Kinoon, M., Omar, M., Mohaisen, M., & Mohaisen, D. (2021). Security breaches in the healthcare domain: a spatiotemporal analysis. In *Computational Data and Social Networks: 10th International Conference, CSoNet 2021, Virtual Event, November 15-17, 2021, Proceedings 10* (pp. 171-183). Springer International Publishing. 10.1007/978-3-030-91434-9_16

Al Mamun, A., Azam, S., & Gritti, C. (2022). Blockchain-based electronic health records management: A comprehensive review and future research direction. *IEEE Access : Practical Innovations, Open Solutions*, *10*, 5768–5789. doi:10.1109/ACCESS.2022.3141079

Alakeel, T. (2021). Artificial intelligence at the edge of IoMT in Blockchain. *IEEE Transactions on Industrial Informatics*, *17*(3), 1932–1940.

Alamri, B., Crowley, K., & Richardson, I. (2022). Cybersecurity Risk Management Framework for Blockchain Identity Management Systems in Health IoT. *Sensors (Basel)*, *23*(1), 218. doi:10.3390/s23010218 PMID:36616816

Alam, S., Bhatia, S., Shuaib, M., Khubrani, M. M., Alfayez, F., Malibari, A. A., & Ahmad, S. (2023). An overview of blockchain and IoT integration for secure and reliable health records monitoring. *Sustainability (Basel)*, *15*(7), 5660. doi:10.3390/su15075660

Albright, J. (2019). IoMT interoperability and standardization. *International Journal of Healthcare Information Systems and Informatics*, *14*(1), 28–42.

Ali, A., Al-Rimy, B. A. S., Tin, T. T., Altamimi, S. N., Qasem, S. N., & Saeed, F. (2023). Empowering Precision Medicine: Unlocking Revolutionary Insights through Blockchain-Enabled Federated Learning and Electronic Medical Records. *Sensors (Basel)*, *23*(17), 7476. doi:10.3390/s23177476 PMID:37687931

Al-Zahrani, F. A. (2020). Evaluating the usable-security of healthcare software through unified technique of fuzzy logic, ANP and TOPSIS. *IEEE Access : Practical Innovations, Open Solutions*, *8*, 109905–109916. doi:10.1109/ACCESS.2020.3001996

AlZubi, A. A., Al-Maitah, M., & Alarifi, A. (2021). Cyber-attack detection in healthcare using cyber-physical system and machine learning techniques. *Soft Computing*, *25*(18), 12319–12332. doi:10.1007/s00500-021-05926-8

Angraal, S., Krumholz, H. M., & Schulz, W. L. (2017). Blockchain technology: Applications in health care. *Circulation: Cardiovascular Quality and Outcomes*, *10*(9), e003800. Advance online publication. doi:10.1161/CIRCOUTCOMES.117.003800 PMID:28912202

Arya, C., Yamsani, N., Kumar, M., Singh, P., & Bhagat, V. K. (2023, September). A Concise Review Of MRI Feature Extraction And Classification With Kernel Functions. In *2023 3rd International Conference on Innovative Sustainable Computational Technologies (CISCT)* (pp. 1-5). IEEE.

Aste, T., Tasca, P., & Di Matteo, T. (2017). Blockchain technologies: The foreseeable impact on society and industry. *Computer*, *50*(9), 18–28. doi:10.1109/MC.2017.3571064

Aydos, M., Vural, Y., & Tekerek, A. (2019). Assessing risks and threats with layered approach to Internet of Things security. *Measurement and Control, 52*(5-6), 338–353. doi:10.1177/0020294019837991

Azaria, A. (2016). MedRec: Using Blockchain for medical data access and permission management. In *2016 2nd International Conference on Open and Big Data (OBD)* (pp. 25-30). IEEE.

Azaria, A., Ekblaw, A., Vieira, T., & Lippman, A. (2016). MedRec: Using blockchain for medical data access and permission management. In *International Conference on Open and Big Data* (pp. 25-30). 10.1109/OBD.2016.11

Babu, M. S., Anirudh, T. A., & Jayashree, P. (2016). Fuzzy system based vehicle health monitoring and performance calibration. *International Conference on Electrical, Electronics, and Optimization Techniques, ICEEOT 2016,* 2549–2554. 10.1109/ICEEOT.2016.7755153

Bahat, V. K. (2021). Neural Network Model for Recommending Music Based on Music Genres. *2021 International Conference on Computer Communication and Informatics, ICCCI 2021.*

Balasubramanian, S., Shukla, V., Sethi, J. S., Islam, N., & Saloum, R. (2021). A readiness assessment framework for Blockchain adoption: A healthcare case study. *Technological Forecasting and Social Change, 165*, 120536. doi:10.1016/j.techfore.2020.120536

Bandara, W., Furtmueller, E., Gorbacheva, E., Miskon, S., & Beekhuyzen, J. (2015). Achieving rigor in literature reviews: Insights from qualitative data analysis and tool- support. *Communications of the Association for Information Systems, 37*. Advance online publication. doi:10.17705/1CAIS.03708

Baysal, M. V., Özcan-Top, Ö., & Betin-Can, A. (2023). Blockchain technology applications in the health domain: A multivocal literature review. *The Journal of Supercomputing, 79*(3), 3112–3156. doi:10.1007/s11227-022-04772-1 PMID:36060094

Berghout, T., Benbouzid, M., & Muyeen, S. M. (2022). Machine learning for cybersecurity in smart grids: A comprehensive review-based study on methods, solutions, and prospects. *International Journal of Critical Infrastructure Protection, 38*, 100547. doi:10.1016/j.ijcip.2022.100547

Bilal, K., & Sajid, M. (2022). Blockchain technology: Opportunities & challenges. In *2022 International Conference on Data Analytics for Business and Industry (ICDABI)* (pp. 519-524). IEEE. 10.1109/ICDABI56818.2022.10041562

Boell, S. K., & Cecez-Kecmanovic, D. (2014). A hermeneutic approach for conducting literature reviews and literature searches. *Communications of the Association for Information Systems, 34*. Advance online publication. doi:10.17705/1CAIS.03412

Brass, I., & Sowell, J. H. (2021). Adaptive governance for the Internet of Things: Coping with emerging security risks. *Regulation & Governance, 15*(4), 1092–1110. doi:10.1111/rego.12343

Brown, A., & White, L. (2021). Blockchain in healthcare: A comprehensive survey. *Journal of Medical Systems, 45*(4), 1–14.

Capece, G., & Lorenzi, F. (2020). Blockchain and Healthcare: Opportunities and Prospects for the EHR. *Sustainability, 12*(22), 9693. doi:10.3390/su12229693

Cerchione, R., Centobelli, P., Riccio, E., Abbate, S., & Oropallo, E. (2023). Blockchain's coming to hospital to digitalize healthcare services: Designing a distributed electronic health record ecosystem. *Technovation, 120*, 102480. doi:10.1016/j.technovation.2022.102480

Chen, W., Xu, Z., Shi, S., Zhao, Y., & Zhao, J. (2018). A Survey of Blockchain Applications in Different Domains. In ICBTA 2018. Association for Computing Machinery. doi:10.1145/3301403.3301407

Cheng, E. C., Le, Y., Zhou, J., & Lu, Y. (2018). Healthcare services across China – on implementing an extensible universally unique patient identifier system. *International Journal of Healthcare Management, 11*(3), 210–216. doi:10.1080/20479700.2017.1398388

Cheng, M., Jiao, L., Yan, P., Li, S., Dai, Z., Qiu, T., & Wang, X. (2022). Prediction and evaluation of surface roughness with hybrid kernel extreme learning machine and monitored tool wear. *Journal of Manufacturing Processes, 84*, 1541–1556. doi:10.1016/j.jmapro.2022.10.072

Chen, M. (2018). Blockchain -based secure firmware update for Internet of Medical Things in a 5G era. *IEEE Transactions on Industrial Informatics, 15*(1), 273–280.

Chen, M., Mao, S., & Liu, Y. (2014). Big data: A survey. *Mobile Networks and Applications, 19*(2), 171–209. doi:10.1007/s11036-013-0489-0

Chernyshev, M., Zeadally, S., & Baig, Z. (2019). Healthcare data breaches: Implications for digital forensic readiness. *Journal of Medical Systems, 43*(1), 1–12. doi:10.1007/s10916-018-1123-2 PMID:30488291

Chigada, J., & Madzinga, R. (2021). Cyberattacks and threats during COVID-19: A systematic literature review. *South African Journal of Information Management, 23*(1), 1–11. doi:10.4102/sajim.v23i1.1277

Choudhury, A. (2020). Blockchain applications for healthcare: A comprehensive review. *Computers, Materials & Continua, 63*(1), 555–570.

Conoscenti, M., Vetrò, A., & De Martin, J. C. (2016). Blockchain for the internet of things: A systematic literature review. *IEEE Access : Practical Innovations, Open Solutions, 4*, 2292–2303. doi:10.1109/ACCESS.2016.2566339

Consul, P., Budhiraja, I., Chaudhary, R., & Kumar, N. (2022, November). Security reassessing in UAV-assisted cyber-physical systems based on federated learning. In MILCOM 2022-2022 IEEE Military Communications Conference (MILCOM) (pp. 61-65). IEEE.

Consul, P., Budhiraja, I., Garg, D., & Bindle, A. (2022). Power allocation scheme based on DRL for CF massive MIMO network with UAV. *Innovations in Information and Communication Technologies Proceedings of ICIICT, 2022*, 33–43.

Croman, K. (2016). On scaling decentralized blockchains: (A position paper). In J. Clark, S. Meiklejohn, P. Y. A. Ryan, D. Wallach, M. Brenner, & K. Rohloff (Eds.), *Financial Cryptography and Data Security* (Vol. 9604, pp. 106–125). Springer Berlin Heidelberg. doi:10.1007/978-3-662-53357-4_8

Czekster, R. M., Grace, P., Marcon, C., Hessel, F., & Cazella, S. C. (2023). Challenges and Opportunities for Conducting Dynamic Risk Assessments in Medical IoT. *Applied Sciences (Basel, Switzerland)*, *13*(13), 7406. doi:10.3390/app13137406

Dabas, P., Bhati, S., Kumar, S., Upreti, K., & Shaik, N. (2023, November). A Hybrid Edge-Cloud Computing Approach for Energy-Efficient Surveillance Using Deep Reinforcement Learning. In *2023 3rd International Conference on Technological Advancements in Computational Sciences (ICTACS)* (pp. 432-438). IEEE.

Dagher, G. G., Marella, P. B., & Malluhi, Q. M. (2018). MedChain: Efficient blockchain-based healthcare system with decentralized access control. *Journal of Medical Systems*, *42*(7), 130. PMID:29876661

Dagher, G. G., Mohler, J., Milojkovic, M., & Marella, P. B. (2018). Ancile: Privacy-preserving framework for access control and interoperability of electronic health records using blockchain technology. *Sustainable Cities and Society*, *39*, 283–297. doi:10.1016/j.scs.2018.02.014

Danzi, P., Kalor, A. E., Stefanovic, C., & Popovski, P. (2018). Analysis of the communication traffic for blockchain synchronization of IoT devices. *2018 IEEE International Conference on Communications (ICC)*, 1–7. 10.1109/ICC.2018.8422485

de Bienassis, K., Fujisawa, R., Hashiguchi, T. C. O., Klazinga, N., & Oderkirk, J. (2022). *Health data and governance developments in relation to COVID-19: How OECD countries are adjusting health data systems for the new normal*. Academic Press.

De Filippi, P., Mannan, M., & Reijers, W. (2020, August). Blockchain as a confidence machine: The problem of trust & challenges of governance. *Technology in Society*, *62*, 101284. doi:10.1016/j.techsoc.2020.101284

Demertzi, V., Demertzis, S., & Demertzis, K. (2023). An Overview of Cyber Threats, Attacks and Countermeasures on the Primary Domains of Smart Cities. *Applied Sciences (Basel, Switzerland)*, *13*(2), 790. doi:10.3390/app13020790

Dinh, T. T. A., Liu, R., Zhang, M., Chen, G., Ooi, B. C., & Wang, J. (2018). Untangling blockchain: A data processing view of blockchain systems. *IEEE Transactions on Knowledge and Data Engineering*, *30*(7), 1366–1385. doi:10.1109/TKDE.2017.2781227

Dinh, T. T. A., Wang, J., Chen, G., Liu, R., Ooi, B. C., & Tan, K.-L. (2017). BLOCKBENCH: a framework for analyzing private blockchains. *Proceedings of the 2017 ACM International Conference on Management of Data*, 1085–100. 10.1145/3035918.3064033

Ducas, E., & Wilner, A. (2017). The security and financial implications of blockchain technologies: Regulating emerging technologies in Canada. *International Journal (Toronto, Ont.)*, *72*(4), 538–562. doi:10.1177/0020702017741909

Du, J., Wang, S., & Fang, Y. (2019). A novel blockchain-based privacy-preserving EHR sharing scheme for healthcare 4.0. *IEEE Access : Practical Innovations, Open Solutions*, *7*, 13519–13527.

Eberhardt, J., & Tai, S. (2017). On or off the blockchain? Insights on off-chaining computation and data. In F. De Paoli, S. Schulte, & E. Broch Johnsen (Eds.), *Service-Oriented and Cloud Computing* (Vol. 10465). Springer International Publishing. doi:10.1007/978-3-319-67262-5_1

Edemekong, P. F., Haydel, M. J., Boyer, J., & Bogdan, B. (2020). *Health insurance portability and accountability act* (HIPAA). StatPearls.

Efanov, D., & Roschin, P. (2018). The all-pervasiveness of the blockchain technology. *Procedia Comput Sci, 123*, 116–21. https://doi.org/.procs.2018.01.019 doi:10.1016/j

Ekblaw, A., Azaria, A., Halamka, J. D., & Lippman, A. (2016). A case study for blockchain in healthcare: "MedRec" prototype for electronic health records and medical research data. In *Proceedings of IEEE Open & Big Data Conference (OBD)* (pp. 1-8). IEEE.

Elhoseny, M., Thilakarathne, N. N., Alghamdi, M. I., Mahendran, R. K., Gardezi, A. A., Weerasinghe, H., & Welhenge, A. (2021). Security and privacy issues in medical internet of things: Overview, countermeasures, challenges and future directions. *Sustainability (Basel)*, *13*(21), 11645. doi:10.3390/su132111645

Engelhardt, M. A. (2017). Hitching healthcare to the chain: An introduction to blockchain technology in the healthcare sector. *Technology Innovation Management Review*, *7*(10), 22–34. doi:10.22215/timreview/1111

Fang, B., Mei, G., Yuan, X., Wang, L., Wang, Z., & Wang, J. (2021). Visual SLAM for robot navigation in healthcare facility. *Pattern Recognition*, *113*, 107822. doi:10.1016/j.patcog.2021.107822 PMID:33495660

FDA. (2019). *IBM and the FDA: A new partnership for using secure Blockchain in healthcare*. U.S. Food and Drug Administration.

Ferreira, B., Rodrigues, J., Leitao, J., & Domingos, H. (2015). Privacy-preserving content-based image retrieval in the cloud. *2015 IEEE 34th Symposium on Reliable Distributed Systems (SRDS)*, 11–20. 10.1109/SRDS.2015.27

Fletcher, G. (2018). The Internet of Things in healthcare: An overview. *Journal of the British Institute of Radiology*, *91*(1084), 20170327.

Gai, K., Choo, K.-K. R., & Zhu, L. (2018). Blockchain-enabled reengineering of cloud datacenters. *IEEE Cloud Comput*, *5*(6), 21–25. doi:10.1109/MCC.2018.064181116

Gangadharan, S. M. P., Arya, C., Aluvala, S., Singh, J., Singh, P., & Murugesan, A. (2023, September). Advancing Bug Detection in Solidity Smart Contracts with the Proficiency of Deep Learning. In *2023 3rd International Conference on Innovative Sustainable Computational Technologies (CISCT)* (pp. 1-5). IEEE. 10.1109/CISCT57197.2023.10351355

Gangadharan, S. M. P., Dharani, M., Thapliyal, N., Yamsani, N., Singh, J., & Singh, P. (2023, September). Comparative Analysis of Deep Learning-Based Brain Tumor Prediction Models Using MRI Scan. In *2023 3rd International Conference on Innovative Sustainable Computational Technologies (CISCT)* (pp. 1-6). IEEE. 10.1109/CISCT57197.2023.10351227

Geetha, S. K., Kanakaprabha, S., Devipriya, A., Brindha, D., & Vetrimani, E. (2023). Implementation of a Blockchain Based Attendance Tracking System. *2023 International Conference on Computer Communication and Informatics (ICCCI)*, 1-5. 10.1109/ICCCI56745.2023.10128438

Gharat, A., Aher, P., Chaudhari, P., & Alte, B. (2021). A framework for secure storage and sharing of electronic health records using blockchain technology. *ITM Web of Conferences*, *40*, 03037.

Ghazal, S. (2019). Security and privacy in the Internet of Medical Things (IoMT). *IEEE Internet of Things Journal*, *6*(3), 4360–4369.

Goel, U., Ruhl, R., & Zavarsky, P. (2019, May). Using healthcare authority and patient blockchains to develop a tamper-proof record tracking system. In *2019 IEEE 5th intl conference on big data security on cloud (BigDataSecurity), IEEE Intl conference on high performance and smart computing,(HPSC) and IEEE Intl conference on intelligent data and security (IDS)* (pp. 25-30). IEEE. 10.1109/BigDataSecurity-HPSC-IDS.2019.00016

Gordon, W. J., & Catalini, C. (2018). Blockchain technology for healthcare: Facilitating the transition to patient-driven interoperability. *Computational and Structural Biotechnology Journal*, *16*, 224–230. doi:10.1016/j.csbj.2018.06.003 PMID:30069284

Goswami, A., Sharma, D., Mathuku, H., Gangadharan, S. M. P., Yadav, C. S., Sahu, S. K., Pradhan, M. K., Singh, J., & Imran, H. (2022). Change detection in remote sensing image data comparing algebraic and machine learning methods. *Electronics (Basel)*, *11*(3), 431. doi:10.3390/electronics11030431

Gupta, D., Rani, S., Raza, S., Faseeh Qureshi, N. M., Mansour, R. F., & Ragab, M. (2023). Security paradigm for remote health monitoring edge devices in internet of things. *Journal of King Saud University. Computer and Information Sciences*, (6), 101478. Advance online publication. doi:10.1016/j.jksuci.2022.12.020

Gupta, M. (2021). PR wallet based blockchain access protocol to secure EHRs. In *Blockchain and IoT Integration* (pp. 65–76). Auerbach Publications. doi:10.1201/9781003094210-4

Gupta, R., Tanwar, S., Al-Turjman, F., Italiya, P., Nauman, A., & Kim, S. W. (2020). Smart Contract Privacy Protection Using AI in Cyber-Physical Systems: Tools, Techniques and Challenges. *IEEE Access : Practical Innovations, Open Solutions*, *8*, 24746–24772. doi:10.1109/ACCESS.2020.2970576

Gupta, R., Tanwar, S., Tyagi, S., Kumar, N., Obaidat, M. S., & Sadoun, B. (2019). HaBiTs: Blockchain-based telesurgery framework for healthcare 4.0. In *International Conference on Computer, Information and Telecommunication Systems, CITS* (pp. 1–5). 10.1109/CITS.2019.8862127

Haddad, A., Habaebi, M. H., Islam, M. R., Hasbullah, N. F., & Zabidi, S. A. (2022). Systematic review on ai-blockchain based e-healthcare records management systems. *IEEE Access : Practical Innovations, Open Solutions*, *10*, 94583–94615. doi:10.1109/ACCESS.2022.3201878

Haddad, P., & Aziz, A. (2019). A novel blockchain framework for data sharing in EHRs. *Journal of Ambient Intelligence and Humanized Computing*, *10*(12), 4753–4763.

Halamka, J. (2020). Ethical considerations in Blockchain and healthcare. *Blockchain in Healthcare Today*, *3*, 1–5.

Hamdani, S. W. A., Abbas, H., Janjua, A. R., Shahid, W. B., Amjad, M. F., Malik, J., Murtaza, M. H., Atiquzzaman, M., & Khan, A. W. (2021). Cybersecurity standards in the context of operating system: Practical aspects, analysis, and comparisons. *ACM Computing Surveys*, *54*(3), 1–36. doi:10.1145/3442480

Hammi, M. T., Hammi, B., Bellot, P., & Serhrouchni, A. (2018). Bubbles of Trust: A decentralized blockchain-based authentication system for IoT. *Computers & Security*, *78*, 126–142. doi:10.1016/j.cose.2018.06.004

Hashemi, S., & Zarei, M. (2021). Internet of Things backdoors: Resource management issues, security challenges, and detection methods. *Transactions on Emerging Telecommunications Technologies*, *32*(2), e4142. doi:10.1002/ett.4142

Hevner, A. R., March, S. T., Park, J., & Ram, S. (2004). Design science in information systems research. *MIS Q*, *28*(1), 75–105. http://misq.org/design-science-in-information-systems-research.html?SID=shpier0675mhpes3hkfagcqee1

Hovenga, E., Grain, H., & Beale, T. (2022). Fragmented global standards development organisations. In *Roadmap to Successful Digital Health Ecosystems* (pp. 65–96). Academic Press., doi:10.1016/B978-0-12-823413-6.00025-2

Hoy, M. B. (2017). An introduction to the blockchain and its implications for libraries and medicine. *Medical Reference Services Quarterly*, *36*(3), 273–279. doi:10.1080/02763869.2017.1332261 PMID:28714815

Huang, B., Liu, Z., Chen, J., Liu, A., Liu, Q., & He, Q. (2017). Behavior pattern clustering in blockchain networks. *Multimedia Tools and Applications*, *76*(19), 20099–20110. doi:10.1007/s11042-017-4396-4

Hu, R., Chen, K., Chen, W., Wang, Q., & Luo, H. (2021). Estimation of construction waste generation based on an improved on-site measurement and SVM-based prediction model: A case of commercial buildings in China. *Waste Management (New York, N.Y.)*, *126*, 791–799. doi:10.1016/j.wasman.2021.04.012 PMID:33894559

Hussain, M. (2020). Blockchain and IoMT-enabled healthcare: Opportunities and challenges. *Journal of Medical Systems*, *44*(2), 35.

Ibarra, J., Jahankhani, H., & Beavers, J. (2020). Biohacking capabilities and threat/attack vectors. *Cyber Defence in the Age of AI, Smart Societies and Augmented Humanity*, 117-131. doi:10.1007/978-3-030-35746-7_7

Ienca, M. (2018). The rise of Blockchain in healthcare. *The Lancet. Oncology*, *19*(12), e720. PMID:30507438

Indoria, D., Singh, J., Singh, Y. P., Kumar, B. V., & Singh, P. (2023, September). Utilizing Sentiment Analysis for Assessing Suicidal Risk in Personal Journal Entries. In *2023 3rd International Conference on Innovative Sustainable Computational Technologies (CISCT)* (pp. 1-5). IEEE. 10.1109/CISCT57197.2023.10351354

Ioannis, S. & Konstanti. (2019, November). Blockchain and Brand Loyalty Programs: A Short Review of Applications and Challenges. *Procedia of Economics and Business Administration.*

Iqbal, M. F., Asim, M., & Umair, M. (2019). A blockchain based framework for healthcare data sharing with patients consent. *IEEE Access : Practical Innovations, Open Solutions*, *7*, 114002–114011.

Jabarulla, M. Y., & Lee, H. N. (2021, August). A blockchain and artificial intelligence-based, patient-centric healthcare system for combating the COVID-19 pandemic: Opportunities and applications. In Healthcare (Vol. 9, No. 8, p. 1019). MDPI. doi:10.3390/healthcare9081019

Jahanbin, P., Sharma, R. S., Wingreen, S. T., Kshetri, N., & Choo, K. K. R. (2023). Towards CRISP-BC: 3TIC specification framework for Blockchain use-cases. *IET Blockchain*, *3*(3), 159–168. doi:10.1049/blc2.12038

Javaid, M., Haleem, A., Singh, R. P., & Suman, R. (2023). Towards insighting cybersecurity for healthcare domains: A comprehensive review of recent practices and trends. *Cyber Security and Applications*, *100016*. Advance online publication. doi:10.1016/j.csa.2023.100016

Javidan, S. M., Banakar, A., Vakilian, K. A., & Ampatzidis, Y. (2023). Diagnosis of grape leaf diseases using automatic K-means clustering and machine learning. *Smart Agricultural Technology*, *3*, 100081. doi:10.1016/j.atech.2022.100081

Johnson, S. (2020). Security and privacy in electronic health records: A review of current healthcare data breaches. *Health Informatics Journal*, *26*(2), 74–86.

Jones, P., & Johnson, R. (2018). Electronic health records: The good, the bad, and the ugly. *Healthcare Informatics Research*, *24*(1), 55–63.

Kamble, S., Gunasekaran, A., & Arha, H. (2019, April). Understanding the Blockchain technology adoption in supply chains-Indian context. *International Journal of Production Research*, *57*(7), 2009–2033. doi:10.1080/00207543.2018.1518610

Kamishima, Y., Inoue, N., & Shinoda, K. (2013). Event detection in consumer videos using GMM supervectors and SVMs. *EURASIP Journal on Image and Video Processing, 2013*(1), 1–13. doi:10.1186/1687-5281-2013-51

Kandasamy, K., Srinivas, S., Achuthan, K., & Rangan, V. P. (2020). IoT cyber risk: A holistic analysis of cyber risk assessment frameworks, risk vectors, and risk ranking process. *EURASIP Journal on Information Security, 2020*(1), 1–18. doi:10.1186/s13635-020-00111-0

Kang, D., Devi, S. A., Felix, A., Narayanamoorthy, S., Kalaiselvan, S., Balaenu, D., & Ahmadian, A. (2022). Intuitionistic fuzzy MAUT-BW Delphi method for medication service robot selection during COVID-19. *Operations Research Perspectives, 9*, 100258. doi:10.1016/j.orp.2022.100258

Kang, J. M., Ryu, S. Y., & Kim, D. (2018). A survey of mobile blockchain: Architecture, consensus, and network. *Journal of Communications and Networks (Seoul), 20*(4), 393–402.

Karahanna, E., Adela, C., Liu, Q. B., & Serrano, C. (2019). Capitalizing on health information technology to enable advantage in U.S. Hospitals. *Management Information Systems Quarterly, 43*(1), 113–140. doi:10.25300/MISQ/2019/12743

Kaur, H., & Sharma, S. (2021). Interoperability in the Internet of Medical Things: Challenges, opportunities, and standardization. *Journal of Ambient Intelligence and Humanized Computing, 12*(1), 205–227.

Khalid, M. I., Ahmed, M., & Kim, J. (2023). Enhancing data protection in dynamic consent management systems: Formalizing privacy and security definitions with differential privacy, decentralization, and Zero-Knowledge proofs. *Sensors (Basel), 23*(17), 7604. doi:10.3390/s23177604 PMID:37688060

Khan, M. A., & Salah, K. (2018). IoT security: Review, blockchain solutions, and open challenges. *Future Generation Computer Systems, 82*, 395–411. doi:10.1016/j.future.2017.11.022

Kim, H., Kim, E., Yun, S. J., Kang, M. G., Shin, H. I., Oh, B. M., & Seo, H. G. (2022). Robot-assisted gait training with auditory and visual cues in Parkinson's disease: A randomized controlled trial. *Annals of Physical and Rehabilitation Medicine, 65*(3), 101620. doi:10.1016/j.rehab.2021.101620 PMID:34896605

Kim, M. G., Lee, A. R., Kwon, H. J., Kim, J. W., & Kim, I. K. (2018). Sharing medical questionnaires based on blockchain. In *2018 IEEE International Conference on Bioinformatics and Biomedicine (BIBM)* (pp. 2767–2769). 10.1109/BIBM.2018.8621154

Kioskli, K., Fotis, T., & Mouratidis, H. (2021, August). The landscape of cybersecurity vulnerabilities and challenges in healthcare: Security standards and paradigm shift recommendations. In *Proceedings of the 16th International Conference on Availability, Reliability and Security* (pp. 1-9). 10.1145/3465481.3470033

Kleinaki, A.-S., Mytis-Gkometh, P., Drosatos, G., Efraimidis, P. S., & Kaldoudi, E. (2018). A blockchain-based notarization service for biomedical knowledge retrieval. *Computational and Structural Biotechnology Journal, 16*, 288–297. doi:10.1016/j.csbj.2018.08.002 PMID:30181840

Kohli, R., & Tan, S. S.-L. (2016). Electronic health records: How can IS researchers contribute to transforming healthcare? [Mar.]. *Management Information Systems Quarterly*, *40*(3), 553–573. doi:10.25300/MISQ/2016/40.3.02

Krawiec, R. J. (2019). Secure and privacy-preserving data sharing for mobile health systems. *IEEE Transactions on Industrial Informatics*, *15*(9), 5555–5562.

Krolovits, P. (2019). The Estonian E-health system—10 years of development. *Studies in Health Technology and Informatics*, *262*, 160–163.

Ktari, J., Frikha, T., Ben Amor, N., Louraidh, L., Elmannai, H., & Hamdi, M. (2022). IoMT-Based Platform for E-Health Monitoring Based on the Blockchain. *Electronics (Basel)*, *11*(15), 2314. doi:10.3390/electronics11152314

Kuo, T. T. (2019). A Blockchain -based telemedicine system for remote healthcare services. *Journal of Medical Internet Research*, *21*(2), e10286.

Kuo, T. T., Kim, H. E., & Ohno-Machado, L. (2016). Blockchain distributed ledger technologies for biomedical and health care applications. *Journal of the American Medical Informatics Association : JAMIA*. PMID:29016974

Kuo, T.-T., Kim, H.-E., & Ohno-Machado, L. (2017, November). Blockchain distributed ledger technologies for biomedical and health care applications. *Journal of the American Medical Informatics Association : JAMIA*, *24*(6), 1211–1220. doi:10.1093/jamia/ocx068 PMID:29016974

Levy, Y., & Ellis, T. J. (2006). A systems approach to conduct an effective literature review in support of information systems research. *Info Sci Int J Emerg Transdiscipl*, *9*, 181–212. doi:10.28945/479

Li, H., Zhu, X., Lyu, L., Guo, Z., & Wu, D. (2018). A secure privacy-preserving key management scheme for blockchain-based electronic health records system. *IEEE Access : Practical Innovations, Open Solutions*, *6*, 44849–44859.

Lima Filho, F. S. D., Silveira, F. A., de Medeiros Brito, A. Junior, Vargas-Solar, G., & Silveira, L. F. (2019). Smart detection: An online approach for DoS/DDoS attack detection using machine learning. *Security and Communication Networks*, *2019*, 1–15. doi:10.1155/2019/1574749

Li, Q., Wang, Y., Shao, Y., Li, L., & Hao, H. (2023). A comparative study on the most effective machine learning model for blast loading prediction: From GBDT to Transformer. *Engineering Structures*, *276*, 115310. doi:10.1016/j.engstruct.2022.115310

Liu, B., Yu, X. L., Chen, S., Xu, X., & Zhu, L. (2017). Blockchain based data integrity service framework for IoT data. *2017 IEEE International Conference on Web Services*, 468–75. 10.1109/ICWS.2017.54

Logambigai, R., & Suresh Babu, C. V. (2024). Blockchain Empowerment for Securing IoT, Sensory Data in Next-Gen Intelligent Systems. In S. Sharma, A. Prakash, & V. Sugumaran (Eds.), *Developments Towards Next Generation Intelligent Systems for Sustainable Development* (pp. 1–34). IGI Global. doi:10.4018/979-8-3693-5643-2.ch001

Lu, W., Swaminathan, A., Varna, A. L., & Wu, M. (2009). *Enabling search over encrypted multimedia databases*. doi:10.1117/12.806980

Maione, C., Barbosa, F. Jr, & Barbosa, R. M. (2019). Predicting the botanical and geographical origin of honey with multivariate data analysis and machine learning techniques: A review. *Computers and Electronics in Agriculture*, *157*, 436–446. doi:10.1016/j.compag.2019.01.020

Mall, S. (2023). Heart diagnosis using deep neural network. In *2023 International Conference on Computational Intelligence and Knowledge Economy (ICCIKE)* (pp. 7-12). IEEE. 10.1109/ICCIKE58312.2023.10131696

Mandal, S., & Khan, D. A. (2020, September). A Study of security threats in cloud: Passive impact of COVID-19 pandemic. In *2020 International Conference on Smart Electronics and Communication (ICOSEC)* (pp. 837-842). IEEE. 10.1109/ICOSEC49089.2020.9215374

Mars, M. (2020). Telemedicine: A new frontier in the provision of health care services. *International Journal of Telemedicine and Applications*, *2020*, 2406829.

Mehta, P., Gupta, R., & Tanwar, S. (2020). Blockchain envisioned UAV networks: Challenges, solutions, and comparisons. *Computer Communications*, *151*, 518–538. doi:10.1016/j.comcom.2020.01.023

Menezes, A. J., Van Oorschot, P. C., & Vanstone, S. A. (1997). *Handbook of applied cryptography*. CRC Press.

Meng, L., & Chen, L. (2021). Reviewing the ISO/IEC standard for timestamping services. *IEEE Communications Standards Magazine*, *5*(3), 20–25. doi:10.1109/MCOMSTD.011.2000083

Meng, L., & Chen, L. (2022, September). A Blockchain-Based Long-Term Time-Stamping Scheme. In *European Symposium on Research in Computer Security* (pp. 3-24). Cham: Springer International Publishing. 10.1007/978-3-031-17140-6_1

Mettler, M. (2016). Blockchain technology in healthcare: The revolution starts here. *Proceedings of the IEEE*, *104*(2), 58–59.

Mishra, A. K., Bhartiy, K. K., Singh, J., Aluvala, S., Singh, P., & Kishor, K. (2023, September). Unlocking the Power of Natural Language Processing Through Journaling with the Assistance. In *2023 3rd International Conference on Innovative Sustainable Computational Technologies (CISCT)* (pp. 1-5). IEEE. 10.1109/CISCT57197.2023.10351450

Mishra, S., Kwong, J. C., Chan, A. K., & Baral, S. D. (2020). Understanding heterogeneity to inform the public health response to COVID-19 in Canada. *Canadian Medical Association Journal*, *192*(25), E684–E685. doi:10.1503/cmaj.201112 PMID:32493741

Mohsin, A., Jararweh, Y., Al-Ayyoub, M., Gupta, B. B., & Gupta, B. (2018). BCDS-health: Permissioned blockchain-based system for secure and efficient sharing of electronic health records. *Future Generation Computer Systems*, *86*, 1106–1116.

Mougayar, W. (2016). *The Business Blockchain: Promise, Practice, and Application of the Next Internet Technology*. Wiley.

Mukherjee, P., & Singh, D. (2020). The opportunities of blockchain in health 4.0. *Blockchain Technology for Industry 4.0: Secure, Decentralized, Distributed and Trusted Industry Environment*, 149-164. doi:10.1007/978-981-15-1137-0_8

Myklebust, T., Onshus, T. E., Lindskog, S., Ottermo, M. V., & Bodsberg, L. (2021). Data safety, sources, and data flow in the offshore industry. In *Proceedings of the 31st European Safety and Reliability Conference*. Research Publishing Services. 10.3850/978-981-18-2016-8_099-cd

Nigam, D., Patel, S. N., Raj Vincent, P. M., Srinivasan, K., & Arunmozhi, S. (2022). Biometric authentication for intelligent and privacy-preserving healthcare systems. *Journal of Healthcare Engineering, 2022*, 1–15. Advance online publication. doi:10.1155/2022/1789996 PMID:35368929

Novo, O. (2018). Blockchain meets IoT: An architecture for scalable access management in IoT. *IEEE Internet of Things Journal*, *5*(2), 1184–1195. doi:10.1109/JIOT.2018.2812239

Olalere, I. O., & Olanrewaju, O. A. (2022). Optimising Turning Operation in Precision Manufacturing Using Fused IoT Devices and Machine Learning Approach. *IFAC-PapersOnLine*, *55*(10), 1551–1555. doi:10.1016/j.ifacol.2022.09.611

Ouaddah, A., Elkalam, A. A., & Ouahman, A. A. (2017). *Towards a novel privacy-preserving access control model based on blockchain technology in IoT. In 2017 IEEE international conference on cloud computing technology and science*. CloudCom.

Pahl, C., El Ioini, N., & Helmer, S. (2018). A decision framework for blockchain platforms for IoT and edge computing. *Proceedings of the 3rd International Conference on Internet of Things, Big Data and Security*, 105–13. 10.5220/0006688601050113

Pandey, P., Pandey, S. C., & Kumar, U. (2020). Security issues of internet of things in health-care sector: An analytical approach. *Advancement of Machine Intelligence in Interactive Medical Image Analysis*, 307-329. doi:10.1007/978-981-15-1100-4_15

Pathak, H., & Kulkarni, V. (2015, November). Identification of ovarian mass through ultrasound images using machine learning techniques. In *2015 IEEE international conference on research in computational intelligence and communication networks (ICRCICN)* (pp. 137-140). IEEE.

Pereraa, S., Nanayakkaraa, S., Rodrigoa, M. N. N., Senaratnea, S., & Wein, R. (2020). Blockchain technology: Is it hype or real in the construction industry? *Journal of Industrial Information Integration, 17*, 100–125. doi:10.1016/j.jii.2020.100125

Perwej, Y., Akhtar, N., Kulshrestha, N., & Mishra, P. (2022). A Methodical Analysis of Medical Internet of Things (MIoT) Security and Privacy in Current and Future Trends. *Journal of Emerging Technologies and Innovative Research*, *9*(1), d346–d371.

Peters, G. W., & Panayi, E. (2016). Understanding modern banking ledgers through blockchain technologies: future of transaction processing and smart contracts on the internet of money. In P. Tasca, T. Aste, L. Pelizzon, & N. Perony (Eds.), *Banking Beyond Banks and Money* (pp. 239–278). Springer International Publishing. doi:10.1007/978-3-319-42448-4_13

Pilares, I. C. A., Azam, S., Akbulut, S., Jonkman, M., & Shanmugam, B. (2022). Addressing the challenges of electronic health records using blockchain and ipfs. *Sensors (Basel)*, *22*(11), 4032. doi:10.3390/s22114032 PMID:35684652

Pilkington, M. (2016). Blockchain technology: principles and applications. *Research Handbook on Digital Transformations*, 1-33.

Pommeranz, A., & Raykova, M. (2018). Efficient arguments for ethereum smart contracts. In *Advances in Cryptology – CRYPTO 2018* (pp. 667–699). Springer.

Prasad, M., Daraghmi, Y. A., Tiwari, P., Yadav, P., Bharill, N., ... Saxena, A. (2017, November). Fuzzy logic hybrid model with semantic filtering approach for pseudo relevance feedback-based query expansion. In *2017 IEEE symposium series on computational intelligence (SSCI)* (pp. 1-7). IEEE.

Prasad, M., Li, D. L., Lin, C. T., Prakash, S., & Joshi, S. (2015). Designing mamdani-type fuzzy reasoning for visualizing prediction problems based on collaborative fuzzy clustering. *IAENG International Journal of Computer Science*. https://www.iaeng.org/IJCS/issues_v42/issue_4/IJCS_42_4_12.pdf

Prodanoff, Z., White-Williams, C., & Chi, H. (2021). Regulations and standards aware framework for recording of mhealth app vulnerabilities. *International Journal of E-Health and Medical Communications*, *12*(3), 1–16. doi:10.4018/IJEHMC.20210501.oa1

Qiu, T., Zhang, R., & Gao, Y. (2019). Ripple vs. SWIFT: Transforming cross border remittance using blockchain technology. *Procedia Computer Science*, *147*, 428–434. doi:10.1016/j.procs.2019.01.260

Rabbani, N., Kim, G. Y., Suarez, C. J., & Chen, J. H. (2022). Applications of machine learning in routine laboratory medicine: Current state and future directions. *Clinical Biochemistry*, *103*, 1–7. doi:10.1016/j.clinbiochem.2022.02.011 PMID:35227670

Rahim, F. A., Ahmad, N. A., Magalingam, P., Jamil, N., Cob, Z. C., & Salahudin, L. (2023). Cybersecurity Vulnerabilities in Smart Grids with Solar Photovoltaic: A Threat Modelling and Risk Assessment Approach. *International Journal of Sustainable Construction Engineering and Technology*, *14*(3), 210–220. doi:10.30880/ijscet.2023.14.03.018

Randma, R. (2018). Use of Blockchain technology to support trust in e-health. *Proceedings of the 21st European Conference on Digital Government*, 479-486.

Rani Hemamalini, R., Vinodhini, R., Shanthini, B., Partheeban, P., Charumathy, M., & Cornelius, K. (2022). Air quality monitoring and forecasting using smart drones and recurrent neural network for sustainable development in Chennai city. *Sustainable Cities and Society*, *85*(April), 104077. doi:10.1016/j.scs.2022.104077

Ray, P. P., Chowhan, B., Kumar, N., & Almogren, A. (2021). BIoTHR: Electronic health record servicing scheme in IoT-blockchain ecosystem. *IEEE Internet of Things Journal*, *8*(13), 10857–10872. doi:10.1109/JIOT.2021.3050703

Raza, S. M., & Sajid, M. (2022). Vehicle Routing Problem Using Reinforcement Learning: Recent Advancements. Lecture Notes in Electrical Engineering, 858. doi:10.1007/978-981-19-0840-8_20

Reegu, F. A., Abas, H., Gulzar, Y., Xin, Q., Alwan, A. A., Jabbari, A., Sonkamble, R. G., & Dziyauddin, R. A. (2023). Blockchain-Based Framework for Interoperable Electronic Health Records for an Improved Healthcare System. *Sustainability (Basel)*, *15*(8), 6337. doi:10.3390/su15086337

Reyna, A., Martín, C., Chen, J., Soler, E., & Díaz, M. (2018, November). On blockchain and its integration with IoT. Challenges and opportunities. *Future Generation Computer Systems*, *88*, 173–190. doi:10.1016/j.future.2018.05.046

Roehrs, A., da Costa, C. A., & Righi, R. R. (2016). OmniPHR: A distributed architecture model to integrate personal health records. In *2016 IEEE 29th International Symposium on Computer-Based Medical Systems (CBMS)* (pp. 459-464). IEEE.

Roehrs, A., da Costa, C. A., da Rosa Righi, R., & da Silva, D. S. (2017). OmniPHR: A distributed architecture model to integrate personal health records. *Journal of Biomedical Informatics*, *71*, 70–81. doi:10.1016/j.jbi.2017.05.012 PMID:28545835

Roman-Belmonte, J. M., De la Corte-Rodriguez, H., & Rodriguez-Merchan, E. C. (2018). How blockchain technology can change medicine. *Postgraduate Medicine*, *130*(4), 420–427. doi:10.1080/00325481.2018.1472996 PMID:29727247

Sadiku, M. N. O., Eze, K. G., & Musa, S. M. (2018). Blockchain Technology in Healthcare. *International Journal of Advances in Scientific Research and Engineering*, *4*(5). Advance online publication. doi:10.31695/IJASRE.2018.32723

Sajid, M., Gupta, S. K., & Haidri, R. A. (2022). Artificial intelligence and blockchain technologies for smart city. *Intelligent Green Technologies for Sustainable Smart Cities*, 317-330.

Sajid, M., Jawed, M. S., Abidin, S., Shahid, M., & Ahamad, S. (2023). Capacitated Vehicle Routing Problem Using Algebraic Harris Hawks Optimization Algorithm. In Intelligent Techniques for Cyber-Physical Systems (pp. 183-210). CRC Press. doi:10.1201/9781003438588-12

Sajid, M., Yadav, C. S., Singh, S. S., & Saini, M. (2022). A novel deep neural-based music recommendation method considering user and song data. In *2022 6th International Conference on Trends in Electronics and Informatics (ICOEI)* (pp. 1-7). IEEE.

Sajid, M., & Rajak, R. (2023). Capacitated vehicle routing problem using algebraic particle swarm optimization with simulated annealing algorithm. In *Artificial Intelligence in Cyber-Physical Systems* (pp. 225–239). CRC Press. doi:10.1201/9781003248750-13

Samanthula, B. K., & Parikh, R. B. (2020). A Blockchain based EHR sharing and access control scheme for COVID-19 pandemic. *Journal of Medical Systems*, *44*(8), 1–11.

Sami UllahH.AslamS.ArjomandN. (2020). Blockchain in Healthcare and Medicine: A Contemporary Research of Applications, Challenges, and Future Perspectives. *Cryptography and Security*. arXiv:2004.06795 [cs.CR].

Seh, A. H., Zarour, M., Alenezi, M., Sarkar, A. K., Agrawal, A., Kumar, R., & Ahmad Khan, R. (2020, May). Healthcare data breaches: insights and implications. In Healthcare (Vol. 8, No. 2, p. 133). MDPI. doi:10.3390/healthcare8020133

Sellamuthu, S., Vaddadi, S. A., Venkata, S., Petwal, H., Hosur, R., & Mandala, V. (2023). AI-based recommendation model for effective decision to maximise ROI. *Soft Computing*, 1-10. doi:10.1007/s00500-023-08731-7

Semantha, F. H., Azam, S., Shanmugam, B., & Yeo, K. C. (2023). PbDinEHR: A Novel Privacy by Design Developed Framework Using Distributed Data Storage and Sharing for Secure and Scalable Electronic Health Records Management. *Journal of Sensor and Actuator Networks*, *12*(2), 36. doi:10.3390/jsan12020036

Semantha, F. H., Azam, S., Shanmugam, B., Yeo, K. C., & Beeravolu, A. R. (2021). A conceptual framework to ensure privacy in patient record management system. *IEEE Access : Practical Innovations, Open Solutions*, *9*, 165667–165689. doi:10.1109/ACCESS.2021.3134873

Semantha, F. H., Azam, S., Yeo, K. C., & Shanmugam, B. (2020). A systematic literature review on privacy by design in the healthcare sector. *Electronics (Basel)*, *9*(3), 452. doi:10.3390/electronics9030452

Shah, S. M., & Khan, R. A. (2020). Secondary use of electronic health record: Opportunities and challenges. *IEEE Access : Practical Innovations, Open Solutions*, *8*, 136947–136965. doi:10.1109/ACCESS.2020.3011099

Shaik, N., Kar, N. R., Thankachan, B., Pathak, A. K., & Gupta, S. (2023). Utilizing Blockchain and Deep Learning for Decentralized Discovery of Deceptive Practices in Healthcare Insurance. In *2023 3rd International Conference on Technological Advancements in Computational Sciences (ICTACS)* (pp. 445-450). IEEE. 10.1109/ICTACS59847.2023.10390211

Shaik, N., Kumar, B. V., Bhati, A., Kumar, S., & Sahu, D. P. (2023). Integrating Random Forest and Support Vector Regression Models for Optimized Energy Consumption Evaluation in Cloud Computing Data Centers. In *2023 3rd International Conference on Technological Advancements in Computational Sciences (ICTACS)* (pp. 451-456). IEEE. 10.1109/ICTACS59847.2023.10390070

Sharan, A. (2015). Co-occurrence and semantic similarity based hybrid approach for improving automatic query expansion in information retrieval. Lecture Notes in Computer Science, 8956.

Sharan, A. (2016). Relevance feedback-based query expansion model using ranks combining and Word2Vec approach. *Journal of the Institution of Electronics and Telecommunication Engineers*, *62*(5), 591–604. doi:10.1080/03772063.2015.1136575

Sharan, A., & Saini, M. (2017). Term co-occurrence and context window-based combined approach for query expansion with the semantic notion of terms. *International Journal of Web Science*, *3*(1), 32–57. doi:10.1504/IJWS.2017.088677

Sharif, M. H. U., & Mohammed, M. A. (2022). A literature review of financial losses statistics for cyber security and future trend. *World Journal of Advanced Research and Reviews*, *15*(1), 138–156. doi:10.30574/wjarr.2022.15.1.0573

Sharma, A., Sarishma, Tomar, R., Chilamkurti, N., & Kim, B.-G. (1609). Blockchain-based smart contracts for Internet of Medical Things in e-Healthcare. *Electronics (Basel)*, *9*(10), 1609. doi:10.3390/electronics9101609

Sharma, N., Mangla, M., Mohanty, S. N., Gupta, D., Tiwari, P., Shorfuzzaman, M., & Rawashdeh, M. (2021). A smart ontology-based IoT framework for remote patient monitoring. *Biomedical Signal Processing and Control*, *68*(March), 102717. doi:10.1016/j.bspc.2021.102717

Sharma, R., Zhang, C., Wingreen, S. C., Kshetri, N., & Zahid, A. (2020). Design of blockchain-based precision health-care using soft systems methodology. *Industrial Management & Data Systems*, *120*(3), 608–632. doi:10.1108/IMDS-07-2019-0401

Shrier, A. A., Zhong, J. L., & Chaves, G. (2018). *Unlocking blockchain's potential in health and life sciences*. Deloitte University Press.

Shuaib, K., Abdella, J., Sallabi, F., & Serhani, M. A. (2022). Secure decentralized electronic health records sharing system based on blockchains. *Journal of King Saud University. Computer and Information Sciences*, *34*(8), 5045–5058. doi:10.1016/j.jksuci.2021.05.002

Shusterman, D., & Krawiec, R. J. (2017). Utilizing blockchain technology for personal health records. *Journal of Health & Medical Informatics*, *8*(1), 261.

Singh Faujdar, D., Sahay, S., Singh, T., Jindal, H., & Kumar, R. (2019). Public health information systems for primary health care in India: A situational analysis study. *Journal of Family Medicine and Primary Care*, *8*(11), 3640–3646. doi:10.4103/jfmpc.jfmpc_808_19 PMID:31803666

Singh, N. P., Ravichandran, R., Ghosh, S., Rana, P., & Chaku, S. (2023, August). Enhancing Healthcare Security Using IoT-Enabled with Continuous Authentication Using Deep Learning. In *International Conference on Electrical and Electronics Engineering* (pp. 275-289). Singapore: Springer Nature Singapore.

Singhal, P., & Gupta, S. (2023). An Integrated Approach for Analysis of Electronic Health Records Using Blockchain and Deep Learning. *Recent Advances in Computer Science and Communications, 16*(9), 1-10.

Singh, I., & Singh, Y. A. S. H. I. K. (2022). Cyber-Security Knowledge and Practice of Nurses in Private Hospitals in Northern Durban, Kwazulu-Natal. *Journal of Theoretical and Applied Information Technology, 100*(1), 246–267.

Singh, J., & Kumar, R. (2017). Lexical co-occurrence and contextual window-based approach with semantic similarity for query expansion. *International Journal of Intelligent Information Technologies, 13*(3), 57–78. doi:10.4018/IJIIT.2017070104

Singh, J., & Sharan, A. (2018). Rank fusion and semantic genetic notion based automatic query expansion model. *Swarm and Evolutionary Computation, 38*, 295–308. doi:10.1016/j.swevo.2017.09.007

Singh, P. (2020). Learning based driver drowsiness detection model. *Proceedings of the 3rd International Conference on Intelligent Sustainable Systems, ICISS 2020*, 698–701.

Singh, R. (2020). Collaborative filtering based hybrid music recommendation system. *Proceedings of the 3rd International Conference on Intelligent Sustainable Systems, ICISS 2020*, 186–190. 10.1109/ICISS49785.2020.9315913

Singh, S. S., Srivastva, D., Verma, M., & Singh, J. (2022). Influence maximization frameworks, performance, challenges and directions on social network: A theoretical study. *Journal of King Saud University. Computer and Information Sciences, 34*(9), 7570–7603. doi:10.1016/j.jksuci.2021.08.009

Sivathanu, G., Wright, C. P., & Zadok, E. (2005). Ensuring data integrity in storage: techniques and applications. *Proceedings of the 2005 ACM workshop on Storage security and survivability - StorageSS '05*, 26. . Fairfax, VA, USA.10.1145/1103780.1103784

Smith, J. (2019). The Internet of Medical Things: A review of recent contributions and a future perspective. *IEEE Internet of Things Journal, 6*(2), 1614–1626.

Sreeraj, R., Singh, A., & Anbarasu, V. (2021). Preserving EMR records using blockchain. *Annals of the Romanian Society for Cell Biology, 25*(6), 5344–5350.

Srivastava, S., Pant, M., Jauhar, S. K., & Nagar, A. K. (2022). Analyzing the Prospects of Blockchain in Healthcare Industry. *Computational and Mathematical Methods in Medicine, 2022*, 1–24. Advance online publication. doi:10.1155/2022/3727389 PMID:36506597

Suresh Babu, C. V. & Das, S. (2023). Impact of Blockchain Technology on the Stock Market. In K. Mehta, R. Sharma, & P. Yu (Eds.), *Revolutionizing Financial Services and Markets Through FinTech and Blockchain* (pp. 44-59). IGI Global. doi:10.4018/978-1-6684-8624-5.ch004

Suresh Babu, C. V. & Pal, A. (2023). Securing Decentralized Finance Through Blockchain Technologies. In R. Thanigaivelan, S. Kaliappan, & C. Jegadheesan (Eds.), *Cyber-Physical Systems and Supporting Technologies for Industrial Automation* (pp. 351-372). IGI Global. https://doi.org/ doi:10.4018/978-1-6684-9267-3.ch020

Suresh Babu, C. V., Purushothaman, R., Anusha, K., & Shri Sakthi. (2023). Smart Gesture Controlled Systems Using IoT. In V. Thayananthan (Ed.), *AI-Based Digital Health Communication for Securing Assistive Systems* (pp. 114-133). IGI Global. doi:10.4018/978-1-6684-8938-3.ch006

Suresh Babu, C. V., Akshayah, N. S., & Maclin Vinola, P. (2024). Artificial Intelligence in Healthcare: Assessing Impacts, Challenges, and Recommendations for Achieving Healthcare Independence. In N. Geada & G. Jamil (Eds.), *Perspectives on Artificial Intelligence in Times of Turbulence: Theoretical Background to Applications* (pp. 61–80). IGI Global. doi:10.4018/978-1-6684-9814-9.ch005

Suresh Babu, C. V., & Praveen, S. (2023). Swarm Intelligence and Evolutionary Machine Learning Algorithms for COVID-19: Pandemic and Epidemic Review. In A. Suresh Kumar, U. Kose, S. Sharma, & S. Jerald Nirmal Kumar (Eds.), *Dynamics of Swarm Intelligence Health Analysis for the Next Generation* (pp. 83–103). IGI Global. doi:10.4018/978-1-6684-6894-4.ch005

Suresh Babu, C. V., & Yadavamuthiah, K. (2023). Cyber Physical Systems Design Challenges in the Areas of Mobility, Healthcare, Energy, and Manufacturing. In R. Thanigaivelan, S. Kaliappan, & C. Jegadheesan (Eds.), *Cyber-Physical Systems and Supporting Technologies for Industrial Automation* (pp. 131–151). IGI Global., doi:10.4018/978-1-6684-9267-3.ch007

Swaminathan, A. (2007). Confidentiality-preserving rank-ordered search. *Proceedings of the 2007 ACM workshop on Storage security and survivability - StorageSS '07*, 7. 10.1145/1314313.1314316

Swan, M. (2015). Blockchain: blueprint for a new economy. O'Reilly.

Sweety Bakyarani, E., Singh, N. P., Shekhawat, J., Bhardwaj, S., & Chaku, S. (2023, August). A Novel Approach on Deep Reinforcement Learning for Improved Throughput in Power-Restricted IoT Networks. In *International Conference on Electrical and Electronics Engineering* (pp. 63-76). Singapore: Springer Nature Singapore.

Świtała, K. (2023, May). Medical Data in the Digital Era-Legal Challenges Related to Providing Information Security, Applying GDPR and Respecting the Professional Secrecy. In *2023 46th MIPRO ICT and Electronics Convention (MIPRO)* (pp. 1457-1466). IEEE. 10.23919/MIPRO57284.2023.10159891

Tang, Q. (2021). A Blockchain -based decentralized privacy-preserving EHR sharing scheme. *IEEE Access : Practical Innovations, Open Solutions*, *9*, 31142–31152.

Tanwar, S., Parekh, K., & Evans, R. (2020). Blockchain-based electronic healthcare record system for healthcare 4.0 applications. *Journal of Information Security and Applications*, *50*, 102407. doi:10.1016/j.jisa.2019.102407

Taylor, P. J., Dargahi, T., Dehghantanha, A., Parizi, R. M., & Choo, K.-K. R. (2019). A systematic literature review of blockchain cyber security. *Digital Communications and Networks*. Advance online publication. doi:10.1016/j.dcan.2019.01.005

Thantharate, P., & Thantharate, A. (2023). ZeroTrustBlock: Enhancing Security, Privacy, and Interoperability of Sensitive Data through ZeroTrust Permissioned Blockchain. *Big Data and Cognitive Computing*, *7*(4), 165. doi:10.3390/bdcc7040165

Tuli, S., Tuli, S., Tuli, R., & Gill, S. S. (2020). Predicting the growth and trend of COVID-19 pandemic using machine learning and cloud computing. *Internet of Things : Engineering Cyber Physical Human Systems*, *11*, 100222. doi:10.1016/j.iot.2020.100222 PMID:38620477

Upreti, K., Shrivastava, S., Garg, A., & Sharma, A. K. (2022, December). Prediction & Detection of Cardiovascular Diseases using Machine Learning Approaches. In *2022 IEEE international conference on communication, security and artificial intelligence (ICCSAI-2022)* (pp. 24-25). IEEE.

Vellappally, S., Al Kheraif, A. A., Anil, S., & Wahba, A. A. (2019). IoT medical tooth mounted sensor for monitoring teeth and food level using bacterial optimization along with adaptive deep learning neural network. Measurement. *Measurement*, *135*, 672–677. doi:10.1016/j.measurement.2018.11.078

Verma, M. (2024). AI-Based Data Analytics for E-Rendering Frameworks. In Architecture and Technological Advancements of Education 4.0 (pp. 276-291). IGI Global.

Vest, J. R., & Gamm, L. D. (2010). Health information exchange: persistent challenges and new strategies: table. *Journal of the American Medical Informatics Association : JAMIA*, *17*(3), 288–294. doi:10.1136/jamia.2010.003673 PMID:20442146

Webster, J., & Watson, R. T. (2002). Analyzing the past to prepare for the future: Writing a literature review. *Management Information Systems Quarterly*, *26*(2), xiii–xxii.

Xu, R., & Zhu, Y. (2018). Patient self-controlled medical record based on blockchain technology. *Journal of Medical Systems*, *42*(8), 1–9.

Yaacoub, J. P. A., Noura, M., Noura, H. N., Salman, O., Yaacoub, E., Couturier, R., & Chehab, A. (2020). Securing internet of medical things systems: Limitations, issues and recommendations. *Future Generation Computer Systems*, *105*, 581–606. doi:10.1016/j.future.2019.12.028

Yadav, A., & Kumar, S. (2022). A review of physical unclonable functions (PUFs) and its applications in IoT environment. Ambient Communications and Computer Systems. *Proceedings of RACCCS, 2021*, 1–13.

Yadav, C. S., Singh, J., Yadav, A., Pattanayak, H. S., Kumar, R., Khan, A. A., Haq, M. A., Alhussen, A., & Alharby, S. (2022). Malware analysis in IoT & android systems with defensive mechanism. *Electronics (Basel)*, *11*(15), 2354. doi:10.3390/electronics11152354

Yaqoob, I., Salah, K., Jayaraman, R., & Al-Hammadi, Y. (2021). Blockchain for healthcare data management: Opportunities, challenges, and future recommendations. *Neural Computing & Applications*, 1–16. doi:10.1007/s00521-020-05519-w

Yaqoob, T., Abbas, H., & Atiquzzaman, M. (2019). Security vulnerabilities, attacks, countermeasures, and regulations of networked medical devices-A review. *IEEE Communications Surveys and Tutorials*, *21*(4), 3723–3768. doi:10.1109/COMST.2019.2914094

Yin, J., Lamp, J., Cameron, K., Wurtz, R., & Chen, H. (2017). A blockchain framework for patient-centered health records and sharing behavior consent. In *International conference on security and privacy in communication systems* (pp. 25-44). Academic Press.

Yin, J., Srinivasan, S., Wang, K., & Jiang, Z. (2018). A blockchain-based framework for data sharing with fine-grained access control in decentralized storage systems. *Journal of Parallel and Distributed Computing, 118*, 112–123.

Yin, S., Nong, G., Shao, L., & Zhang, W. (2019). An access control method of electronic medical records based on blockchain technology. *Future Generation Computer Systems, 95*, 511–517.

Yin, S., Xia, Q., Niu, J., Sun, L., & Wang, J. (2019). ACES: An efficient access control scheme based on attribute certificate for blockchain in electronic health record system. *IEEE Access : Practical Innovations, Open Solutions, 7*, 54847–54857.

Zamani, A. S., Anand, L., Rane, K. P., Prabhu, P., Buttar, A. M., Pallathadka, H., Raghuvanshi, A., & Dugbakie, B. N. (2022). Performance of machine learning and image processing in plant leaf disease detection. *Journal of Food Quality, 2022*, 1–7. doi:10.1155/2022/1598796

Zhang, P., Walker, M. A., White, J., Schmidt, D. C., & Lenz, G. (2017). Metrics for assessing blockchain-based healthcare decentralized apps. *2017 IEEE 19th International Conference on e-Health Networking, Applications and Services (Healthcom),* 1–4. 10.1109/HealthCom.2017.8210842

Zhang, P., White, J., Schmidt, D. C., & Lenz, G. (2020). Blockchain technology use cases in healthcare: A systematic review. *Journal of Medical Systems, 44*(7), 1–14. PMID:32462430

Zohrevand, P., & Beznosov, K. (2017). A systematic literature review on blockchain technology for secure sharing of medical electronic records. In *2017 IEEE 19th International Conference on e-Health Networking, Applications and Services (Healthcom)* (pp. 1-6). IEEE.

Zohrevand, P., & Beznosov, K. (2018). Personal health records: Privacy and security considerations for mobile apps. *International Journal of Medical Informatics, 112*, 54–71.

Zyskind, G., & Nathan, O. A. (2015). Decentralizing privacy: using blockchain to protect personal data. 2015 IEEE Security and Privacy Workshops, 180–4. doi:10.1109/SPW.2015.27

Related References

To continue our tradition of advancing information science and technology research, we have compiled a list of recommended IGI Global readings. These references will provide additional information and guidance to further enrich your knowledge and assist you with your own research and future publications.

Aasi, P., Rusu, L., & Vieru, D. (2017). The Role of Culture in IT Governance Five Focus Areas: A Literature Review. *International Journal of IT/Business Alignment and Governance, 8*(2), 42-61. https://doi.org/ doi:10.4018/IJITBAG.2017070103

Abdrabo, A. A. (2018). Egypt's Knowledge-Based Development: Opportunities, Challenges, and Future Possibilities. In A. Alraouf (Ed.), *Knowledge-Based Urban Development in the Middle East* (pp. 80–101). Hershey, PA: IGI Global. doi:10.4018/978-1-5225-3734-2.ch005

Abu Doush, I., & Alhami, I. (2018). Evaluating the Accessibility of Computer Laboratories, Libraries, and Websites in Jordanian Universities and Colleges. *International Journal of Information Systems and Social Change*, *9*(2), 44–60. doi:10.4018/IJISSC.2018040104

Abu Seman, S. A., & Ramayah, T. (2017). Are We Ready to App?: A Study on mHealth Apps, Its Future, and Trends in Malaysia Context. In J. Pelet (Ed.), *Mobile Platforms, Design, and Apps for Social Commerce* (pp. 69–83). Hershey, PA: IGI Global. doi:10.4018/978-1-5225-2469-4.ch005

Adegbore, A. M., Quadri, M. O., & Oyewo, O. R. (2018). A Theoretical Approach to the Adoption of Electronic Resource Management Systems (ERMS) in Nigerian University Libraries. In A. Tella & T. Kwanya (Eds.), *Handbook of Research on Managing Intellectual Property in Digital Libraries* (pp. 292–311). Hershey, PA: IGI Global. doi:10.4018/978-1-5225-3093-0.ch015

Adeleke, I. T., & Abdul, Q. B. (2020). Opinions on Cyber Security, Electronic Health Records, and Medical Confidentiality: Emerging Issues on Internet of Medical Things From Nigeria. In P. Pankajavalli & G. Karthick (Eds.), *Incorporating the Internet of Things in Healthcare Applications and Wearable Devices* (pp. 199–211). IGI Global. https://doi.org/10.4018/978-1-7998-1090-2.ch012

Afolabi, O. A. (2018). Myths and Challenges of Building an Effective Digital Library in Developing Nations: An African Perspective. In A. Tella & T. Kwanya (Eds.), *Handbook of Research on Managing Intellectual Property in Digital Libraries* (pp. 51–79). Hershey, PA: IGI Global. doi:10.4018/978-1-5225-3093-0.ch004

Agarwal, P., Kurian, R., & Gupta, R. K. (2022). Additive Manufacturing Feature Taxonomy and Placement of Parts in AM Enclosure. In S. Salunkhe, H. Hussein, & J. Davim (Eds.), *Applications of Artificial Intelligence in Additive Manufacturing* (pp. 138–176). IGI Global. https://doi.org/10.4018/978-1-7998-8516-0.ch007

Aggarwal, S., & Azad, V. (2017). A Hybrid System Based on FMM and MLP to Diagnose Heart Disease. In S. Bhattacharyya, S. De, I. Pan, & P. Dutta (Eds.), *Intelligent Multidimensional Data Clustering and Analysis* (pp. 293–325). Hershey, PA: IGI Global. doi:10.4018/978-1-5225-1776-4.ch011

Al-Alawi, A. I., Al-Hammam, A. H., Al-Alawi, S. S., & AlAlawi, E. I. (2021). The Adoption of E-Wallets: Current Trends and Future Outlook. In Y. Albastaki, A. Razzaque, & A. Sarea (Eds.), *Innovative Strategies for Implementing FinTech in Banking* (pp. 242–262). IGI Global. https://doi.org/10.4018/978-1-7998-3257-7.ch015

Al-Busaidi, S. S. (2018). Interdisciplinary Relationships Between Medicine and Social Sciences. In M. Al-Suqri, A. Al-Kindi, S. AlKindi, & N. Saleem (Eds.), *Promoting Interdisciplinarity in Knowledge Generation and Problem Solving* (pp. 124–137). Hershey, PA: IGI Global. doi:10.4018/978-1-5225-3878-3.ch009

Al Kareh, T., & Thoumy, M. (2018). The Impact of Health Information Digitization on the Physiotherapist-Patient Relationship: A Pilot Study of the Lebanese Community. *International Journal of Healthcare Information Systems and Informatics, 13*(2), 29–53. doi:10.4018/IJHISI.2018040103

Alenzuela, R. (2017). Research, Leadership, and Resource-Sharing Initiatives: The Role of Local Library Consortia in Access to Medical Information. In S. Ram (Ed.), *Library and Information Services for Bioinformatics Education and Research* (pp. 199–211). Hershey, PA: IGI Global. doi:10.4018/978-1-5225-1871-6.ch012

Ali, S., Samie, A. U., Ali, A., Bhat, A. H., Mir, T., & Prasad, B. V. (2020). Mental Health: A Global Issue Affecting the Pattern of Life in Kashmir. In S. Taukeni (Ed.), *Biopsychosocial Perspectives and Practices for Addressing Communicable and Non-Communicable Diseases* (pp. 18–29). IGI Global. https://doi.org/10.4018/978-1-7998-2139-7.ch002

Almpani, S., Stefaneas, P., Boley, H., Mitsikas, T., & Frangos, P. (2019). A Rule-Based Model for Compliance of Medical Devices Applied to the European Market. *International Journal of Extreme Automation and Connectivity in Healthcare*, *1*(2), 56–78. https://doi.org/10.4018/IJEACH.2019070104

Alnakhi, W. K. (2021). Medical Travel and Public Health: Definitions, Frameworks, and Future Research. In M. Singh & S. Kumaran (Eds.), *Growth of the Medical Tourism Industry and Its Impact on Society: Emerging Research and Opportunities* (pp. 74–94). IGI Global. https://doi.org/10.4018/978-1-7998-3427-4.ch004

Alsharo, M. (2017). Attitudes Towards Cloud Computing Adoption in Emerging Economies. *International Journal of Cloud Applications and Computing*, *7*(3), 44–58. doi:10.4018/IJCAC.2017070102

Amer, T. S., & Johnson, T. L. (2017). Information Technology Progress Indicators: Research Employing Psychological Frameworks. In A. Mesquita (Ed.), *Research Paradigms and Contemporary Perspectives on Human-Technology Interaction* (pp. 168–186). Hershey, PA: IGI Global. doi:10.4018/978-1-5225-1868-6.ch008

Ameri, H., Alizadeh, S., & Noughabi, E. A. (2017). Application of Data Mining Techniques in Clinical Decision Making: A Literature Review and Classification. In E. Noughabi, B. Raahemi, A. Albadvi, & B. Far (Eds.), *Handbook of Research on Data Science for Effective Healthcare Practice and Administration* (pp. 257–295). Hershey, PA: IGI Global. doi:10.4018/978-1-5225-2515-8.ch012

Anand, S. (2017). Medical Image Enhancement Using Edge Information-Based Methods. In B. Singh (Ed.), *Computational Tools and Techniques for Biomedical Signal Processing* (pp. 123–148). Hershey, PA: IGI Global. doi:10.4018/978-1-5225-0660-7.ch006

Andreeva, A., & Yolova, G. (2021). Liability in Labor Legislation: New Challenges Related to the Use of Artificial Intelligence. In B. Vassileva & M. Zwilling (Eds.), *Responsible AI and Ethical Issues for Businesses and Governments* (pp. 214–232). IGI Global. https://doi.org/10.4018/978-1-7998-4285-9.ch012

Anohah, E. (2017). Paradigm and Architecture of Computing Augmented Learning Management System for Computer Science Education. *International Journal of Online Pedagogy and Course Design*, *7*(2), 60–70. doi:10.4018/IJOPCD.2017040105

Anohah, E., & Suhonen, J. (2017). Trends of Mobile Learning in Computing Education from 2006 to 2014: A Systematic Review of Research Publications. *International Journal of Mobile and Blended Learning*, *9*(1), 16–33. doi:10.4018/IJMBL.2017010102

Anton, J. L., Soriano, J. V., Martinez, M. I., & Garcia, F. B. (2018). Comprehensive E-Learning Appraisal System. In M. Khosrow-Pour, D.B.A. (Ed.), Encyclopedia of Information Science and Technology, Fourth Edition (pp. 5787-5799). Hershey, PA: IGI Global. https://doi.org/ doi:10.4018/978-1-5225-2255-3.ch503

Arbaiza, C. S., Huerta, H. V., & Rodriguez, C. R. (2021). Contributions to the Technological Adoption Model for the Peruvian Agro-Export Sector. *International Journal of E-Adoption*, *13*(1), 1–17. https://doi.org/10.4018/IJEA.2021010101

Aslan, F. (2021). Could There Be an Alternative Method of Media Literacy in Promoting Health in Children and Adolescents? Media Literacy and Health Promotion. In G. Sarı (Eds.), *Handbook of Research on Representing Health and Medicine in Modern Media* (pp. 191-199). IGI Global. https://doi.org/10.4018/978-1-7998-6825-5.ch013

Atzori, B., Hoffman, H. G., Vagnoli, L., Messeri, A., & Grotto, R. L. (2018). Virtual Reality as Distraction Technique for Pain Management in Children and Adolescents. In M. Khosrow-Pour, D.B.A. (Ed.), Encyclopedia of Information Science and Technology, Fourth Edition (pp. 5955-5965). Hershey, PA: IGI Global. doi:10.4018/978-1-5225-2255-3.ch518

Audibert, M., Mathonnat, J., Pélissier, A., & Huang, X. X. (2018). The Impact of the New Rural Cooperative Medical Scheme on Township Hospitals' Utilization and Income Structure in Weifang Prefecture, China. In I. Management Association (Ed.), Health Economics and Healthcare Reform: Breakthroughs in Research and Practice (pp. 109-121). Hershey, PA: IGI Global. https://doi.org/ doi:10.4018/978-1-5225-3168-5.ch007

Aulia, A., & Pratiti, B. (2022). Cyberchondria and Medical Student Syndrome: An Anxious Path to Be an Anxiety Healer? In H. Aker & M. Aiken (Eds.), *Handbook of Research on Cyberchondria, Health Literacy, and the Role of Media in Society's Perception of Medical Information* (pp. 98–113). IGI Global. https://doi.org/10.4018/978-1-7998-8630-3.ch006

Babu, A., & Ayyappan, S. (2017). A Methodological Evaluation of Crypto-Watermarking System for Medical Images. In C. Bhatt & S. Peddoju (Eds.), *Cloud Computing Systems and Applications in Healthcare* (pp. 189–217). Hershey, PA: IGI Global. doi:10.4018/978-1-5225-1002-4.ch010

Bailey, E. K. (2017). Applying Learning Theories to Computer Technology Supported Instruction. In M. Grassetti & S. Brookby (Eds.), *Advancing Next-Generation Teacher Education through Digital Tools and Applications* (pp. 61–81). Hershey, PA: IGI Global. doi:10.4018/978-1-5225-0965-3.ch004

Baker, J. D. (2021). Introduction to Machine Learning as a New Methodological Framework for Performance Assessment. In M. Bocarnea, B. Winston, & D. Dean (Eds.), *Handbook of Research on Advancements in Organizational Data Collection and Measurements: Strategies for Addressing Attitudes, Beliefs, and Behaviors* (pp. 326–342). IGI Global. https://doi.org/10.4018/978-1-7998-7665-6.ch021

Bakke, A. (2017). Ethos in E-Health: From Informational to Interactive Websites. In M. Folk & S. Apostel (Eds.), *Establishing and Evaluating Digital Ethos and Online Credibility* (pp. 85–103). Hershey, PA: IGI Global. doi:10.4018/978-1-5225-1072-7.ch005

Bali, S. (2018). Enhancing the Reach of Health Care Through Telemedicine: Status and New Possibilities in Developing Countries. In U. Pandey & V. Indrakanti (Eds.), *Open and Distance Learning Initiatives for Sustainable Development* (pp. 339–354). Hershey, PA: IGI Global. doi:10.4018/978-1-5225-2621-6.ch019

Balls-Berry, J. E., & Albold, C. (2019). Asynchronous Education for Graduate Medical Trainees to Reduce Health Disparities and Address Social Determinants of Health: Online Education for Graduate Medical Trainees. In E. Demiroz & S. Waldman (Eds.), *Optimizing Medical Education With Instructional Technology* (pp. 1–20). IGI Global. https://doi.org/10.4018/978-1-5225-6289-4.ch001

Banerjee, S., Sing, T. Y., Chowdhury, A. R., & Anwar, H. (2018). Let's Go Green: Towards a Taxonomy of Green Computing Enablers for Business Sustainability. In M. Khosrow-Pour (Ed.), *Green Computing Strategies for Competitive Advantage and Business Sustainability* (pp. 89–109). Hershey, PA: IGI Global. doi:10.4018/978-1-5225-5017-4.ch005

Barrett, T. E. (2018). Essentials for Education and Training for Tomorrow's Physicians. In C. Smith (Ed.), *Exploring the Pressures of Medical Education From a Mental Health and Wellness Perspective* (pp. 230–252). Hershey, PA: IGI Global. doi:10.4018/978-1-5225-2811-1.ch010

Basham, R. (2018). Information Science and Technology in Crisis Response and Management. In M. Khosrow-Pour, D.B.A. (Ed.), Encyclopedia of Information Science and Technology, Fourth Edition (pp. 1407-1418). Hershey, PA: IGI Global. doi:10.4018/978-1-5225-2255-3.ch121

Batyashe, T., & Iyamu, T. (2018). Architectural Framework for the Implementation of Information Technology Governance in Organisations. In M. Khosrow-Pour, D.B.A. (Ed.), Encyclopedia of Information Science and Technology, Fourth Edition (pp. 810-819). Hershey, PA: IGI Global. doi:10.4018/978-1-5225-2255-3.ch070

Bazan, V., Jax, M. D., & Zwischenberger, J. B. (2020). Alice in Simulation-Land: Surgical Simulation in Medical Education. In R. Gotian, Y. Kang, & J. Safdieh (Eds.), *Handbook of Research on the Efficacy of Training Programs and Systems in Medical Education* (pp. 449–458). IGI Global. https://doi.org/10.4018/978-1-7998-1468-9.ch023

Beaudoin, S. (2019). The Hidden Face of Medical Intervention. In C. Albuquerque (Eds.), *Emerging Trends and Innovations in Privacy and Health Information Management* (pp. 188-211). IGI Global. https://doi.org/10.4018/978-1-5225-8470-4.ch008

Bekleyen, N., & Çelik, S. (2017). Attitudes of Adult EFL Learners towards Preparing for a Language Test via CALL. In D. Tafazoli & M. Romero (Eds.), *Multiculturalism and Technology-Enhanced Language Learning* (pp. 214–229). Hershey, PA: IGI Global. doi:10.4018/978-1-5225-1882-2.ch013

Bergeron, F., Croteau, A., Uwizeyemungu, S., & Raymond, L. (2017). A Framework for Research on Information Technology Governance in SMEs. In S. De Haes & W. Van Grembergen (Eds.), *Strategic IT Governance and Alignment in Business Settings* (pp. 53–81). Hershey, PA: IGI Global. doi:10.4018/978-1-5225-0861-8.ch003

Bernardes, O., Amorim, V., & Usman, B. (2021). The Good, the Bad, and the Ugly: Don't Blame COVID-19 for Health System Inefficiencies. In J. Santos, & I. Pereira (Ed.), *Management and Marketing for Improved Competitiveness and Performance in the Healthcare Sector* (pp. 115-139). IGI Global. https://doi.org/10.4018/978-1-7998-7263-4.ch006

Berrahal, S., & Boudriga, N. (2017). The Risks of Wearable Technologies to Individuals and Organizations. In A. Marrington, D. Kerr, & J. Gammack (Eds.), *Managing Security Issues and the Hidden Dangers of Wearable Technologies* (pp. 18–46). Hershey, PA: IGI Global. doi:10.4018/978-1-5225-1016-1.ch002

Bhardwaj, M., Shukla, N., & Sharma, A. (2021). Improvement and Reduction of Clustering Overhead in Mobile Ad Hoc Network With Optimum Stable Bunching Algorithm. In S. Kumar, M. Trivedi, P. Ranjan, & A. Punhani (Eds.), *Evolution of Software-Defined Networking Foundations for IoT and 5G Mobile Networks* (pp. 139–158). IGI Global. https://doi.org/10.4018/978-1-7998-4685-7.ch008

Bhargava, P. (2018). Blended Learning: An Effective Application to Clinical Teaching. In S. Tang & C. Lim (Eds.), *Preparing the Next Generation of Teachers for 21st Century Education* (pp. 302–320). Hershey, PA: IGI Global. doi:10.4018/978-1-5225-4080-9.ch018

Bhatt, G. D., Wang, Z., & Rodger, J. A. (2017). Information Systems Capabilities and Their Effects on Competitive Advantages: A Study of Chinese Companies. *Information Resources Management Journal, 30*(3), 41–57. doi:10.4018/IRMJ.2017070103

Bhattacharya, A. (2021). Blockchain, Cybersecurity, and Industry 4.0. In A. Tyagi, G. Rekha, & N. Sreenath (Eds.), *Opportunities and Challenges for Blockchain Technology in Autonomous Vehicles* (pp. 210–244). IGI Global. https://doi.org/10.4018/978-1-7998-3295-9.ch013

Bhyan, P., Shrivastava, B., & Kumar, N. (2022). Requisite Sustainable Development Contemplating Buildings: Economic and Environmental Sustainability. In A. Hussain, K. Tiwari, & A. Gupta (Eds.), *Addressing Environmental Challenges Through Spatial Planning* (pp. 269–288). IGI Global. https://doi.org/10.4018/978-1-7998-8331-9.ch014

Bird, J. L. (2017). Writing Healing Narratives. In V. Bryan & J. Bird (Eds.), *Healthcare Community Synergism between Patients, Practitioners, and Researchers* (pp. 1–28). Hershey, PA: IGI Global. doi:10.4018/978-1-5225-0640-9.ch001

Boido, C., Davico, P., & Spallone, R. (2021). Digital Tools Aimed to Represent Urban Survey. In M. Khosrow-Pour D.B.A. (Ed.), *Encyclopedia of Information Science and Technology, Fifth Edition* (pp. 1181-1195). IGI Global. https://doi.org/10.4018/978-1-7998-3479-3.ch082

Borkar, P. S., Chanana, P. U., Atwal, S. K., Londe, T. G., & Dalal, Y. D. (2021). The Replacement of HMI (Human-Machine Interface) in Industry Using Single Interface Through IoT. In R. Raut & A. Mihovska (Eds.), *Examining the Impact of Deep Learning and IoT on Multi-Industry Applications* (pp. 195–208). IGI Global. https://doi.org/10.4018/978-1-7998-7511-6.ch011

Bougoulias, K., Kouris, I., Prasinos, M., Giokas, K., & Koutsouris, D. (2017). Ob/Gyn EMR Software: A Solution for Obstetricians and Gynecologists. In A. Moumtzoglou (Ed.), *Design, Development, and Integration of Reliable Electronic Healthcare Platforms* (pp. 101–111). Hershey, PA: IGI Global. doi:10.4018/978-1-5225-1724-5.ch006

Bouslimi, R., Ayadi, M. G., & Akaichi, J. (2018). Medical Image Retrieval in Healthcare Social Networks. *International Journal of Healthcare Information Systems and Informatics, 13*(2), 13–28. doi:10.4018/IJHISI.2018040102

Bouzaabia, O., Bouzaabia, R., & Mejri, K. (2017). Role of Internet in the Development of Medical Tourism Service in Tunisia. In A. Capatina & E. Rancati (Eds.), *Key Challenges and Opportunities in Web Entrepreneurship* (pp. 211–241). Hershey, PA: IGI Global. doi:10.4018/978-1-5225-2466-3.ch009

Brahmane, A. V., & Krishna, C. B. (2021). Rider Chaotic Biography Optimization-driven Deep Stacked Auto-encoder for Big Data Classification Using Spark Architecture: Rider Chaotic Biography Optimization. *International Journal of Web Services Research, 18*(3), 42–62. https://doi.org/10.4018/ijwsr.2021070103

Brown-Jackson, K. L. (2018). Telemedicine and Telehealth: Academics Engaging the Community in a Call to Action. In S. Burton (Ed.), *Engaged Scholarship and Civic Responsibility in Higher Education* (pp. 166–193). Hershey, PA: IGI Global. doi:10.4018/978-1-5225-3649-9.ch008

Burcoff, A., & Shamir, L. (2017). Computer Analysis of Pablo Picasso's Artistic Style. *International Journal of Art, Culture and Design Technologies, 6*(1), 1–18. doi:10.4018/IJACDT.2017010101

Bwalya, K. J. (2017). Next Wave of Tele-Medicine: Virtual Presence of Medical Personnel. In K. Moahi, K. Bwalya, & P. Sebina (Eds.), *Health Information Systems and the Advancement of Medical Practice in Developing Countries* (pp. 168–180). Hershey, PA: IGI Global. doi:10.4018/978-1-5225-2262-1.ch010

Byker, E. J. (2017). I Play I Learn: Introducing Technological Play Theory. In C. Martin & D. Polly (Eds.), *Handbook of Research on Teacher Education and Professional Development* (pp. 297–306). Hershey, PA: IGI Global. doi:10.4018/978-1-5225-1067-3.ch016

Calongne, C. M., Stricker, A. G., Truman, B., & Arenas, F. J. (2017). Cognitive Apprenticeship and Computer Science Education in Cyberspace: Reimagining the Past. In A. Stricker, C. Calongne, B. Truman, & F. Arenas (Eds.), *Integrating an Awareness of Selfhood and Society into Virtual Learning* (pp. 180–197). Hershey, PA: IGI Global. doi:10.4018/978-1-5225-2182-2.ch013

Carneiro, A. D. (2017). Defending Information Networks in Cyberspace: Some Notes on Security Needs. In M. Dawson, D. Kisku, P. Gupta, J. Sing, & W. Li (Eds.), Developing Next-Generation Countermeasures for Homeland Security Threat Prevention (pp. 354-375). Hershey, PA: IGI Global. https://doi.org/ doi:10.4018/978-1-5225-0703-1.ch016

Carvalho, W. F., & Zarate, L. (2021). Causal Feature Selection. In A. Azevedo & M. Santos (Eds.), *Integration Challenges for Analytics, Business Intelligence, and Data Mining* (pp. 145-160). IGI Global. https://doi.org/10.4018/978-1-7998-5781-5.ch007

Celik, G. (2018). Determining Headache Diseases With Genetic Algorithm. In U. Kose, G. Guraksin, & O. Deperlioglu (Eds.), *Nature-Inspired Intelligent Techniques for Solving Biomedical Engineering Problems* (pp. 249–262). Hershey, PA: IGI Global. doi:10.4018/978-1-5225-4769-3.ch012

Chakraborty, S., Chatterjee, S., Ashour, A. S., Mali, K., & Dey, N. (2018). Intelligent Computing in Medical Imaging: A Study. In N. Dey (Ed.), *Advancements in Applied Metaheuristic Computing* (pp. 143–163). Hershey, PA: IGI Global. doi:10.4018/978-1-5225-4151-6.ch006

Chandra, L., Downey, C. L., Svavarsdottir, H. S., Skinner, H., & Young, A. L. (2020). Gender Equity in Medical Leadership. In M. Bellini & V. Papalois (Eds.), *Gender Equity in the Medical Profession* (pp. 94–109). IGI Global. https://doi.org/10.4018/978-1-5225-9599-1.ch007

Chandran, S. (2019). Medical Data Storage and Compression. In A. Swarnambiga (Ed.), *Medical Image Processing for Improved Clinical Diagnosis* (pp. 140–154). IGI Global. https://doi.org/10.4018/978-1-5225-5876-7.ch007

Chase, J. P., & Yan, Z. (2017). Affect in Statistics Cognition. In *Assessing and Measuring Statistics Cognition in Higher Education Online Environments: Emerging Research and Opportunities* (pp. 144–187). Hershey, PA: IGI Global. doi:10.4018/978-1-5225-2420-5.ch005

Chatterjee, A., Roy, S., & Shrivastava, R. (2021). A Machine Learning Approach to Prevent Cancer. In G. Rani & P. Tiwari (Eds.), *Handbook of Research on Disease Prediction Through Data Analytics and Machine Learning* (pp. 112–141). IGI Global. https://doi.org/10.4018/978-1-7998-2742-9.ch007

Chavez, A., & Kovarik, C. (2017). Open Source Technology for Medical Practice in Developing Countries. In K. Moahi, K. Bwalya, & P. Sebina (Eds.), *Health Information Systems and the Advancement of Medical Practice in Developing Countries* (pp. 33–59). Hershey, PA: IGI Global. doi:10.4018/978-1-5225-2262-1.ch003

Chen, S., Traba, C., Lamba, S., & Soto-Greene, M. (2020). Professional and Career Development of Medical Students. In R. Gotian, Y. Kang, & J. Safdieh (Eds.), *Handbook of Research on the Efficacy of Training Programs and Systems in Medical Education* (pp. 305–326). IGI Global. https://doi.org/10.4018/978-1-7998-1468-9.ch016

Chien, G. C., Haroutunian, A., England, B., & Candido, K. D. (2019). Optimizing Medical Education With Instructional Technology: Technology to Optimize Teaching Human Anatomy. In E. Demiroz & S. Waldman (Eds.), *Optimizing Medical Education With Instructional Technology* (pp. 71–78). IGI Global. https://doi.org/10.4018/978-1-5225-6289-4.ch005

Choudhari, R. H. (2021). Multidimensional Impact of Climate Change on Human Reproduction and Fertility: A Medical Perspective on Changing Dynamics. In K. Wani, & N. Naha (Eds.), *Climate Change and Its Impact on Fertility* (pp. 278-315). IGI Global. https://doi.org/10.4018/978-1-7998-4480-8.ch014

Cifci, M. A. (2021). Optimizing WSNs for CPS Using Machine Learning Techniques. In A. Luhach & A. Elçi (Eds.), *Artificial Intelligence Paradigms for Smart Cyber-Physical Systems* (pp. 204–228). IGI Global. https://doi.org/10.4018/978-1-7998-5101-1.ch010

Cimermanova, I. (2017). Computer-Assisted Learning in Slovakia. In D. Tafazoli & M. Romero (Eds.), *Multiculturalism and Technology-Enhanced Language Learning* (pp. 252–270). Hershey, PA: IGI Global. doi:10.4018/978-1-5225-1882-2.ch015

Cipolla-Ficarra, F. V., & Cipolla-Ficarra, M. (2018). Computer Animation for Ingenious Revival. In F. Cipolla-Ficarra, M. Ficarra, M. Cipolla-Ficarra, A. Quiroga, J. Alma, & J. Carré (Eds.), *Technology-Enhanced Human Interaction in Modern Society* (pp. 159–181). Hershey, PA: IGI Global. doi:10.4018/978-1-5225-3437-2.ch008

Ciufudean, C. (2018). Innovative Formalism for Biological Data Analysis. In M. Khosrow-Pour, D.B.A. (Ed.), Encyclopedia of Information Science and Technology, Fourth Edition (pp. 1814-1824). Hershey, PA: IGI Global. doi:10.4018/978-1-5225-2255-3.ch158

Cockrell, S., Damron, T. S., Melton, A. M., & Smith, A. D. (2018). Offshoring IT. In M. Khosrow-Pour, D.B.A. (Ed.), Encyclopedia of Information Science and Technology, Fourth Edition (pp. 5476-5489). Hershey, PA: IGI Global. https://doi.org/ doi:10.4018/978-1-5225-2255-3.ch476

Coffey, J. W. (2018). Logic and Proof in Computer Science: Categories and Limits of Proof Techniques. In J. Horne (Ed.), *Philosophical Perceptions on Logic and Order* (pp. 218–240). Hershey, PA: IGI Global. doi:10.4018/978-1-5225-2443-4.ch007

Colaguori, R., & Danesi, M. (2017). Medical Semiotics: A Revisitation and an Exhortation. *International Journal of Semiotics and Visual Rhetoric*, *1*(1), 11–18. doi:10.4018/IJSVR.2017010102

Cole, A. W., & Salek, T. A. (2017). Adopting a Parasocial Connection to Overcome Professional Kakoethos in Online Health Information. In M. Folk & S. Apostel (Eds.), *Establishing and Evaluating Digital Ethos and Online Credibility* (pp. 104–120). Hershey, PA: IGI Global. doi:10.4018/978-1-5225-1072-7.ch006

Dale, M. (2017). Re-Thinking the Challenges of Enterprise Architecture Implementation. In M. Tavana (Ed.), *Enterprise Information Systems and the Digitalization of Business Functions* (pp. 205–221). Hershey, PA: IGI Global. doi:10.4018/978-1-5225-2382-6.ch009

Das, A., & Mohanty, M. N. (2021). An Useful Review on Optical Character Recognition for Smart Era Generation. In A. Tyagi (Ed.), *Multimedia and Sensory Input for Augmented, Mixed, and Virtual Reality* (pp. 1–41). IGI Global. https://doi.org/10.4018/978-1-7998-4703-8.ch001

Dash, A. K., & Mohapatra, P. (2021). A Survey on Prematurity Detection of Diabetic Retinopathy Based on Fundus Images Using Deep Learning Techniques. In S. Saxena & S. Paul (Eds.), *Deep Learning Applications in Medical Imaging* (pp. 140–155). IGI Global. https://doi.org/10.4018/978-1-7998-5071-7.ch006

De Maere, K., De Haes, S., & von Kutzschenbach, M. (2017). CIO Perspectives on Organizational Learning within the Context of IT Governance. *International Journal of IT/Business Alignment and Governance, 8*(1), 32-47. https://doi.org/doi:10.4018/IJITBAG.2017010103

Demir, K., Çaka, C., Yaman, N. D., İslamoğlu, H., & Kuzu, A. (2018). Examining the Current Definitions of Computational Thinking. In H. Ozcinar, G. Wong, & H. Ozturk (Eds.), *Teaching Computational Thinking in Primary Education* (pp. 36–64). Hershey, PA: IGI Global. doi:10.4018/978-1-5225-3200-2.ch003

Deng, X., Hung, Y., & Lin, C. D. (2017). Design and Analysis of Computer Experiments. In S. Saha, A. Mandal, A. Narasimhamurthy, S. V, & S. Sangam (Eds.), Handbook of Research on Applied Cybernetics and Systems Science (pp. 264-279). Hershey, PA: IGI Global. doi:10.4018/978-1-5225-2498-4.ch013

Denner, J., Martinez, J., & Thiry, H. (2017). Strategies for Engaging Hispanic/Latino Youth in the US in Computer Science. In Y. Rankin & J. Thomas (Eds.), *Moving Students of Color from Consumers to Producers of Technology* (pp. 24–48). Hershey, PA: IGI Global. doi:10.4018/978-1-5225-2005-4.ch002

Deperlioglu, O. (2018). Intelligent Techniques Inspired by Nature and Used in Biomedical Engineering. In U. Kose, G. Guraksin, & O. Deperlioglu (Eds.), *Nature-Inspired Intelligent Techniques for Solving Biomedical Engineering Problems* (pp. 51–77). Hershey, PA: IGI Global. doi:10.4018/978-1-5225-4769-3.ch003

Desai, K. P., Shah, M. A., Lapasia, M. C., Patil, S. A., & Pathak, S. P. (2022). Applied Intelligence for Mental Health Detection: ManoVaidya – A Mental Health Therapist. In A. Thakare, S. Wagh, M. Bhende, A. Anter, & X. Gao (Eds.), *Handbook of Research on Applied Intelligence for Health and Clinical Informatics* (pp. 80–91). IGI Global. https://doi.org/10.4018/978-1-7998-7709-7.ch005

Devi, A. (2017). Cyber Crime and Cyber Security: A Quick Glance. In R. Kumar, P. Pattnaik, & P. Pandey (Eds.), *Detecting and Mitigating Robotic Cyber Security Risks* (pp. 160–171). Hershey, PA: IGI Global. doi:10.4018/978-1-5225-2154-9.ch011

Dey, N., & Ashour, A. S. (2018). Meta-Heuristic Algorithms in Medical Image Segmentation: A Review. In N. Dey (Ed.), *Advancements in Applied Metaheuristic Computing* (pp. 185–203). Hershey, PA: IGI Global. doi:10.4018/978-1-5225-4151-6.ch008

Dey, N., Ashour, A. S., & Althoupety, A. S. (2017). Thermal Imaging in Medical Science. In V. Santhi (Ed.), *Recent Advances in Applied Thermal Imaging for Industrial Applications* (pp. 87–117). Hershey, PA: IGI Global. doi:10.4018/978-1-5225-2423-6.ch004

Dhaya, R., & Kanthavel, R. (2022). Futuristic Research Perspectives of IoT Platforms. In D. Jeya Mala (Ed.), *Integrating AI in IoT Analytics on the Cloud for Healthcare Applications* (pp. 258–275). IGI Global. doi:10.4018/978-1-7998-9132-1.ch015

Di Virgilio, F., Camillo, A. A., & Camillo, I. C. (2017). The Impact of Social Network on Italian Users' Behavioural Intention for the Choice of a Medical Tourist Destination. *International Journal of Tourism and Hospitality Management in the Digital Age, 1*(1), 36–49. doi:10.4018/IJTHMDA.2017010103

Dobani, F., Pennington, M. L., Coe, E., Morrison, P., & Gulliver, S. B. (2020). Bridging the Gaps: Toward Effective Collaboration Between Peer Supporters and Behavioral Health Professionals. In C. Bowers, D. Beidel, & M. Marks (Eds.), *Mental Health Intervention and Treatment of First Responders and Emergency Workers* (pp. 190–204). IGI Global. https://doi.org/10.4018/978-1-5225-9803-9.ch011

Dogra, A. K., & Dogra, P. (2017). The Medical Tourism Industry in the BRIC Nations: An Indian Analysis. In M. Dhiman (Ed.), *Opportunities and Challenges for Tourism and Hospitality in the BRIC Nations* (pp. 320–336). Hershey, PA: IGI Global. doi:10.4018/978-1-5225-0708-6.ch020

Doublestein, B. A., Lee, W. T., & Pfohl, R. M. (2020). Overview of Professionalism Competence: Bringing Balance to the Medical Education Continuum. In R. Selladurai, C. Hobson, R. Selladurai, & A. Greer (Eds.), *Evaluating Challenges and Opportunities for Healthcare Reform* (pp. 215–231). IGI Global. https://doi.org/10.4018/978-1-7998-2949-2.ch010

Doyle, D. J., & Fahy, P. J. (2018). Interactivity in Distance Education and Computer-Aided Learning, With Medical Education Examples. In M. Khosrow-Pour, D.B.A. (Ed.), Encyclopedia of Information Science and Technology, Fourth Edition (pp. 5829-5840). Hershey, PA: IGI Global. https://doi.org/ doi:10.4018/978-1-5225-2255-3.ch507

Drowos, J. L., & Wood, S. K. (2017). Preparing Future Physicians to Adapt to the Changing Health Care System: Promoting Humanism through Curricular Design. In V. Bryan & J. Bird (Eds.), *Healthcare Community Synergism between Patients, Practitioners, and Researchers* (pp. 106–125). Hershey, PA: IGI Global. doi:10.4018/978-1-5225-0640-9.ch006

Dulam, K. (2017). Medical Patents and Impact on Availability and Affordability of Essential Medicines in India. In R. Aggarwal & R. Kaur (Eds.), *Patent Law and Intellectual Property in the Medical Field* (pp. 41–57). Hershey, PA: IGI Global. doi:10.4018/978-1-5225-2414-4.ch003

Dutta, P. (2017). Decision Making in Medical Diagnosis via Distance Measures on Interval Valued Fuzzy Sets. *International Journal of System Dynamics Applications*, *6*(4), 63–83. doi:10.4018/IJSDA.2017100104

Dutta, P. (2021). Medical Pre-Screening of Common Diseases: An Interval-Valued Fuzzy Set Approach. In A. Azar & N. Kamal (Eds.), *Handbook of Research on Modeling, Analysis, and Control of Complex Systems* (pp. 267–292). IGI Global. https://doi.org/10.4018/978-1-7998-5788-4.ch011

Dwivedi, M. K., Pandey, S. K., & Singh, P. K. (2021). Public Health Surveillance System: Infectious Diseases. In D. Yadav, A. Bansal, M. Bhatia, M. Hooda, & J. Morato (Eds.), *Diagnostic Applications of Health Intelligence and Surveillance Systems* (pp. 201–220). IGI Global. https://doi.org/10.4018/978-1-7998-6527-8.ch010

Eklund, P. (2021). Reinforcement Learning in Social Media Marketing. In B. Christiansen & T. Škrinjarić (Eds.), *Handbook of Research on Applied AI for International Business and Marketing Applications* (pp. 30–48). IGI Global. https://doi.org/10.4018/978-1-7998-5077-9.ch003

El Ghandour, N., Benaissa, M., & Lebbah, Y. (2021). An Integer Linear Programming-Based Method for the Extraction of Ontology Alignment. *International Journal of Information Technology and Web Engineering*, *16*(2), 25–44. https://doi.org/10.4018/IJITWE.2021040102

El Guemhioui, K., & Demurjian, S. A. (2017). Semantic Reconciliation of Electronic Health Records Using Semantic Web Technologies. *International Journal of Information Technology and Web Engineering*, *12*(2), 26–48. doi:10.4018/IJITWE.2017040102

Elias, N. I., & Walker, T. W. (2017). Factors that Contribute to Continued Use of E-Training among Healthcare Professionals. In F. Topor (Ed.), *Handbook of Research on Individualism and Identity in the Globalized Digital Age* (pp. 403–429). Hershey, PA: IGI Global. doi:10.4018/978-1-5225-0522-8.ch018

Etim, A., Etim, D. N., & Scott, J. (2020). Mobile Health and Telemedicine: Awareness, Adoption and Importance of Health Study. *International Journal of Healthcare Information Systems and Informatics*, *15*(1), 81–96. https://doi.org/10.4018/IJHISI.2020010105

Fino, E., & Hanna-Khalil, B. (2020). Psychometric Post-Examination Analysis in Medical Education Training Programs. In R. Gotian, Y. Kang, & J. Safdieh (Eds.), *Handbook of Research on the Efficacy of Training Programs and Systems in Medical Education* (pp. 221–242). IGI Global. https://doi.org/10.4018/978-1-7998-1468-9.ch012

Fishback, J. L., & Klein, R. M. (2019). Collaborative Learning for Histopathology Education. In E. Demiroz & S. Waldman (Eds.), *Optimizing Medical Education With Instructional Technology* (pp. 177–193). IGI Global. https://doi.org/10.4018/978-1-5225-6289-4.ch010

Fisher, J. (2018). Sociological Perspectives on Improving Medical Diagnosis Emphasizing CAD. In M. Khosrow-Pour, D.B.A. (Ed.), Encyclopedia of Information Science and Technology, Fourth Edition (pp. 1017-1024). Hershey, PA: IGI Global. doi:10.4018/978-1-5225-2255-3.ch088

Fisher, R. L. (2018). Computer-Assisted Indian Matrimonial Services. In M. Khosrow-Pour, D.B.A. (Ed.), Encyclopedia of Information Science and Technology, Fourth Edition (pp. 4136-4145). Hershey, PA: IGI Global. doi:10.4018/978-1-5225-2255-3.ch358

Franco Santos, D., Branco Silva, A. R., Novo, M. D., & Vaz de Almeida, C. (2022). Medical Burnout: Is Mindfulness an Effective Coping Strategy? In S. Gupta (Ed.), *Handbook of Research on Clinical Applications of Meditation and Mindfulness-Based Interventions in Mental Health* (pp. 184–194). IGI Global. https://doi.org/10.4018/978-1-7998-8682-2.ch012

Frank, E. M. (2018). Healthcare Education: Integrating Simulation Technologies. In V. Bryan, A. Musgrove, & J. Powers (Eds.), *Handbook of Research on Human Development in the Digital Age* (pp. 163–182). Hershey, PA: IGI Global. doi:10.4018/978-1-5225-2838-8.ch008

Galiautdinov, R. (2021). Nonlinear Filtering in Artificial Neural Network Applications in Business and Engineering. In Q. Do (Ed.), *Artificial Neural Network Applications in Business and Engineering* (pp. 1–23). IGI Global. https://doi.org/10.4018/978-1-7998-3238-6.ch001

Gambhir, P. (2021). Enhancing Mental Health: A Role for Technology. In A. Hooke (Ed.), *Technological Breakthroughs and Future Business Opportunities in Education, Health, and Outer Space* (pp. 264–269). IGI Global. https://doi.org/10.4018/978-1-7998-6772-2.ch017

Garcia-Santa, N., San Miguel, B., & Ugai, T. (2019). Converging Semantic Knowledge and Deep Learning for Medical Coding. *International Journal of Privacy and Health Information Management, 7*(2), 33–52. https://doi.org/10.4018/IJPHIM.2019070103

Gardner-McCune, C., & Jimenez, Y. (2017). Historical App Developers: Integrating CS into K-12 through Cross-Disciplinary Projects. In Y. Rankin & J. Thomas (Eds.), *Moving Students of Color from Consumers to Producers of Technology* (pp. 85–112). Hershey, PA: IGI Global. doi:10.4018/978-1-5225-2005-4.ch005

Garg, P. K. (2021). The Internet of Things-Based Technologies. In S. Kumar, M. Trivedi, P. Ranjan, & A. Punhani (Eds.), *Evolution of Software-Defined Networking Foundations for IoT and 5G Mobile Networks* (pp. 37–65). IGI Global. https://doi.org/10.4018/978-1-7998-4685-7.ch003

Garg, T., & Bharti, M. (2021). Congestion Control Protocols for UWSNs. In N. Goyal, L. Sapra, & J. Sandhu (Eds.), *Energy-Efficient Underwater Wireless Communications and Networking* (pp. 85–100). IGI Global. https://doi.org/10.4018/978-1-7998-3640-7.ch006

Garner, G. (2018). Foundations for Yoga Practice in Rehabilitation. In S. Telles & N. Singh (Eds.), *Research-Based Perspectives on the Psychophysiology of Yoga* (pp. 263–307). Hershey, PA: IGI Global. doi:10.4018/978-1-5225-2788-6.ch015

Garrote Andújar, S. A., Araújo Vila, N., Brea, J. A., & de Araújo, A. F. (2021). Medical Tourism: Analysis and Expectations Worldwide. In A. Borges & P. Rodrigues (Eds.), *New Techniques for Brand Management in the Healthcare Sector* (pp. 84–102). IGI Global. https://doi.org/10.4018/978-1-7998-3034-4.ch006

Gauttier, S. (2021). A Primer on Q-Method and the Study of Technology. In M. Khosrow-Pour D.B.A. (Eds.), *Encyclopedia of Information Science and Technology, Fifth Edition* (pp. 1746-1756). IGI Global. https://doi.org/10.4018/978-1-7998-3479-3.ch120

Gavurová, B., Kováč, V., & Šoltés, M. (2018). Medical Equipment and Economic Determinants of Its Structure and Regulation in the Slovak Republic. In M. Khosrow-Pour, D.B.A. (Ed.), Encyclopedia of Information Science and Technology, Fourth Edition (pp. 5841-5852). Hershey, PA: IGI Global. doi:10.4018/978-1-5225-2255-3.ch508

Ge, X., Wang, Q., Huang, K., Law, V., & Thomas, D. C. (2017). Designing Simulated Learning Environments and Facilitating Authentic Learning Experiences in Medical Education. In J. Stefaniak (Ed.), *Advancing Medical Education Through Strategic Instructional Design* (pp. 77–100). Hershey, PA: IGI Global. doi:10.4018/978-1-5225-2098-6.ch004

Gewald, H., & Gewald, C. (2018). Inhibitors of Physicians' Use of Mandatory Hospital Information Systems (HIS). *International Journal of Healthcare Information Systems and Informatics, 13*(1), 29–44. doi:10.4018/IJHISI.2018010103

Ghafele, R., & Gibert, B. (2018). Open Growth: The Economic Impact of Open Source Software in the USA. In M. Khosrow-Pour (Ed.), *Optimizing Contemporary Application and Processes in Open Source Software* (pp. 164–197). Hershey, PA: IGI Global. doi:10.4018/978-1-5225-5314-4.ch007

Ghobakhloo, M., & Azar, A. (2018). Information Technology Resources, the Organizational Capability of Lean-Agile Manufacturing, and Business Performance. *Information Resources Management Journal, 31*(2), 47–74. doi:10.4018/IRMJ.2018040103

Ghosh, D., & Dinda, S. (2017). Health Infrastructure and Economic Development in India. In R. Das (Ed.), *Social, Health, and Environmental Infrastructures for Economic Growth* (pp. 99–119). Hershey, PA: IGI Global. doi:10.4018/978-1-5225-2364-2.ch006

Ghosh, K., & Sen, K. C. (2017). The Potential of Crowdsourcing in the Health Care Industry. In N. Wickramasinghe (Ed.), *Handbook of Research on Healthcare Administration and Management* (pp. 418–427). Hershey, PA: IGI Global. doi:10.4018/978-1-5225-0920-2.ch024

Gikandi, J. W. (2017). Computer-Supported Collaborative Learning and Assessment: A Strategy for Developing Online Learning Communities in Continuing Education. In J. Keengwe & G. Onchwari (Eds.), *Handbook of Research on Learner-Centered Pedagogy in Teacher Education and Professional Development* (pp. 309–333). Hershey, PA: IGI Global. doi:10.4018/978-1-5225-0892-2.ch017

Gokhale, A. A., & Machina, K. F. (2017). Development of a Scale to Measure Attitudes toward Information Technology. In L. Tomei (Ed.), *Exploring the New Era of Technology-Infused Education* (pp. 49–64). Hershey, PA: IGI Global. doi:10.4018/978-1-5225-1709-2.ch004

Gonzalez-Urquijo, M., Macias-Rodriguez, Y., & Davila-Rivas, J. A. (2022). The Role of Telemedicine and Globalization in Medical Education. In M. Lopez (Ed.), *Advancing Health Education With Telemedicine* (pp. 288–295). IGI Global. https://doi.org/10.4018/978-1-7998-8783-6.ch015

Gopalan, V., Chan, E., & Ho, D. T. (2018). Deliberate Self-Harm and Suicide Ideology in Medical Students. In C. Smith (Ed.), *Exploring the Pressures of Medical Education From a Mental Health and Wellness Perspective* (pp. 122–143). Hershey, PA: IGI Global. doi:10.4018/978-1-5225-2811-1.ch005

Goswami, J. K., Jalal, S., Negi, C. S., & Jalal, A. S. (2022). A Texture Features-Based Robust Facial Expression Recognition. *International Journal of Computer Vision and Image Processing, 12*(1), 1–15. https://doi.org/10.4018/IJCVIP.2022010103

Goswami, N. (2021). Effects of Spaceflight, Aging, and Bedrest on Falls: Aging Meets Spaceflight! In P. Eklund (Ed.), *Integrated Care and Fall Prevention in Active and Healthy Aging* (pp. 91–106). IGI Global. https://doi.org/10.4018/978-1-7998-4411-2.ch005

Goswami, S., Dey, U., Roy, P., Ashour, A., & Dey, N. (2017). Medical Video Processing: Concept and Applications. In N. Dey, A. Ashour, & P. Patra (Eds.), *Feature Detectors and Motion Detection in Video Processing* (pp. 1–17). Hershey, PA: IGI Global. doi:10.4018/978-1-5225-1025-3.ch001

Goswami, S., Mahanta, K., Goswami, S., Jigdung, T., & Devi, T. P. (2018). Ageing and Cancer: The Epigenetic Basis, Alternative Treatment, and Care. In B. Prasad & S. Akbar (Eds.), *Handbook of Research on Geriatric Health, Treatment, and Care* (pp. 206–235). Hershey, PA: IGI Global. doi:10.4018/978-1-5225-3480-8.ch012

Gouva, M. I. (2017). The Psychological Impact of Medical Error on Patients, Family Members, and Health Professionals. In M. Riga (Ed.), *Impact of Medical Errors and Malpractice on Health Economics, Quality, and Patient Safety* (pp. 171–196). Hershey, PA: IGI Global. doi:10.4018/978-1-5225-2337-6.ch007

Gündüz, U., & Pembecioğlu, N. (2021). Case Study of Gender and Career Choices: Being and Becoming Medical People. In G. Sarı (Ed.), *Handbook of Research on Representing Health and Medicine in Modern Media* (pp. 269-307). IGI Global. https://doi.org/10.4018/978-1-7998-6825-5.ch018

Gupta, A. (2021). Artificial Intelligence Approaches to Detect Neurodegenerative Disease From Medical Records: A Perspective. In G. Rani & P. Tiwari (Eds.), *Handbook of Research on Disease Prediction Through Data Analytics and Machine Learning* (pp. 254–267). IGI Global. https://doi.org/10.4018/978-1-7998-2742-9.ch013

Gürcü, M., & Tengilimoğlu, D. (2017). Health Tourism-Based Destination Marketing. In A. Bayraktar & C. Uslay (Eds.), *Strategic Place Branding Methodologies and Theory for Tourist Attraction* (pp. 308–331). Hershey, PA: IGI Global. doi:10.4018/978-1-5225-0579-2.ch015

Gürsel, G. (2017). For Better Healthcare Mining Health Data. In S. Bhattacharyya, S. De, I. Pan, & P. Dutta (Eds.), *Intelligent Multidimensional Data Clustering and Analysis* (pp. 135–158). Hershey, PA: IGI Global. doi:10.4018/978-1-5225-1776-4.ch006

Gyaase, P. O., Darko-Lartey, R., William, H., & Borkloe, F. (2017). Towards an Integrated Electronic Medical Records System for Quality Healthcare in Ghana: An Exploratory Factor Analysis. *International Journal of Computers in Clinical Practice*, *2*(2), 38–55. doi:10.4018/IJCCP.2017070103

Hafeez-Baig, A., Gururajan, R., & Wickramasinghe, N. (2017). Readiness as a Novel Construct of Readiness Acceptance Model (RAM) for the Wireless Handheld Technology. In N. Wickramasinghe (Ed.), *Handbook of Research on Healthcare Administration and Management* (pp. 578–595). Hershey, PA: IGI Global. doi:10.4018/978-1-5225-0920-2.ch035

Hagle, H. N., Liu, Y., Murphy, D. M., & Krom, L. (2022). Innovative Adaptation of Training and Technical Assistance: Education for the Behavioral Health Workforce. In C. Ford & K. Garza (Eds.), *Handbook of Research on Updating and Innovating Health Professions Education: Post-Pandemic Perspectives* (pp. 239–264). IGI Global. https://doi.org/10.4018/978-1-7998-7623-6.ch011

Halis, M., & Halis, M. (2021). The Relationship Between Organizational Culture and Organizational Commitment: A Research in Private Health Institutions. In G. Sarı (Ed.), *Handbook of Research on Representing Health and Medicine in Modern Media* (pp. 308-329). IGI Global. https://doi.org/10.4018/978-1-7998-6825-5.ch019

Halis, M., Tepret, S., Çamlibel, Z., & Halis, M. (2021). Competitiveness in Medical Tourism: An Evaluation on Kocaeli Medical Tourism Market. In G. Sarı (Ed.), *Handbook of Research on Representing Health and Medicine in Modern Media* (pp. 239-268). IGI Global. https://doi.org/10.4018/978-1-7998-6825-5.ch017

Hanafizadeh, P., Ghandchi, S., & Asgarimehr, M. (2017). Impact of Information Technology on Lifestyle: A Literature Review and Classification. *International Journal of Virtual Communities and Social Networking*, *9*(2), 1–23. doi:10.4018/IJVCSN.2017040101

Hanel, P. (2017). Is China Catching Up?: Health-Related Applications of Biotechnology. In T. Bas & J. Zhao (Eds.), *Comparative Approaches to Biotechnology Development and Use in Developed and Emerging Nations* (pp. 465–520). Hershey, PA: IGI Global. doi:10.4018/978-1-5225-1040-6.ch016

Hartman, A., & Brown, S. (2017). Synergism through Therapeutic Visual Arts. In V. Bryan & J. Bird (Eds.), *Healthcare Community Synergism between Patients, Practitioners, and Researchers* (pp. 29–48). Hershey, PA: IGI Global. doi:10.4018/978-1-5225-0640-9.ch002

Haseski, H. İ., Ilic, U., & Tuğtekin, U. (2018). Computational Thinking in Educational Digital Games: An Assessment Tool Proposal. In H. Ozcinar, G. Wong, & H. Ozturk (Eds.), *Teaching Computational Thinking in Primary Education* (pp. 256–287). Hershey, PA: IGI Global. doi:10.4018/978-1-5225-3200-2.ch013

Heck, A. J., Cross, C. E., & Tatum, V. Y. (2020). Early Medical Education Readiness Interventions: Enhancing Undergraduate Preparedness. In R. Gotian, Y. Kang, & J. Safdieh (Eds.), *Handbook of Research on the Efficacy of Training Programs and Systems in Medical Education* (pp. 283–304). IGI Global. https://doi.org/10.4018/978-1-7998-1468-9.ch015

Hee, W. J., Jalleh, G., Lai, H., & Lin, C. (2017). E-Commerce and IT Projects: Evaluation and Management Issues in Australian and Taiwanese Hospitals. *International Journal of Public Health Management and Ethics*, *2*(1), 69–90. doi:10.4018/IJPHME.2017010104

Hemant, B., Arasappa, R. G. I., Udupa, K., & Varambally, S. (2021). Yoga for Mental Health Disorders: Research and Practice. In S. Telles & R. Gupta (Eds.), *Handbook of Research on Evidence-Based Perspectives on the Psychophysiology of Yoga and Its Applications* (pp. 179–198). IGI Global. https://doi.org/10.4018/978-1-7998-3254-6.ch011

Herdeiro, M. T., Gouveia, N., & Roque, F. (2021). Clinical Research and Regulatory Affairs: Skills and Tools in Pharmacy Education. In I. Figueiredo & A. Cavaco (Eds.), *Pedagogies for Pharmacy Curricula* (pp. 160–184). IGI Global. https://doi.org/10.4018/978-1-7998-4486-0.ch008

Hernandez, A. A. (2017). Green Information Technology Usage: Awareness and Practices of Philippine IT Professionals. *International Journal of Enterprise Information Systems, 13*(4), 90–103. doi:10.4018/IJEIS.2017100106

Hernandez, M. A., Marin, E. C., Garcia-Rodriguez, J., Azorin-Lopez, J., & Cazorla, M. (2017). Automatic Learning Improves Human-Robot Interaction in Productive Environments: A Review. *International Journal of Computer Vision and Image Processing, 7*(3), 65–75. doi:10.4018/IJCVIP.2017070106

Hirota, A. (2021). Design of Narrative Creation in Innovation: "Signature Story" and Two Types of Pivots. In T. Ogata & J. Ono (Eds.), *Bridging the Gap Between AI, Cognitive Science, and Narratology With Narrative Generation* (pp. 363–376). IGI Global. https://doi.org/10.4018/978-1-7998-4864-6.ch012

Hond, D., Asgari, H., Jeffery, D., & Newman, M. (2021). An Integrated Process for Verifying Deep Learning Classifiers Using Dataset Dissimilarity Measures. *International Journal of Artificial Intelligence and Machine Learning, 11*(2), 1–21. https://doi.org/10.4018/IJAIML.289536

Horne-Popp, L. M., Tessone, E. B., & Welker, J. (2018). If You Build It, They Will Come: Creating a Library Statistics Dashboard for Decision-Making. In L. Costello & M. Powers (Eds.), *Developing In-House Digital Tools in Library Spaces* (pp. 177–203). Hershey, PA: IGI Global. doi:10.4018/978-1-5225-2676-6.ch009

Hosoda, M., & Hosoda, M. (2019). Supporting Patient-led Initiatives to Improve Healthcare: An Investigation of Cancer and ME/CFS Support Groups and Prefectural Medical Councils in Japan. *International Journal of Patient-Centered Healthcare, 9*(2), 44–56. https://doi.org/10.4018/IJPCH.20190701.oa2

Hu, H., Hu, P. J., & Al-Gahtani, S. S. (2017). User Acceptance of Computer Technology at Work in Arabian Culture: A Model Comparison Approach. In M. Khosrow-Pour (Ed.), *Handbook of Research on Technology Adoption, Social Policy, and Global Integration* (pp. 205–228). Hershey, PA: IGI Global. doi:10.4018/978-1-5225-2668-1.ch011

Huang, C., Sun, Y., & Fuh, C. (2022). Vehicle License Plate Recognition With Deep Learning. In C. Chen, W. Yang, & L. Chen (Eds.), *Technologies to Advance Automation in Forensic Science and Criminal Investigation* (pp. 161-219). IGI Global. https://doi.org/10.4018/978-1-7998-8386-9.ch009

Ifinedo, P. (2017). Using an Extended Theory of Planned Behavior to Study Nurses' Adoption of Healthcare Information Systems in Nova Scotia. *International Journal of Technology Diffusion*, *8*(1), 1–17. doi:10.4018/IJTD.2017010101

Ilie, V., & Sneha, S. (2018). A Three Country Study for Understanding Physicians' Engagement With Electronic Information Resources Pre and Post System Implementation. *Journal of Global Information Management*, *26*(2), 48–73. doi:10.4018/JGIM.2018040103

Ilo, P. I., Nkiko, C., Ugwu, C. I., Ekere, J. N., Izuagbe, R., & Fagbohun, M. O. (2021). Prospects and Challenges of Web 3.0 Technologies Application in the Provision of Library Services. In M. Khosrow-Pour D.B.A. (Ed.), *Encyclopedia of Information Science and Technology, Fifth Edition* (pp. 1767-1781). IGI Global. https://doi.org/10.4018/978-1-7998-3479-3.ch122

Inoue-Smith, Y. (2017). Perceived Ease in Using Technology Predicts Teacher Candidates' Preferences for Online Resources. *International Journal of Online Pedagogy and Course Design*, *7*(3), 17–28. doi:10.4018/IJOPCD.2017070102

Iqbal, S., Ahmad, S., & Willis, I. (2017). Influencing Factors for Adopting Technology Enhanced Learning in the Medical Schools of Punjab, Pakistan. *International Journal of Information and Communication Technology Education*, *13*(3), 27–39. doi:10.4018/IJICTE.2017070103

Islam, A. Y. (2017). Technology Satisfaction in an Academic Context: Moderating Effect of Gender. In A. Mesquita (Ed.), *Research Paradigms and Contemporary Perspectives on Human-Technology Interaction* (pp. 187–211). Hershey, PA: IGI Global. doi:10.4018/978-1-5225-1868-6.ch009

Jagdale, S. C., Hable, A. A., & Chabukswar, A. R. (2021). Protocol Development in Clinical Trials for Healthcare Management. In M. Khosrow-Pour D.B.A. (Ed.), *Encyclopedia of Information Science and Technology, Fifth Edition* (pp. 1797-1814). IGI Global. https://doi.org/10.4018/978-1-7998-3479-3.ch124

Jagiello, K., Sosnowska, A., Mikolajczyk, A., & Puzyn, T. (2017). Nanomaterials in Medical Devices: Regulations' Review and Future Perspectives. *Journal of Nanotoxicology and Nanomedicine*, *2*(2), 1–11. doi:10.4018/JNN.2017070101

Jagtap, R., Phulare, K., Kurhade, M., & Gawande, K. S. (2021). Healthcare Conversational Chatbot for Medical Diagnosis. In B. Patil & M. Vohra (Eds.), *Handbook of Research on Engineering, Business, and Healthcare Applications of Data Science and Analytics* (pp. 401–415). IGI Global. https://doi.org/10.4018/978-1-7998-3053-5.ch020

Jamil, G. L., & Jamil, C. C. (2017). Information and Knowledge Management Perspective Contributions for Fashion Studies: Observing Logistics and Supply Chain Management Processes. In G. Jamil, A. Soares, & C. Pessoa (Eds.), *Handbook of Research on Information Management for Effective Logistics and Supply Chains* (pp. 199–221). Hershey, PA: IGI Global. doi:10.4018/978-1-5225-0973-8.ch011

Jamil, M. I., & Almunawar, M. N. (2021). Importance of Digital Literacy and Hindrance Brought About by Digital Divide. In M. Khosrow-Pour D.B.A. (Ed.), *Encyclopedia of Information Science and Technology, Fifth Edition* (pp. 1683-1698). IGI Global. https://doi.org/10.4018/978-1-7998-3479-3.ch116

Janakova, M. (2018). Big Data and Simulations for the Solution of Controversies in Small Businesses. In M. Khosrow-Pour, D.B.A. (Ed.), Encyclopedia of Information Science and Technology, Fourth Edition (pp. 6907-6915). Hershey, PA: IGI Global. doi:10.4018/978-1-5225-2255-3.ch598

Janosek, D. M. (2022). What Is the "Public Good" in a Pandemic? Who Decides?: Policy Makers and the Need for Leadership in Society's Perception of Medical Information. In H. Aker & M. Aiken (Eds.), *Handbook of Research on Cyberchondria, Health Literacy, and the Role of Media in Society's Perception of Medical Information* (pp. 1–15). IGI Global. https://doi.org/10.4018/978-1-7998-8630-3.ch001

Jena, T. K. (2018). Skill Training Process in Medicine Through Distance Mode. In U. Pandey & V. Indrakanti (Eds.), *Optimizing Open and Distance Learning in Higher Education Institutions* (pp. 228–243). Hershey, PA: IGI Global. doi:10.4018/978-1-5225-2624-7.ch010

Jhawar, A., & Garg, S. K. (2018). Logistics Improvement by Investment in Information Technology Using System Dynamics. In A. Azar & S. Vaidyanathan (Eds.), *Advances in System Dynamics and Control* (pp. 528–567). Hershey, PA: IGI Global. doi:10.4018/978-1-5225-4077-9.ch017

Joseph, V., & Miller, J. M. (2018). Medical Students' Perceived Stigma in Seeking Care: A Cultural Perspective. In C. Smith (Ed.), *Exploring the Pressures of Medical Education From a Mental Health and Wellness Perspective* (pp. 44–67). Hershey, PA: IGI Global. doi:10.4018/978-1-5225-2811-1.ch002

Joyce, B. L., & Swanberg, S. M. (2017). Using Backward Design for Competency-Based Undergraduate Medical Education. In J. Stefaniak (Ed.), *Advancing Medical Education Through Strategic Instructional Design* (pp. 53–76). Hershey, PA: IGI Global. doi:10.4018/978-1-5225-2098-6.ch003

Kalder, M., & Kostev, K. (2021). Epidemiology of Gynaecological and Breast Cancers: Incidence, Survival, and Mental Health. In K. Dinas, S. Petousis, M. Kalder, & G. Mavromatidis (Eds.), *Handbook of Research on Oncological and Endoscopical Dilemmas in Modern Gynecological Clinical Practice* (pp. 1–21). IGI Global. https://doi.org/10.4018/978-1-7998-4213-2.ch001

Kalelioğlu, F., Gülbahar, Y., & Doğan, D. (2018). Teaching How to Think Like a Programmer: Emerging Insights. In H. Ozcinar, G. Wong, & H. Ozturk (Eds.), *Teaching Computational Thinking in Primary Education* (pp. 18–35). Hershey, PA: IGI Global. doi:10.4018/978-1-5225-3200-2.ch002

Kaljo, K., & Jacques, L. (2018). Flipping the Medical School Classroom. In M. Khosrow-Pour, D.B.A. (Ed.), Encyclopedia of Information Science and Technology, Fourth Edition (pp. 5800-5809). Hershey, PA: IGI Global. doi:10.4018/978-1-5225-2255-3.ch504

Kamberi, S. (2017). A Girls-Only Online Virtual World Environment and its Implications for Game-Based Learning. In A. Stricker, C. Calongne, B. Truman, & F. Arenas (Eds.), *Integrating an Awareness of Selfhood and Society into Virtual Learning* (pp. 74–95). Hershey, PA: IGI Global. doi:10.4018/978-1-5225-2182-2.ch006

Kamel, S., & Rizk, N. (2017). ICT Strategy Development: From Design to Implementation – Case of Egypt. In C. Howard & K. Hargiss (Eds.), *Strategic Information Systems and Technologies in Modern Organizations* (pp. 239–257). Hershey, PA: IGI Global. doi:10.4018/978-1-5225-1680-4.ch010

Kamel, S. H. (2018). The Potential Role of the Software Industry in Supporting Economic Development. In M. Khosrow-Pour, D.B.A. (Ed.), Encyclopedia of Information Science and Technology, Fourth Edition (pp. 7259-7269). Hershey, PA: IGI Global. doi:10.4018/978-1-5225-2255-3.ch631

Kang, H., Kang, Y., & Kim, J. (2022). Improved Fall Detection Model on GRU Using PoseNet. *International Journal of Software Innovation*, *10*(2), 1–11. https://doi.org/10.4018/IJSI.289600

Kankam, P. K. (2021). Employing Case Study and Survey Designs in Information Research. *Journal of Information Technology Research*, *14*(1), 167–177. https://doi.org/10.4018/JITR.2021010110

Karanfiloglu, M. (2021). The Role of Social Media Use in Health Communication: Digitized Health Communication During COVID-19 Pandemic. In G. Sarı (Eds.), *Handbook of Research on Representing Health and Medicine in Modern Media* (pp. 84-104). IGI Global. https://doi.org/10.4018/978-1-7998-6825-5.ch006

Karas, V., & Schuller, B. W. (2021). Deep Learning for Sentiment Analysis: An Overview and Perspectives. In F. Pinarbasi & M. Taskiran (Eds.), *Natural Language Processing for Global and Local Business* (pp. 97–132). IGI Global. https://doi.org/10.4018/978-1-7998-4240-8.ch005

Karthikeyan, P., Vasuki, S., & Karthik, K. (2019). Non-Subsampled Contourlet Transform-Based Effective Denoising of Medical Images: Denoising of Medical Images Using Contourlet. In A. Swarnambiga (Ed.), *Medical Image Processing for Improved Clinical Diagnosis* (pp. 155–183). IGI Global. https://doi.org/10.4018/978-1-5225-5876-7.ch008

Kashyap, R., & Rahamatkar, S. (2019). Medical Image Segmentation: An Advanced Approach. In S. Paul, P. Bhattacharya, & A. Bit (Eds.), *Early Detection of Neurological Disorders Using Machine Learning Systems* (pp. 292–321). IGI Global. https://doi.org/10.4018/978-1-5225-8567-1.ch015

Kasina, H., Bahubalendruni, M. V., & Botcha, R. (2017). Robots in Medicine: Past, Present and Future. *International Journal of Manufacturing, Materials, and Mechanical Engineering*, *7*(4), 44–64. doi:10.4018/IJMMME.2017100104

Katehakis, D. G. (2018). Electronic Medical Record Implementation Challenges for the National Health System in Greece. *International Journal of Reliable and Quality E-Healthcare*, *7*(1), 16–30. doi:10.4018/IJRQEH.2018010102

Katehakis, D. G., & Kouroubali, A. (2022). Digital Transformation Challenges for the Development of Quality Electronic Medical Records in Greece. In A. Moumtzoglou (Ed.), *Quality of Healthcare in the Aftermath of the COVID-19 Pandemic* (pp. 112–134). IGI Global. https://doi.org/10.4018/978-1-7998-9198-7.ch007

Kaufman, L. M. (2022). Reimagining the Magic of the Workshop Model. In T. Driscoll III, (Ed.), *Designing Effective Distance and Blended Learning Environments in K-12* (pp. 89–109). IGI Global. https://doi.org/10.4018/978-1-7998-6829-3.ch007

Kaur, P. D., & Sharma, P. (2017). Success Dimensions of ICTs in Healthcare. In B. Singh (Ed.), *Computational Tools and Techniques for Biomedical Signal Processing* (pp. 149–173). Hershey, PA: IGI Global. doi:10.4018/978-1-5225-0660-7.ch007

Kaushik, P. (2018). Comorbidity of Medical and Psychiatric Disorders in Geriatric Population: Treatment and Care. In B. Prasad & S. Akbar (Eds.), *Handbook of Research on Geriatric Health, Treatment, and Care* (pp. 448–474). Hershey, PA: IGI Global. doi:10.4018/978-1-5225-3480-8.ch025

Kawata, S. (2018). Computer-Assisted Parallel Program Generation. In M. Khosrow-Pour, D.B.A. (Ed.), Encyclopedia of Information Science and Technology, Fourth Edition (pp. 4583-4593). Hershey, PA: IGI Global. doi:10.4018/978-1-5225-2255-3.ch398

Khachane, M. Y. (2017). Organ-Based Medical Image Classification Using Support Vector Machine. *International Journal of Synthetic Emotions*, *8*(1), 18–30. doi:10.4018/IJSE.2017010102

Kharb, L., & Singh, P. (2021). Role of Machine Learning in Modern Education and Teaching. In S. Verma & P. Tomar (Ed.), *Impact of AI Technologies on Teaching, Learning, and Research in Higher Education* (pp. 99-123). IGI Global. https://doi.org/10.4018/978-1-7998-4763-2.ch006

Kharbanda, V., Madaan, R., & Bhatia, K. K. (2021). Incautious Usage of Social Media: Impact on Emotional Intelligence and Health Concerns. In D. Yadav, A. Bansal, M. Bhatia, M. Hooda, & J. Morato (Eds.), *Diagnostic Applications of Health Intelligence and Surveillance Systems* (pp. 172–186). IGI Global. https://doi.org/10.4018/978-1-7998-6527-8.ch008

Khari, M., Shrivastava, G., Gupta, S., & Gupta, R. (2017). Role of Cyber Security in Today's Scenario. In R. Kumar, P. Pattnaik, & P. Pandey (Eds.), *Detecting and Mitigating Robotic Cyber Security Risks* (pp. 177–191). Hershey, PA: IGI Global. doi:10.4018/978-1-5225-2154-9.ch013

Khekare, G., & Sheikh, S. (2021). Autonomous Navigation Using Deep Reinforcement Learning in ROS. *International Journal of Artificial Intelligence and Machine Learning*, *11*(2), 63–70. https://doi.org/10.4018/IJAIML.20210701.oa4

Khouja, M., Rodriguez, I. B., Ben Halima, Y., & Moalla, S. (2018). IT Governance in Higher Education Institutions: A Systematic Literature Review. *International Journal of Human Capital and Information Technology Professionals*, *9*(2), 52–67. doi:10.4018/IJHCITP.2018040104

Kiourt, C., Pavlidis, G., Koutsoudis, A., & Kalles, D. (2017). Realistic Simulation of Cultural Heritage. *International Journal of Computational Methods in Heritage Science*, *1*(1), 10–40. doi:10.4018/IJCMHS.2017010102

Kirci, P. (2018). Intelligent Techniques for Analysis of Big Data About Healthcare and Medical Records. In N. Shah & M. Mittal (Eds.), *Handbook of Research on Promoting Business Process Improvement Through Inventory Control Techniques* (pp. 559–582). Hershey, PA: IGI Global. doi:10.4018/978-1-5225-3232-3.ch029

Kldiashvili, E. (2018). Cloud Approach for the Medical Information System: MIS on Cloud. In M. Khosrow-Pour (Ed.), *Incorporating Nature-Inspired Paradigms in Computational Applications* (pp. 238–261). Hershey, PA: IGI Global. doi:10.4018/978-1-5225-5020-4.ch008

Ko, H., Mesicek, L., Choi, J., Choi, J., & Hwang, S. (2018). A Study on Secure Contents Strategies for Applications With DRM on Cloud Computing. *International Journal of Cloud Applications and Computing*, *8*(1), 143–153. doi:10.4018/IJCAC.2018010107

Komendziński, T., Mikołajewska, E., & Mikołajewski, D. (2018). Cross-Cultural Decision-Making in Healthcare: Theory and Practical Application in Real Clinical Conditions. In A. Rosiek-Kryszewska & K. Leksowski (Eds.), *Healthcare Administration for Patient Safety and Engagement* (pp. 276–298). Hershey, PA: IGI Global. doi:10.4018/978-1-5225-3946-9.ch015

Konecny, L. T. (2018). Medical School Wellness Initiatives. In C. Smith (Ed.), *Exploring the Pressures of Medical Education From a Mental Health and Wellness Perspective* (pp. 209–228). Hershey, PA: IGI Global. doi:10.4018/978-1-5225-2811-1.ch009

Köse, U. (2017). An Augmented-Reality-Based Intelligent Mobile Application for Open Computer Education. In G. Kurubacak & H. Altinpulluk (Eds.), *Mobile Technologies and Augmented Reality in Open Education* (pp. 154–174). Hershey, PA: IGI Global. doi:10.4018/978-1-5225-2110-5.ch008

Kromrei, H., Solomonson, W. L., & Juzych, M. S. (2017). Teaching Residents How to Teach. In J. Stefaniak (Ed.), *Advancing Medical Education Through Strategic Instructional Design* (pp. 164–185). Hershey, PA: IGI Global. doi:10.4018/978-1-5225-2098-6.ch008

Kulkarni, S., Savyanavar, A., Kulkarni, P., Stranieri, A., & Ghorpade, V. (2018). Framework for Integration of Medical Image and Text-Based Report Retrieval to Support Radiological Diagnosis. In M. Kolekar & V. Kumar (Eds.), *Biomedical Signal and Image Processing in Patient Care* (pp. 86–122). Hershey, PA: IGI Global. doi:10.4018/978-1-5225-2829-6.ch006

Kumar, A., & Sarkar, B. K. (2018). Performance Analysis of Nature-Inspired Algorithms-Based Bayesian Prediction Models for Medical Data Sets. In U. Singh, A. Tiwari, & R. Singh (Eds.), *Soft-Computing-Based Nonlinear Control Systems Design* (pp. 134–155). Hershey, PA: IGI Global. doi:10.4018/978-1-5225-3531-7.ch007

Labbadi, W., & Akaichi, J. (2017). Efficient Algorithm for Answering Fuzzy Medical Requests in Pervasive Healthcare Information Systems. *International Journal of Healthcare Information Systems and Informatics, 12*(2), 46–64. doi:10.4018/IJHISI.2017040103

Lagumdzija, A., & Swing, V. K. (2017). Health, Digitalization, and Individual Empowerment. In F. Topor (Ed.), *Handbook of Research on Individualism and Identity in the Globalized Digital Age* (pp. 380–402). Hershey, PA: IGI Global. doi:10.4018/978-1-5225-0522-8.ch017

Lahmiri, S. (2018). Information Technology Outsourcing Risk Factors and Provider Selection. In M. Gupta, R. Sharman, J. Walp, & P. Mulgund (Eds.), *Information Technology Risk Management and Compliance in Modern Organizations* (pp. 214–228). Hershey, PA: IGI Global. doi:10.4018/978-1-5225-2604-9.ch008

Lakkad, A. K., Bhadaniya, R. D., Shah, V. N., & Lavanya, K. (2021). Complex Events Processing on Live News Events Using Apache Kafka and Clustering Techniques. *International Journal of Intelligent Information Technologies, 17*(1), 39–52. https://doi.org/10.4018/IJIIT.2021010103

Lamey, T. W., & Davidson-Shivers, G. V. (2017). Instructional Strategies and Sequencing. In J. Stefaniak (Ed.), *Advancing Medical Education Through Strategic Instructional Design* (pp. 30–52). Hershey, PA: IGI Global. doi:10.4018/978-1-5225-2098-6.ch002

Landriscina, F. (2017). Computer-Supported Imagination: The Interplay Between Computer and Mental Simulation in Understanding Scientific Concepts. In I. Levin & D. Tsybulsky (Eds.), *Digital Tools and Solutions for Inquiry-Based STEM Learning* (pp. 33–60). Hershey, PA: IGI Global. doi:10.4018/978-1-5225-2525-7.ch002

Lara López, G. (2021). Virtual Reality in Object Location. In A. Negrón & M. Muñoz (Eds.), *Latin American Women and Research Contributions to the IT Field* (pp. 307–324). IGI Global. https://doi.org/10.4018/978-1-7998-7552-9.ch014

Lee, D. C., & Gefen, D. (2020). Promises and Challenges of Medical Patient Healthcare Portals in Underserved Communities: The Case of Einstein Medical Center Philadelphia (EMCP). In R. McHaney, I. Reychev, J. Azuri, M. McHaney, & R. Moshonov (Eds.), *Impacts of Information Technology on Patient Care and Empowerment* (pp. 219–251). IGI Global. https://doi.org/10.4018/978-1-7998-0047-7.ch012

Lee, W. W. (2018). Ethical Computing Continues From Problem to Solution. In M. Khosrow-Pour, D.B.A. (Ed.), Encyclopedia of Information Science and Technology, Fourth Edition (pp. 4884-4897). Hershey, PA: IGI Global. doi:10.4018/978-1-5225-2255-3.ch423

Leon, G. (2017). The Role of Forensic Medicine in Medical Errors. In M. Riga (Ed.), *Impact of Medical Errors and Malpractice on Health Economics, Quality, and Patient Safety* (pp. 144–170). Hershey, PA: IGI Global. doi:10.4018/978-1-5225-2337-6.ch006

Leung, L. Y. (2020). Representation of Gender Equality From the Perspective of the Medical Trainee and its Ripple Effect: Highlighting Gender Inequality in Medical Student Experiences. In M. Bellini & V. Papalois (Eds.), *Gender Equity in the Medical Profession* (pp. 29–50). IGI Global. https://doi.org/10.4018/978-1-5225-9599-1.ch003

Lin, S., Chen, S., & Chuang, S. (2017). Perceived Innovation and Quick Response Codes in an Online-to-Offline E-Commerce Service Model. *International Journal of E-Adoption*, *9*(2), 1–16. doi:10.4018/IJEA.2017070101

Liu, M., Wang, Y., Xu, W., & Liu, L. (2017). Automated Scoring of Chinese Engineering Students' English Essays. *International Journal of Distance Education Technologies*, *15*(1), 52–68. doi:10.4018/IJDET.2017010104

Lopes, M. J., Fonseca, C., & Barbosa, P. (2020). The Individual Care Plan as Electronic Health Record: A Tool for Management, Integration of Care, and Better Health Results. In D. Mendes, C. Fonseca, M. Lopes, J. García-Alonso, & J. Murillo (Eds.), *Exploring the Role of ICTs in Healthy Aging* (pp. 1–12). IGI Global. https://doi.org/10.4018/978-1-7998-1937-0.ch001

Love, L., & McDowelle, D. (2018). Developing a Comprehensive Wellness Program for Medical Students. In C. Smith (Ed.), *Exploring the Pressures of Medical Education From a Mental Health and Wellness Perspective* (pp. 190–208). Hershey, PA: IGI Global. doi:10.4018/978-1-5225-2811-1.ch008

Lovell, K. L. (2017). Development and Evaluation of Neuroscience Computer-Based Modules for Medical Students: Instructional Design Principles and Effectiveness. In J. Stefaniak (Ed.), *Advancing Medical Education Through Strategic Instructional Design* (pp. 262–276). Hershey, PA: IGI Global. doi:10.4018/978-1-5225-2098-6.ch013

Lubin, R., & Hamlin, M. D. (2018). Medical Student Burnout: A Social Cognitive Learning Perspective on Medical Student Mental Health and Wellness. In C. Smith (Ed.), *Exploring the Pressures of Medical Education From a Mental Health and Wellness Perspective* (pp. 92–121). Hershey, PA: IGI Global. doi:10.4018/978-1-5225-2811-1.ch004

Luk, C. Y. (2018). Moving Towards Universal Health Coverage: Challenges for the Present and Future in China. In B. Fong, A. Ng, & P. Yuen (Eds.), *Sustainable Health and Long-Term Care Solutions for an Aging Population* (pp. 19–45). Hershey, PA: IGI Global. doi:10.4018/978-1-5225-2633-9.ch002

Ma, X., Li, X., Zhong, B., Huang, Y., Gu, Y., Wu, M., Liu, Y., & Zhang, M. (2021). A Detector and Evaluation Framework of Abnormal Bidding Behavior Based on Supplier Portrait. *International Journal of Information Technology and Web Engineering, 16*(2), 58–74. https://doi.org/10.4018/IJITWE.2021040104

Mabe, L. K., & Oladele, O. I. (2017). Application of Information Communication Technologies for Agricultural Development through Extension Services: A Review. In T. Tossy (Ed.), *Information Technology Integration for Socio-Economic Development* (pp. 52–101). Hershey, PA: IGI Global. doi:10.4018/978-1-5225-0539-6.ch003

Mackintosh, S. E., & Katsaros, E. (2020). Building Interprofessional Competencies Into Medical Education and Assessment. In S. Waldman & S. Bowlin (Eds.), *Building a Patient-Centered Interprofessional Education Program* (pp. 84–112). IGI Global. https://doi.org/10.4018/978-1-7998-3066-5.ch005

Magalhães, J. L., Quoniam, L., Hartz, Z., Silveira, H., & Rito, P. D. (2022). Knowledge Management in Big Data Times for Global Health: Challenges for Quality in One Health. In J. Lima de Magalhães, Z. Hartz, G. Jamil, H. Silveira, & L. Jamil (Eds.), *Handbook of Research on Essential Information Approaches to Aiding Global Health in the One Health Context* (pp. 149–163). IGI Global. https://doi.org/10.4018/978-1-7998-8011-0.ch008

Mahat, M., & Pettigrew, A. (2017). The Regulatory Environment of Non-Profit Higher Education and Research Institutions and Its Implications for Managerial Strategy: The Case of Medical Education and Research. In L. West & A. Worthington (Eds.), *Handbook of Research on Emerging Business Models and Managerial Strategies in the Nonprofit Sector* (pp. 336–351). Hershey, PA: IGI Global. doi:10.4018/978-1-5225-2537-0.ch017

Mahboub, S. A., Sayed Ali Ahmed, E., & Saeed, R. A. (2021). Smart IDS and IPS for Cyber-Physical Systems. In A. Luhach & A. Elçi (Eds.), *Artificial Intelligence Paradigms for Smart Cyber-Physical Systems* (pp. 109–136). IGI Global. https://doi.org/10.4018/978-1-7998-5101-1.ch006

Maitra, I. K., & Bandhyopadhyaay, S. K. (2017). Adaptive Edge Detection Method towards Features Extraction from Diverse Medical Imaging Technologies. In S. Bhattacharyya, S. De, I. Pan, & P. Dutta (Eds.), *Intelligent Multidimensional Data Clustering and Analysis* (pp. 159–192). Hershey, PA: IGI Global. doi:10.4018/978-1-5225-1776-4.ch007

Mane, V. M., Patki, S., Dhumma, A. V., & Apte, K. J. (2022). Telehealth System for Effective Treatment in COVID-19 Pandemics. In A. Thakare, S. Wagh, M. Bhende, A. Anter, & X. Gao (Eds.), *Handbook of Research on Applied Intelligence for Health and Clinical Informatics* (pp. 328–339). IGI Global. https://doi.org/10.4018/978-1-7998-7709-7.ch019

Mangu, V. P. (2017). Mobile Health Care: A Technology View. In C. Bhatt & S. Peddoju (Eds.), *Cloud Computing Systems and Applications in Healthcare* (pp. 1–18). Hershey, PA: IGI Global. doi:10.4018/978-1-5225-1002-4.ch001

Manirabona, A., Fourati, L. C., & Boudjit, S. (2017). Investigation on Healthcare Monitoring Systems: Innovative Services and Applications. *International Journal of E-Health and Medical Communications*, *8*(1), 1–18. doi:10.4018/IJEHMC.2017010101

Manogaran, G., Thota, C., & Lopez, D. (2018). Human-Computer Interaction With Big Data Analytics. In D. Lopez & M. Durai (Eds.), *HCI Challenges and Privacy Preservation in Big Data Security* (pp. 1–22). Hershey, PA: IGI Global. doi:10.4018/978-1-5225-2863-0.ch001

Margolis, J., Goode, J., & Flapan, J. (2017). A Critical Crossroads for Computer Science for All: "Identifying Talent" or "Building Talent," and What Difference Does It Make? In Y. Rankin & J. Thomas (Eds.), *Moving Students of Color from Consumers to Producers of Technology* (pp. 1–23). Hershey, PA: IGI Global. doi:10.4018/978-1-5225-2005-4.ch001

Martins, C. L., Martinho, D., Marreiros, G., Conceição, L., Faria, L., & Simões de Almeida, R. (2022). Artificial Intelligence in Digital Mental Health. In A. Marques & R. Queirós (Eds.), *Digital Therapies in Psychosocial Rehabilitation and Mental Health* (pp. 201–225). IGI Global. https://doi.org/10.4018/978-1-7998-8634-1.ch010

Marwan, M., Kartit, A., & Ouahmane, H. (2018). A Framework to Secure Medical Image Storage in Cloud Computing Environment. *Journal of Electronic Commerce in Organizations*, *16*(1), 1–16. doi:10.4018/JECO.2018010101

Mason, A., Bhati, S., Jiang, R., & Spencer, E. A. (2020). Medical Tourism Patient Mortality: Considerations From a 10-Year Review of Global News Media Representations. In M. Merviö (Ed.), *Global Issues and Innovative Solutions in Healthcare, Culture, and the Environment* (pp. 206–225). IGI Global. https://doi.org/10.4018/978-1-7998-3576-9.ch011

Masoud, M. P., Nejad, M. K., Darebaghi, H., Chavoshi, M., & Farahani, M. (2018). The Decision Support System and Conventional Method of Telephone Triage by Nurses in Emergency Medical Services: A Comparative Investigation. *International Journal of E-Business Research*, *14*(1), 77–88. doi:10.4018/IJEBR.2018010105

Mathew, N. E., Walter, A., & Eapen, V. (2020). Mental Health Challenges in Children With Intellectual Disabilities. In R. Gopalan (Ed.), *Developmental Challenges and Societal Issues for Individuals With Intellectual Disabilities* (pp. 13–39). IGI Global. https://doi.org/10.4018/978-1-7998-1223-4.ch002

Mazzola, A. (2020). The Social Mandate to Deal With Mental Health: A Comparison Between Interventions in a Mental Health Center, a School, and a Psychoanalytic Office. In S. Padmanaban & C. Subudhi (Eds.), *Psycho-Social Perspectives on Mental Health and Well-Being* (pp. 234–254). IGI Global. https://doi.org/10.4018/978-1-7998-1185-5.ch012

Mazzù, M. F., Benetton, A., Baccelloni, A., & Lavini, L. (2022). A Milk Blockchain-Enabled Supply Chain: Evidence From Leading Italian Farms. In P. De Giovanni (Ed.), *Blockchain Technology Applications in Businesses and Organizations* (pp. 73–98). IGI Global. https://doi.org/10.4018/978-1-7998-8014-1.ch004

Mbale, J. (2018). Computer Centres Resource Cloud Elasticity-Scalability (CRECES): Copperbelt University Case Study. In S. Aljawarneh & M. Malhotra (Eds.), *Critical Research on Scalability and Security Issues in Virtual Cloud Environments* (pp. 48–70). Hershey, PA: IGI Global. doi:10.4018/978-1-5225-3029-9.ch003

McDonald, W. G., Martin, M., & Salzberg, L. D. (2018). From Medical Student to Medical Resident: Graduate Medical Education and Mental Health in the United States. In C. Smith (Ed.), *Exploring the Pressures of Medical Education From a Mental Health and Wellness Perspective* (pp. 145–169). Hershey, PA: IGI Global. doi:10.4018/978-1-5225-2811-1.ch006

McGrowder, D. A., Miller, F. G., Nwokocha, C., Wilson-Clarke, C. F., Anderson, M., Anderson-Jackson, L., Williams, L., & Alexander-Lindo, R. (2021). Medical Herbs and the Treatment of Diabetes Mellitus: Mechanisms of Action. In A. Hussain & S. Behl (Eds.), *Treating Endocrine and Metabolic Disorders With Herbal Medicines* (pp. 48–73). IGI Global. https://doi.org/10.4018/978-1-7998-4808-0.ch003

McKee, J. (2018). The Right Information: The Key to Effective Business Planning. In *Business Architectures for Risk Assessment and Strategic Planning: Emerging Research and Opportunities* (pp. 38–52). Hershey, PA: IGI Global. doi:10.4018/978-1-5225-3392-4.ch003

Meddah, I. H., Remil, N. E., & Meddah, H. N. (2021). Novel Approach for Mining Patterns. *International Journal of Applied Evolutionary Computation, 12*(1), 27–42. https://doi.org/10.4018/IJAEC.2021010103

Medhekar, A. (2017). The Role of Social Media for Knowledge Dissemination in Medical Tourism: A Case of India. In R. Chugh (Ed.), *Harnessing Social Media as a Knowledge Management Tool* (pp. 25–54). Hershey, PA: IGI Global. doi:10.4018/978-1-5225-0495-5.ch002

Medhekar, A. (2020). Digital Health Innovation Enhancing Patient Experience in Medical Travel. In K. Sandhu (Ed.), *Opportunities and Challenges in Digital Healthcare Innovation* (pp. 13–35). IGI Global. https://doi.org/10.4018/978-1-7998-3274-4.ch002

Medhekar, A., & Haq, F. (2018). Urbanization and New Jobs Creation in Healthcare Services in India: Challenges and Opportunities. In U. Benna & I. Benna (Eds.), *Urbanization and Its Impact on Socio-Economic Growth in Developing Regions* (pp. 198–218). Hershey, PA: IGI Global. doi:10.4018/978-1-5225-2659-9.ch010

Mehta, P. (2017). Framework of Indian Healthcare System and its Challenges: An Insight. In V. Bryan & J. Bird (Eds.), *Healthcare Community Synergism between Patients, Practitioners, and Researchers* (pp. 247–271). Hershey, PA: IGI Global. doi:10.4018/978-1-5225-0640-9.ch011

Mendes, E., Sousa, B. B., & Gonçalves, M. (2021). The Role of Technologies in Relationship Management and Internal Marketing: An Approach in the Health Sector. In J. Santos, & I. Pereira (Ed.), *Management and Marketing for Improved Competitiveness and Performance in the Healthcare Sector* (pp. 213-237). IGI Global. https://doi.org/10.4018/978-1-7998-7263-4.ch010

Mensah, I. K., & Mi, J. (2018). Determinants of Intention to Use Local E-Government Services in Ghana: The Perspective of Local Government Workers. *International Journal of Technology Diffusion*, *9*(2), 41–60. doi:10.4018/IJTD.2018040103

Meyer, T. M., & Simen, J. H. (2020). Geriatric Interprofessional Education: A Practical Guide for Health Professions Educators. In S. Waldman & S. Bowlin (Eds.), *Building a Patient-Centered Interprofessional Education Program* (pp. 120–136). IGI Global. https://doi.org/10.4018/978-1-7998-3066-5.ch007

Mi, M. (2017). Informal Learning in Medical Education. In J. Stefaniak (Ed.), *Advancing Medical Education Through Strategic Instructional Design* (pp. 225–244). Hershey, PA: IGI Global. doi:10.4018/978-1-5225-2098-6.ch011

Mishra, K., & Thomas, R. (2022). Low Cost, User-Controlled Peroneal Stimulator for Foot Drop in Patients With Stroke: An Experiment in Indian Rehabilitation Set-Up. In F. Stasolla (Ed.), *Assistive Technologies for Assessment and Recovery of Neurological Impairments* (pp. 279–303). IGI Global. https://doi.org/10.4018/978-1-7998-7430-0.ch014

Mishra, S., & Panda, M. (2019). Artificial Intelligence in Medical Science. In N. Bouchemal (Ed.), *Intelligent Systems for Healthcare Management and Delivery* (pp. 306–330). IGI Global. https://doi.org/10.4018/978-1-5225-7071-4.ch014

Mohamed, J. H. (2018). Scientograph-Based Visualization of Computer Forensics Research Literature. In J. Jeyasekar & P. Saravanan (Eds.), *Innovations in Measuring and Evaluating Scientific Information* (pp. 148–162). Hershey, PA: IGI Global. doi:10.4018/978-1-5225-3457-0.ch010

Montañés-Del Río, M. Á., Cornejo, V. R., Rodríguez, M. R., & Ortiz, J. S. (2021). Gamification of University Subjects: A Case Study for Operations Management. *Journal of Information Technology Research*, *14*(2), 1–29. https://doi.org/10.4018/JITR.2021040101

Moore, R. L., & Johnson, N. (2017). Earning a Seat at the Table: How IT Departments Can Partner in Organizational Change and Innovation. *International Journal of Knowledge-Based Organizations*, *7*(2), 1–12. doi:10.4018/IJKBO.2017040101

Mosadeghrad, A. M., & Woldemichael, A. (2017). Application of Quality Management in Promoting Patient Safety and Preventing Medical Errors. In M. Riga (Ed.), *Impact of Medical Errors and Malpractice on Health Economics, Quality, and Patient Safety* (pp. 91–112). Hershey, PA: IGI Global. doi:10.4018/978-1-5225-2337-6.ch004

Moumtzoglou, A. (2017). Digital Medicine: The Quality Standpoint. In A. Moumtzoglou (Ed.), *Design, Development, and Integration of Reliable Electronic Healthcare Platforms* (pp. 179–195). Hershey, PA: IGI Global. doi:10.4018/978-1-5225-1724-5.ch011

Moumtzoglou, A., & Pouliakis, A. (2018). Population Health Management and the Science of Individuality. *International Journal of Reliable and Quality E-Healthcare, 7*(2), 1–26. doi:10.4018/IJRQEH.2018040101

Mukhtar, W. F., & Abuelyaman, E. S. (2017). Opportunities and Challenges of Big Data in Healthcare. In N. Wickramasinghe (Ed.), *Handbook of Research on Healthcare Administration and Management* (pp. 47–58). Hershey, PA: IGI Global. doi:10.4018/978-1-5225-0920-2.ch004

Mukul, M. K., & Bhattaharyya, S. (2017). Brain-Machine Interface: Human-Computer Interaction. In E. Noughabi, B. Raahemi, A. Albadvi, & B. Far (Eds.), *Handbook of Research on Data Science for Effective Healthcare Practice and Administration* (pp. 417–443). Hershey, PA: IGI Global. doi:10.4018/978-1-5225-2515-8.ch018

Munugala, S., Brar, G. K., Syed, A., Mohammad, A., & Halgamuge, M. N. (2018). The Much Needed Security and Data Reforms of Cloud Computing in Medical Data Storage. In M. Lytras & P. Papadopoulou (Eds.), *Applying Big Data Analytics in Bioinformatics and Medicine* (pp. 99–113). Hershey, PA: IGI Global. doi:10.4018/978-1-5225-2607-0.ch005

Na, L. (2017). Library and Information Science Education and Graduate Programs in Academic Libraries. In L. Ruan, Q. Zhu, & Y. Ye (Eds.), *Academic Library Development and Administration in China* (pp. 218–229). Hershey, PA: IGI Global. doi:10.4018/978-1-5225-0550-1.ch013

Nagpal, G., Bishnoi, G. K., Dhami, H. S., & Vijayvargia, A. (2021). Use of Data Analytics to Increase the Efficiency of Last Mile Logistics for Ecommerce Deliveries. In B. Patil & M. Vohra (Eds.), *Handbook of Research on Engineering, Business, and Healthcare Applications of Data Science and Analytics* (pp. 167–180). IGI Global. https://doi.org/10.4018/978-1-7998-3053-5.ch009

Naha, N., & Manickavachagam, G. (2021). Textile Industry and Health Hazards: Impact of Climate Change Issues and Fertility Potential. In K. Wani, & N. Naha (Ed.), *Climate Change and Its Impact on Fertility* (pp. 42-69). IGI Global. https://doi.org/10.4018/978-1-7998-4480-8.ch003

Nair, L. D. (2019). Childhood Neurodegenerative Disorders. In M. Uddin & M. Amran (Eds.), *Handbook of Research on Critical Examinations of Neurodegenerative Disorders* (pp. 385–412). IGI Global. https://doi.org/10.4018/978-1-5225-5282-6.ch018

Nair, S. M., Ramesh, V., & Tyagi, A. K. (2021). Issues and Challenges (Privacy, Security, and Trust) in Blockchain-Based Applications. In A. Tyagi, G. Rekha, & N. Sreenath (Eds.), *Opportunities and Challenges for Blockchain Technology in Autonomous Vehicles* (pp. 196–209). IGI Global. https://doi.org/10.4018/978-1-7998-3295-9.ch012

Naomi, J. F. M., K., & V., S. (2021). Machine and Deep Learning Techniques in IoT and Cloud. In S. Velayutham (Ed.), *Challenges and Opportunities for the Convergence of IoT, Big Data, and Cloud Computing* (pp. 225-247). IGI Global. https://doi.org/10.4018/978-1-7998-3111-2.ch013

Nath, R., & Murthy, V. N. (2018). What Accounts for the Differences in Internet Diffusion Rates Around the World? In M. Khosrow-Pour, D.B.A. (Ed.), Encyclopedia of Information Science and Technology, Fourth Edition (pp. 8095-8104). Hershey, PA: IGI Global. https://doi.org/ doi:10.4018/978-1-5225-2255-3.ch705

Nayak, S. R., & Mishra, J. (2019). Analysis of Medical Images Using Fractal Geometry. In N. Dey, A. Ashour, H. Kalia, R. Goswami, & H. Das (Eds.), *Histopathological Image Analysis in Medical Decision Making* (pp. 181–201). IGI Global. https://doi.org/10.4018/978-1-5225-6316-7.ch008

Nedelko, Z., & Potocan, V. (2018). The Role of Emerging Information Technologies for Supporting Supply Chain Management. In M. Khosrow-Pour, D.B.A. (Ed.), Encyclopedia of Information Science and Technology, Fourth Edition (pp. 5559-5569). Hershey, PA: IGI Global. doi:10.4018/978-1-5225-2255-3.ch483

Negrini, L., Giang, C., & Bonnet, E. (2022). Designing Tools and Activities for Educational Robotics in Online Learning. In N. Eteokleous & E. Nisiforou (Eds.), *Designing, Constructing, and Programming Robots for Learning* (pp. 202–222). IGI Global. https://doi.org/10.4018/978-1-7998-7443-0.ch010

Netto, J. T., Hartz, Z., & de Magalhães, J. L. (2022). One Health and Information Management Using Big Data in Health: A Brazilian Case Study for COVID-19. In J. Lima de Magalhães, Z. Hartz, G. Jamil, H. Silveira, & L. Jamil (Eds.), *Handbook of Research on Essential Information Approaches to Aiding Global Health in the One Health Context* (pp. 36–51). IGI Global. https://doi.org/10.4018/978-1-7998-8011-0.ch003

Ngafeeson, M. N. (2018). User Resistance to Health Information Technology. In M. Khosrow-Pour, D.B.A. (Ed.), Encyclopedia of Information Science and Technology, Fourth Edition (pp. 3816-3825). Hershey, PA: IGI Global. doi:10.4018/978-1-5225-2255-3.ch331

Ngara, R. (2017). Multiple Voices, Multiple Paths: Towards Dialogue between Western and Indigenous Medical Knowledge Systems. In P. Ngulube (Ed.), *Handbook of Research on Theoretical Perspectives on Indigenous Knowledge Systems in Developing Countries* (pp. 332–358). Hershey, PA: IGI Global. doi:10.4018/978-1-5225-0833-5.ch015

Nguyen, T. T., Giang, N. L., Tran, D. T., Nguyen, T. T., Nguyen, H. Q., Pham, A. V., & Vu, T. D. (2021). A Novel Filter-Wrapper Algorithm on Intuitionistic Fuzzy Set for Attribute Reduction From Decision Tables. *International Journal of Data Warehousing and Mining*, *17*(4), 67–100. https://doi.org/10.4018/IJDWM.2021100104

Nigam, A., & Dewani, P. P. (2022). Consumer Engagement Through Conditional Promotions: An Exploratory Study. *Journal of Global Information Management*, *30*(5), 1–19. https://doi.org/10.4018/JGIM.290364

Nikumbh, D. D., Sayyad, S., Joshi, R. R., Dubey, K. S., Mehta, D. V., & Matta, D. K. (2022). Applied Intelligence for Medical Diagnosing. In A. Thakare, S. Wagh, M. Bhende, A. Anter, & X. Gao (Eds.), *Handbook of Research on Applied Intelligence for Health and Clinical Informatics* (pp. 44–79). IGI Global. https://doi.org/10.4018/978-1-7998-7709-7.ch004

O'Connor, Y., & Heavin, C. (2018). Defining and Characterising the Landscape of eHealth. In M. Khosrow-Pour, D.B.A. (Ed.), Encyclopedia of Information Science and Technology, Fourth Edition (pp. 5864-5875). Hershey, PA: IGI Global. doi:10.4018/978-1-5225-2255-3.ch510

Ochonogor, W. C., & Okite-Amughoro, F. A. (2018). Building an Effective Digital Library in a University Teaching Hospital (UTH) in Nigeria. In A. Tella & T. Kwanya (Eds.), *Handbook of Research on Managing Intellectual Property in Digital Libraries* (pp. 184–204). Hershey, PA: IGI Global. doi:10.4018/978-1-5225-3093-0.ch010

Odagiri, K. (2017). Introduction of Individual Technology to Constitute the Current Internet. In *Strategic Policy-Based Network Management in Contemporary Organizations* (pp. 20–96). Hershey, PA: IGI Global. doi:10.4018/978-1-68318-003-6.ch003

Odia, J. O., & Akpata, O. T. (2021). Role of Data Science and Data Analytics in Forensic Accounting and Fraud Detection. In B. Patil & M. Vohra (Eds.), *Handbook of Research on Engineering, Business, and Healthcare Applications of Data Science and Analytics* (pp. 203–227). IGI Global. https://doi.org/10.4018/978-1-7998-3053-5.ch011

Okike, E. U. (2018). Computer Science and Prison Education. In I. Biao (Ed.), *Strategic Learning Ideologies in Prison Education Programs* (pp. 246–264). Hershey, PA: IGI Global. doi:10.4018/978-1-5225-2909-5.ch012

Olelewe, C. J., & Nwafor, I. P. (2017). Level of Computer Appreciation Skills Acquired for Sustainable Development by Secondary School Students in Nsukka LGA of Enugu State, Nigeria. In C. Ayo & V. Mbarika (Eds.), *Sustainable ICT Adoption and Integration for Socio-Economic Development* (pp. 214–233). Hershey, PA: IGI Global. doi:10.4018/978-1-5225-2565-3.ch010

Olivares, S. L., Cruz, A. G., Cabrera, M. V., Regalado, A. I., & García, J. E. (2017). An Assessment Study of Quality Model for Medical Schools in Mexico. In S. Mukerji & P. Tripathi (Eds.), *Handbook of Research on Administration, Policy, and Leadership in Higher Education* (pp. 404–439). Hershey, PA: IGI Global. doi:10.4018/978-1-5225-0672-0.ch016

Oliveira, M., Maçada, A. C., Curado, C., & Nodari, F. (2017). Infrastructure Profiles and Knowledge Sharing. *International Journal of Technology and Human Interaction*, *13*(3), 1–12. doi:10.4018/IJTHI.2017070101

Omoruyi, E. A., & Omidele, F. (2018). Resident Physician and Medical Academic Faculty Burnout: A Review of Current Literature. In C. Smith (Ed.), *Exploring the Pressures of Medical Education From a Mental Health and Wellness Perspective* (pp. 171–189). Hershey, PA: IGI Global. doi:10.4018/978-1-5225-2811-1.ch007

Otarkhani, A., Shokouhyar, S., & Pour, S. S. (2017). Analyzing the Impact of Governance of Enterprise IT on Hospital Performance: Tehran's (Iran) Hospitals – A Case Study. *International Journal of Healthcare Information Systems and Informatics*, *12*(3), 1–20. doi:10.4018/IJHISI.2017070101

Otunla, A. O., & Amuda, C. O. (2018). Nigerian Undergraduate Students' Computer Competencies and Use of Information Technology Tools and Resources for Study Skills and Habits' Enhancement. In M. Khosrow-Pour, D.B.A. (Ed.), Encyclopedia of Information Science and Technology, Fourth Edition (pp. 2303-2313). Hershey, PA: IGI Global. https://doi.org/ doi:10.4018/978-1-5225-2255-3.ch200

Özçınar, H. (2018). A Brief Discussion on Incentives and Barriers to Computational Thinking Education. In H. Ozcinar, G. Wong, & H. Ozturk (Eds.), *Teaching Computational Thinking in Primary Education* (pp. 1–17). Hershey, PA: IGI Global. doi:10.4018/978-1-5225-3200-2.ch001

Pandey, A., Singh, B., Saini, B. S., & Sood, N. (2019). Medical Data Security Tools and Techniques in E-Health Applications. In B. Singh, B. Saini, D. Singh, & A. Pandey (Eds.), *Medical Data Security for Bioengineers* (pp. 124–131). IGI Global. https://doi.org/10.4018/978-1-5225-7952-6.ch006

Pandey, J. M., Garg, S., Mishra, P., & Mishra, B. P. (2017). Computer Based Psychological Interventions: Subject to the Efficacy of Psychological Services. *International Journal of Computers in Clinical Practice*, *2*(1), 25–33. doi:10.4018/IJCCP.2017010102

Pandkar, S. D., & Paatil, S. D. (2021). Big Data and Knowledge Resource Centre. In S. Dhamdhere (Ed.), *Big Data Applications for Improving Library Services* (pp. 90–106). IGI Global. https://doi.org/10.4018/978-1-7998-3049-8.ch007

Papadopoulou, P., Lytras, M., & Marouli, C. (2018). Bioinformatics as Applied to Medicine: Challenges Faced Moving from Big Data to Smart Data to Wise Data. In M. Lytras & P. Papadopoulou (Eds.), *Applying Big Data Analytics in Bioinformatics and Medicine* (pp. 1–25). Hershey, PA: IGI Global. doi:10.4018/978-1-5225-2607-0.ch001

Paraskou, A., & George, B. P. (2018). An Overview of Reproductive Tourism. In *Legal and Economic Considerations Surrounding Reproductive Tourism: Emerging Research and Opportunities* (pp. 1–17). Hershey, PA: IGI Global. doi:10.4018/978-1-5225-2694-0.ch001

Patro, C. (2017). Impulsion of Information Technology on Human Resource Practices. In P. Ordóñez de Pablos (Ed.), *Managerial Strategies and Solutions for Business Success in Asia* (pp. 231–254). Hershey, PA: IGI Global. doi:10.4018/978-1-5225-1886-0.ch013

Patro, C. S., & Raghunath, K. M. (2017). Information Technology Paraphernalia for Supply Chain Management Decisions. In M. Tavana (Ed.), *Enterprise Information Systems and the Digitalization of Business Functions* (pp. 294–320). Hershey, PA: IGI Global. doi:10.4018/978-1-5225-2382-6.ch014

Paul, P. K. (2018). The Context of IST for Solid Information Retrieval and Infrastructure Building: Study of Developing Country. *International Journal of Information Retrieval Research*, *8*(1), 86–100. doi:10.4018/IJIRR.2018010106

Paul, P. K., & Chatterjee, D. (2018). iSchools Promoting "Information Science and Technology" (IST) Domain Towards Community, Business, and Society With Contemporary Worldwide Trend and Emerging Potentialities in India. In M. Khosrow-Pour, D.B.A. (Ed.), Encyclopedia of Information Science and Technology, Fourth Edition (pp. 4723-4735). Hershey, PA: IGI Global. https://doi.org/ doi:10.4018/978-1-5225-2255-3.ch410

Pereira, S., Silva, L., Machado, J., & Cabral, A. (2020). The Clinical Informatization in Portugal: An Approach to the National Health Service Certification. *International Journal of Reliable and Quality E-Healthcare*, *9*(2), 34–47. https://doi.org/10.4018/IJRQEH.2020040103

Pessoa, C. R., & Marques, M. E. (2017). Information Technology and Communication Management in Supply Chain Management. In G. Jamil, A. Soares, & C. Pessoa (Eds.), *Handbook of Research on Information Management for Effective Logistics and Supply Chains* (pp. 23–33). Hershey, PA: IGI Global. doi:10.4018/978-1-5225-0973-8.ch002

Phuritsabam, B., & Devi, A. B. (2017). Information Seeking Behavior of Medical Scientists at Jawaharlal Nehru Institute of Medical Science: A Study. In S. Ram (Ed.), *Library and Information Services for Bioinformatics Education and Research* (pp. 177–187). Hershey, PA: IGI Global. doi:10.4018/978-1-5225-1871-6.ch010

Pieczka, B. (2018). Management of Risk and Adverse Events in Medical Entities. In A. Rosiek-Kryszewska & K. Leksowski (Eds.), *Healthcare Administration for Patient Safety and Engagement* (pp. 31–46). Hershey, PA: IGI Global. doi:10.4018/978-1-5225-3946-9.ch003

Pineda, R. G. (2018). Remediating Interaction: Towards a Philosophy of Human-Computer Relationship. In M. Khosrow-Pour (Ed.), *Enhancing Art, Culture, and Design With Technological Integration* (pp. 75–98). Hershey, PA: IGI Global. doi:10.4018/978-1-5225-5023-5.ch004

Poduval, J. (2017). Medical Errors: Impact on Health Care Quality. In M. Riga (Ed.), *Impact of Medical Errors and Malpractice on Health Economics, Quality, and Patient Safety* (pp. 33–60). Hershey, PA: IGI Global. doi:10.4018/978-1-5225-2337-6.ch002

Politis, D., Stagiopoulos, P., Aidona, S., Kyriafinis, G., & Constantinidis, I. (2018). Autonomous Learning and Skill Accreditation: A Paradigm for Medical Studies. In A. Kumar (Ed.), *Optimizing Student Engagement in Online Learning Environments* (pp. 266–296). Hershey, PA: IGI Global. doi:10.4018/978-1-5225-3634-5.ch012

Pomares-Quimbaya, A., González, R. A., Sierra, A., Daza, J. C., Muñoz, O., García, A., ... Bohórquez, W. R. (2017). ICT for Enabling the Quality Evaluation of Health Care Services: A Case Study in a General Hospital. In A. Moumtzoglou (Ed.), *Design, Development, and Integration of Reliable Electronic Healthcare Platforms* (pp. 196–210). Hershey, PA: IGI Global. doi:10.4018/978-1-5225-1724-5.ch012

Ponnuswamy, P., Paul, A. S., & Jose, A. B. (2021). Pre-, Peri-, and Post-Natal Risk Factors in ADHD. In R. Gopalan (Ed.), *New Developments in Diagnosing, Assessing, and Treating ADHD* (pp. 43–54). IGI Global. https://doi.org/10.4018/978-1-7998-5495-1.ch003

Pouliakis, A., Margari, N., Karakitsou, E., Archondakis, S., & Karakitsos, P. (2018). Emerging Technologies Serving Cytopathology: Big Data, the Cloud, and Mobile Computing. In I. El Naqa (Ed.), *Emerging Developments and Practices in Oncology* (pp. 114–152). Hershey, PA: IGI Global. doi:10.4018/978-1-5225-3085-5.ch005

Prabha, V. D., & R., R. (2021). Clinical Decision Support Systems: Decision-Making System for Clinical Data. In G. Rani & P. Tiwari (Eds.), *Handbook of Research on Disease Prediction Through Data Analytics and Machine Learning* (pp. 268-280). IGI Global. https://doi.org/10.4018/978-1-7998-2742-9.ch014

Praveenkumar, P., Santhiyadevi, R., & Amirtharajan, R. (2019). Medical Data Are Safe: An Encrypted Quantum Approach. In B. Singh, B. Saini, D. Singh, & A. Pandey (Eds.), *Medical Data Security for Bioengineers* (pp. 142–165). IGI Global. https://doi.org/10.4018/978-1-5225-7952-6.ch008

Punhani, R., Saini, S., Varun, N., & Rustagi, R. (2021). mHealth: A Resolution in Improving Global Health. In D. Yadav, A. Bansal, M. Bhatia, M. Hooda, & J. Morato (Ed.), *Diagnostic Applications of Health Intelligence and Surveillance Systems* (pp. 86-105). IGI Global. https://doi.org/10.4018/978-1-7998-6527-8.ch004

Pushpa, R., & Siddappa, M. (2021). An Optimal Way of VM Placement Strategy in Cloud Computing Platform Using ABCS Algorithm. *International Journal of Ambient Computing and Intelligence*, *12*(3), 16–38. https://doi.org/10.4018/IJACI.2021070102

Qian, Y. (2017). Computer Simulation in Higher Education: Affordances, Opportunities, and Outcomes. In P. Vu, S. Fredrickson, & C. Moore (Eds.), *Handbook of Research on Innovative Pedagogies and Technologies for Online Learning in Higher Education* (pp. 236–262). Hershey, PA: IGI Global. doi:10.4018/978-1-5225-1851-8.ch011

Quintela, A., & Veiga, A. (2022). An Integrated Approach (Social and Health) in the Elderly With Diabetes: An Increase in Health Literacy. In C. Vaz de Almeida & S. Ramos (Eds.), *Handbook of Research on Assertiveness, Clarity, and Positivity in Health Literacy* (pp. 134–142). IGI Global. https://doi.org/10.4018/978-1-7998-8824-6.ch008

Rahman, N. (2017). Lessons from a Successful Data Warehousing Project Management. *International Journal of Information Technology Project Management*, *8*(4), 30–45. doi:10.4018/IJITPM.2017100103

Rahman, N. (2018). Environmental Sustainability in the Computer Industry for Competitive Advantage. In M. Khosrow-Pour (Ed.), *Green Computing Strategies for Competitive Advantage and Business Sustainability* (pp. 110–130). Hershey, PA: IGI Global. doi:10.4018/978-1-5225-5017-4.ch006

Rai, A., Kothari, R., & Singh, D. P. (2017). Assessment of Available Technologies for Hospital Waste Management: A Need for Society. In R. Singh, A. Singh, & V. Srivastava (Eds.), *Environmental Issues Surrounding Human Overpopulation* (pp. 172–188). Hershey, PA: IGI Global. doi:10.4018/978-1-5225-1683-5.ch010

Rajagopalan, S., Janakiraman, S., & Rengarajan, A. (2019). Medical Image Encryption: Microcontroller and FPGA Perspective. In B. Singh, B. Saini, D. Singh, & A. Pandey (Eds.), *Medical Data Security for Bioengineers* (pp. 278–304). IGI Global. https://doi.org/10.4018/978-1-5225-7952-6.ch014

Rajh, A., & Pavetic, T. (2017). Computer Generated Description as the Required Digital Competence in Archival Profession. *International Journal of Digital Literacy and Digital Competence*, *8*(1), 36–49. doi:10.4018/IJDLDC.2017010103

Ramamoorthy, S., & Sivasubramaniam, R. (2018). Image Processing Including Medical Liver Imaging: Medical Image Processing from Big Data Perspective, Ultrasound Liver Images, Challenges. In M. Lytras & P. Papadopoulou (Eds.), *Applying Big Data Analytics in Bioinformatics and Medicine* (pp. 380–392). Hershey, PA: IGI Global. doi:10.4018/978-1-5225-2607-0.ch016

Raman, A., & Goyal, D. P. (2017). Extending IMPLEMENT Framework for Enterprise Information Systems Implementation to Information System Innovation. In M. Tavana (Ed.), *Enterprise Information Systems and the Digitalization of Business Functions* (pp. 137–177). Hershey, PA: IGI Global. doi:10.4018/978-1-5225-2382-6.ch007

Rao, A. P., & Reddy, K. S. (2021). Automated Soil Residue Levels Detecting Device With IoT Interface. In V. Sathiyamoorthi & A. Elci (Eds.), *Challenges and Applications of Data Analytics in Social Perspectives* (Vol. S, pp. 123–135). IGI Global. https://doi.org/10.4018/978-1-7998-2566-1.ch007

Rao, Y. S., Rauta, A. K., Saini, H., & Panda, T. C. (2017). Mathematical Model for Cyber Attack in Computer Network. *International Journal of Business Data Communications and Networking*, *13*(1), 58–65. doi:10.4018/IJBDCN.2017010105

Rapaport, W. J. (2018). Syntactic Semantics and the Proper Treatment of Computationalism. In M. Danesi (Ed.), *Empirical Research on Semiotics and Visual Rhetoric* (pp. 128–176). Hershey, PA: IGI Global. doi:10.4018/978-1-5225-5622-0.ch007

Rathor, G. P., & Gupta, S. K. (2017). Improving Multimodality Image Fusion through Integrate AFL and Wavelet Transform. In V. Tiwari, B. Tiwari, R. Thakur, & S. Gupta (Eds.), *Pattern and Data Analysis in Healthcare Settings* (pp. 143–157). Hershey, PA: IGI Global. doi:10.4018/978-1-5225-0536-5.ch008

Raut, R., Priyadarshinee, P., & Jha, M. (2017). Understanding the Mediation Effect of Cloud Computing Adoption in Indian Organization: Integrating TAM-TOE- Risk Model. *International Journal of Service Science, Management, Engineering, and Technology*, *8*(3), 40–59. doi:10.4018/IJSSMET.2017070103

Rexhepi, H., & Persson, A. (2017). Challenges to Implementing IT Support for Evidence Based Practice Among Nurses and Assistant Nurses: A Qualitative Study. *Journal of Electronic Commerce in Organizations*, *15*(2), 61–76. doi:10.4018/JECO.2017040105

Rezaie, S., Mirabedini, S. J., & Abtahi, A. (2018). Designing a Model for Implementation of Business Intelligence in the Banking Industry. *International Journal of Enterprise Information Systems*, *14*(1), 77–103. doi:10.4018/IJEIS.2018010105

Rezende, D. A. (2018). Strategic Digital City Projects: Innovative Information and Public Services Offered by Chicago (USA) and Curitiba (Brazil). In M. Lytras, L. Daniela, & A. Visvizi (Eds.), *Enhancing Knowledge Discovery and Innovation in the Digital Era* (pp. 204–223). Hershey, PA: IGI Global. doi:10.4018/978-1-5225-4191-2.ch012

Ribeiro, A. D., Ribeiro, L. P., Silva, C. A., & Magalhães-Ribeiro, L. P. (2021). Patient Safety: The Patient's Perspective From Public Sector Health Institutions in the Algarve Region, Portugal. In P. Eklund (Ed.), *Integrated Care and Fall Prevention in Active and Healthy Aging* (pp. 200–222). IGI Global. https://doi.org/10.4018/978-1-7998-4411-2.ch011

Rodrigues, H., & Brochado, A. (2021). Going for Silver-Senior Consumers' Reviews of Medical Tourism. In A. Borges & P. Rodrigues (Eds.), *New Techniques for Brand Management in the Healthcare Sector* (pp. 64–83). IGI Global. https://doi.org/10.4018/978-1-7998-3034-4.ch005

Rodrigues, J. M., Oliveira, F., Ribeiro, C. P., & Santos, R. C. (2022). Mobile Mental Health for Depression Assistance: Research Directions, Obstacles, Advantages, and Disadvantages of Implementing mHealth. In A. Marques & R. Queirós (Eds.), *Digital Therapies in Psychosocial Rehabilitation and Mental Health* (pp. 21–40). IGI Global. https://doi.org/10.4018/978-1-7998-8634-1.ch002

Rodriguez, A., Rico-Diaz, A. J., Rabuñal, J. R., & Gestal, M. (2017). Fish Tracking with Computer Vision Techniques: An Application to Vertical Slot Fishways. In M. S., & V. V. (Eds.), Multi-Core Computer Vision and Image Processing for Intelligent Applications (pp. 74-104). Hershey, PA: IGI Global. https://doi.org/doi:10.4018/978-1-5225-0889-2.ch003

Romero, J. A. (2018). Sustainable Advantages of Business Value of Information Technology. In M. Khosrow-Pour, D.B.A. (Ed.), Encyclopedia of Information Science and Technology, Fourth Edition (pp. 923-929). Hershey, PA: IGI Global. doi:10.4018/978-1-5225-2255-3.ch079

Romero, J. A. (2018). The Always-On Business Model and Competitive Advantage. In N. Bajgoric (Ed.), *Always-On Enterprise Information Systems for Modern Organizations* (pp. 23–40). Hershey, PA: IGI Global. doi:10.4018/978-1-5225-3704-5.ch002

Ros, M., Weaver, L., & Neuwirth, L. S. (2020). Virtual Reality Stereoscopic 180-Degree Video-Based Immersive Environments: Applications for Training Surgeons and Other Medical Professionals. In J. Stefaniak (Ed.), *Cases on Instructional Design and Performance Outcomes in Medical Education* (pp. 92–119). IGI Global. https://doi.org/10.4018/978-1-7998-5092-2.ch005

Rosen, Y. (2018). Computer Agent Technologies in Collaborative Learning and Assessment. In M. Khosrow-Pour, D.B.A. (Ed.), Encyclopedia of Information Science and Technology, Fourth Edition (pp. 2402-2410). Hershey, PA: IGI Global. doi:10.4018/978-1-5225-2255-3.ch209

Rosiek, A. (2018). The Assessment of Actions of the Environment and the Impact of Preventive Medicine for Public Health in Poland. In A. Rosiek-Kryszewska & K. Leksowski (Eds.), *Healthcare Administration for Patient Safety and Engagement* (pp. 106–119). Hershey, PA: IGI Global. doi:10.4018/978-1-5225-3946-9.ch006

Rosiek, A., & Rosiek-Kryszewska, A. (2018). Managed Healthcare: Doctor Life Satisfaction and Its Impact on the Process of Communicating With the Patient. In A. Rosiek-Kryszewska & K. Leksowski (Eds.), *Healthcare Administration for Patient Safety and Engagement* (pp. 244–261). Hershey, PA: IGI Global. doi:10.4018/978-1-5225-3946-9.ch013

Rosiek-Kryszewska, A., & Rosiek, A. (2018). The Involvement of the Patient and his Perspective Evaluation of the Quality of Healthcare. In A. Rosiek-Kryszewska & K. Leksowski (Eds.), *Healthcare Administration for Patient Safety and Engagement* (pp. 121–144). Hershey, PA: IGI Global. doi:10.4018/978-1-5225-3946-9.ch007

Rosiek-Kryszewska, A., & Rosiek, A. (2018). The Impact of Management and Leadership Roles in Building Competitive Healthcare Units. In A. Rosiek-Kryszewska & K. Leksowski (Eds.), *Healthcare Administration for Patient Safety and Engagement* (pp. 13–30). Hershey, PA: IGI Global. doi:10.4018/978-1-5225-3946-9.ch002

Rouzbehani, K. (2017). Health Policy Implementation: Moving Beyond Its Barriers in United States. In N. Wickramasinghe (Ed.), *Handbook of Research on Healthcare Administration and Management* (pp. 541–552). Hershey, PA: IGI Global. doi:10.4018/978-1-5225-0920-2.ch032

Roy, D. (2018). Success Factors of Adoption of Mobile Applications in Rural India: Effect of Service Characteristics on Conceptual Model. In M. Khosrow-Pour (Ed.), *Green Computing Strategies for Competitive Advantage and Business Sustainability* (pp. 211–238). Hershey, PA: IGI Global. doi:10.4018/978-1-5225-5017-4.ch010

Ruffin, T. R., & Hawkins, D. P. (2018). Trends in Health Care Information Technology and Informatics. In M. Khosrow-Pour, D.B.A. (Ed.), Encyclopedia of Information Science and Technology, Fourth Edition (pp. 3805-3815). Hershey, PA: IGI Global. doi:10.4018/978-1-5225-2255-3.ch330

Sadasivam, U. M., & Ganesan, N. (2021). Detecting Fake News Using Deep Learning and NLP. In S. Misra, C. Arumugam, S. Jaganathan, & S. S. (Eds.), *Confluence of AI, Machine, and Deep Learning in Cyber Forensics* (pp. 117-133). IGI Global. https://doi.org/10.4018/978-1-7998-4900-1.ch007

Safari, M. R., & Jiang, Q. (2018). The Theory and Practice of IT Governance Maturity and Strategies Alignment: Evidence From Banking Industry. *Journal of Global Information Management*, *26*(2), 127–146. doi:10.4018/JGIM.2018040106

Sahin, H. B., & Anagun, S. S. (2018). Educational Computer Games in Math Teaching: A Learning Culture. In E. Toprak & E. Kumtepe (Eds.), *Supporting Multiculturalism in Open and Distance Learning Spaces* (pp. 249–280). Hershey, PA: IGI Global. doi:10.4018/978-1-5225-3076-3.ch013

Sajjad, N., Hassan, S., Qadir, J., Ali, R., & Shah, D. (2020). Analyses of the Recycling Potential of Medical Plastic Wastes. In K. Wani, L. Ariana, & S. Zuber (Eds.), *Handbook of Research on Environmental and Human Health Impacts of Plastic Pollution* (pp. 178–199). IGI Global. https://doi.org/10.4018/978-1-5225-9452-9.ch010

Sakalle, A., Tomar, P., Bhardwaj, H., & Sharma, U. (2021). Impact and Latest Trends of Intelligent Learning With Artificial Intelligence. In S. Verma & P. Tomar (Eds.), *Impact of AI Technologies on Teaching, Learning, and Research in Higher Education* (pp. 172-189). IGI Global. https://doi.org/10.4018/978-1-7998-4763-2.ch011

Sala, N. (2021). Virtual Reality, Augmented Reality, and Mixed Reality in Education: A Brief Overview. In D. Choi, A. Dailey-Hebert, & J. Estes (Eds.), *Current and Prospective Applications of Virtual Reality in Higher Education* (pp. 48–73). IGI Global. https://doi.org/10.4018/978-1-7998-4960-5.ch003

Salunkhe, S., Kanagachidambaresan, G., Rajkumar, C., & Jayanthi, K. (2022). Online Detection and Prediction of Fused Deposition Modelled Parts Using Artificial Intelligence. In S. Salunkhe, H. Hussein, & J. Davim (Eds.), *Applications of Artificial Intelligence in Additive Manufacturing* (pp. 194–209). IGI Global. https://doi.org/10.4018/978-1-7998-8516-0.ch009

Sam, S. (2017). Mobile Phones and Expanding Human Capabilities in Plural Health Systems. In K. Moahi, K. Bwalya, & P. Sebina (Eds.), *Health Information Systems and the Advancement of Medical Practice in Developing Countries* (pp. 93–114). Hershey, PA: IGI Global. doi:10.4018/978-1-5225-2262-1.ch006

Samy, V. S., Pramanick, K., Thenkanidiyoor, V., & Victor, J. (2021). Data Analysis and Visualization in Python for Polar Meteorological Data. *International Journal of Data Analytics*, *2*(1), 32–60. https://doi.org/10.4018/IJDA.2021010102

Sanna, A., & Valpreda, F. (2017). An Assessment of the Impact of a Collaborative Didactic Approach and Students' Background in Teaching Computer Animation. *International Journal of Information and Communication Technology Education*, *13*(4), 1–16. doi:10.4018/IJICTE.2017100101

Santos-Trigo, M., Suaste, E., & Figuerola, P. (2018). Technology Design and Routes for Tool Appropriation in Medical Practices. In M. Khosrow-Pour, D.B.A. (Ed.), Encyclopedia of Information Science and Technology, Fourth Edition (pp. 3794-3804). Hershey, PA: IGI Global. doi:10.4018/978-1-5225-2255-3.ch329

Sarivougioukas, J., & Vagelatos, A. (2022). Fused Contextual Data With Threading Technology to Accelerate Processing in Home UbiHealth. *International Journal of Software Science and Computational Intelligence*, *14*(1), 1–14. https://doi.org/10.4018/IJSSCI.285590

Sarivougioukas, J., Vagelatos, A., Parsopoulos, K. E., & Lagaris, I. E. (2018). Home UbiHealth. In M. Khosrow-Pour, D.B.A. (Ed.), Encyclopedia of Information Science and Technology, Fourth Edition (pp. 7765-7774). Hershey, PA: IGI Global. doi:10.4018/978-1-5225-2255-3.ch675

Sarkar, B. K. (2017). Big Data and Healthcare Data: A Survey. *International Journal of Knowledge-Based Organizations*, *7*(4), 50–77. doi:10.4018/IJKBO.2017100104

Sarkar, K., & Li, B. (2021). Deep Learning for Medical Image Segmentation. In S. Saxena & S. Paul (Eds.), *Deep Learning Applications in Medical Imaging* (pp. 40–77). IGI Global. https://doi.org/10.4018/978-1-7998-5071-7.ch002

Savani, M. M. (2021). Commitment Devices for Health: Theory and Evidence on Weight Loss. In V. Mihaila (Ed.), *Behavioral-Based Interventions for Improving Public Policies* (pp. 35–54). IGI Global. https://doi.org/10.4018/978-1-7998-2731-3.ch003

Saxena, K., & Banodha, U. (2017). An Essence of the SOA on Healthcare. In R. Bhadoria, N. Chaudhari, G. Tomar, & S. Singh (Eds.), *Exploring Enterprise Service Bus in the Service-Oriented Architecture Paradigm* (pp. 283–304). Hershey, PA: IGI Global. doi:10.4018/978-1-5225-2157-0.ch018

Saxena, N. (2020). Considerations for Stakeholders of Medical Tourism: A Comprehensive Examination. In S. Paul & S. Kulshreshtha (Eds.), *Global Developments in Healthcare and Medical Tourism* (pp. 23–37). IGI Global. https://doi.org/10.4018/978-1-5225-9787-2.ch002

Scott, A., Martin, A., & McAlear, F. (2017). Enhancing Participation in Computer Science among Girls of Color: An Examination of a Preparatory AP Computer Science Intervention. In Y. Rankin & J. Thomas (Eds.), *Moving Students of Color from Consumers to Producers of Technology* (pp. 62–84). Hershey, PA: IGI Global. doi:10.4018/978-1-5225-2005-4.ch004

Segura-Azuara, N. D., Guzman-Segura, J. G., Guzmán-Segura, N. M., & Guzmán-Segura, J. P. (2022). Disease Awareness Campaigns: Education for Citizenship in Medical Schools. In M. Lopez (Ed.), *Advancing Health Education With Telemedicine* (pp. 113–122). IGI Global. https://doi.org/10.4018/978-1-7998-8783-6.ch006

Sekaran, P. A. (2022). Smart Medical Kit in Chronic Kidney Disease Management. In D. Jeya Mala (Ed.), *Integrating AI in IoT Analytics on the Cloud for Healthcare Applications* (pp. 24–40). IGI Global. https://doi.org/10.4018/978-1-7998-9132-1.ch002

Sen, K., & Ghosh, K. (2018). Incorporating Global Medical Knowledge to Solve Healthcare Problems: A Framework for a Crowdsourcing System. *International Journal of Healthcare Information Systems and Informatics*, *13*(1), 1–14. doi:10.4018/IJHISI.2018010101

Senanayake, B., Tyagi, N., Zhou, X., & Edirippulige, S. (2020). Workforce Readiness and Digital Health Integration. In K. Sandhu (Ed.), *Opportunities and Challenges in Digital Healthcare Innovation* (pp. 170–185). IGI Global. https://doi.org/10.4018/978-1-7998-3274-4.ch010

Shakdher, A., & Pandey, K. (2017). REDAlert+: Medical/Fire Emergency and Warning System using Android Devices. *International Journal of E-Health and Medical Communications*, *8*(1), 37–51. doi:10.4018/IJEHMC.2017010103

Shanmugam, M., Ibrahim, N., Gorment, N. Z., Sugu, R., Dandarawi, T. N., & Ahmad, N. A. (2022). Towards an Integrated Omni-Channel Strategy Framework for Improved Customer Interaction. In P. Lai (Ed.), *Handbook of Research on Social Impacts of E-Payment and Blockchain Technology* (pp. 409–427). IGI Global. https://doi.org/10.4018/978-1-7998-9035-5.ch022

Sharma, A., & Kumar, S. (2021). Network Slicing and the Role of 5G in IoT Applications. In S. Kumar, M. Trivedi, P. Ranjan, & A. Punhani (Eds.), *Evolution of Software-Defined Networking Foundations for IoT and 5G Mobile Networks* (pp. 172–190). IGI Global. https://doi.org/10.4018/978-1-7998-4685-7.ch010

Shekarian, E., Abdul-Rashid, S. H., & Olugu, E. U. (2017). An Integrated Fuzzy VIKOR Method for Performance Management in Healthcare. In M. Tavana, K. Szabat, & K. Puranam (Eds.), *Organizational Productivity and Performance Measurements Using Predictive Modeling and Analytics* (pp. 40–61). Hershey, PA: IGI Global. doi:10.4018/978-1-5225-0654-6.ch003

Shijina, V., & John, S. J. (2017). Multiple Relations and its Application in Medical Diagnosis. *International Journal of Fuzzy System Applications*, *6*(4), 47–62. doi:10.4018/IJFSA.2017100104

Shipley, N., & Chakraborty, J. (2018). Big Data and mHealth: Increasing the Usability of Healthcare Through the Customization of Pinterest – Literary Perspective. In J. Machado, A. Abelha, M. Santos, & F. Portela (Eds.), *Next-Generation Mobile and Pervasive Healthcare Solutions* (pp. 46–66). Hershey, PA: IGI Global. doi:10.4018/978-1-5225-2851-7.ch004

Shridevi, S., & Saleena, B. (2019). Semantic Technologies for Medical Knowledge Representation. In A. Puratchikody, S. Prabu, & A. Umamaheswari (Eds.), *Computer Applications in Drug Discovery and Development* (Vol. 5, pp. 260–275). IGI Global. https://doi.org/10.4018/978-1-5225-7326-5.ch012

Siddoo, V., & Wongsai, N. (2017). Factors Influencing the Adoption of ISO/IEC 29110 in Thai Government Projects: A Case Study. *International Journal of Information Technologies and Systems Approach*, *10*(1), 22–44. doi:10.4018/IJITSA.2017010102

Silveira, C., Hir, M. E., & Chaves, H. K. (2022). An Approach to Information Management as a Subsidy of Global Health Actions: A Case Study of Big Data in Health for Dengue, Zika, and Chikungunya. In J. Lima de Magalhães, Z. Hartz, G. Jamil, H. Silveira, & L. Jamil (Eds.), *Handbook of Research on Essential Information Approaches to Aiding Global Health in the One Health Context* (pp. 219–234). IGI Global. https://doi.org/10.4018/978-1-7998-8011-0.ch012

Simões, A. (2017). Using Game Frameworks to Teach Computer Programming. In R. Alexandre Peixoto de Queirós & M. Pinto (Eds.), *Gamification-Based E-Learning Strategies for Computer Programming Education* (pp. 221–236). Hershey, PA: IGI Global. doi:10.4018/978-1-5225-1034-5.ch010

Simões de Almeida, R. (2022). Mobile Mental Health: Opportunities and Challenges. In A. Marques & R. Queirós (Eds.), *Digital Therapies in Psychosocial Rehabilitation and Mental Health* (pp. 1–20). IGI Global. https://doi.org/10.4018/978-1-7998-8634-1.ch001

Simões de Almeida, R., & da Silva, T. (2022). AI Chatbots in Mental Health: Are We There Yet? In A. Marques & R. Queirós (Eds.), *Digital Therapies in Psychosocial Rehabilitation and Mental Health* (pp. 226–243). IGI Global. https://doi.org/10.4018/978-1-7998-8634-1.ch011

Simões de Almeida, R., & da Silva, T. P. (2022). AI Chatbots in Mental Health: Are We There Yet? In A. Marques & R. Queirós (Eds.), *Digital Therapies in Psychosocial Rehabilitation and Mental Health* (pp. 226–243). IGI Global. https://doi.org/10.4018/978-1-7998-8634-1.ch011

Singh, A., & Dutta, M. K. (2017). A Reversible Data Hiding Scheme for Efficient Management of Tele-Ophthalmological Data. *International Journal of E-Health and Medical Communications*, *8*(3), 38–54. doi:10.4018/IJEHMC.2017070103

Singh, L. K., Khanna, M., Thawkar, S., & Gopal, J. (2021). Robustness for Authentication of the Human Using Face, Ear, and Gait Multimodal Biometric System. *International Journal of Information System Modeling and Design*, *12*(1), 39–72. https://doi.org/10.4018/IJISMD.2021010103

Skourti, P. K., & Pavlakis, A. (2017). The Second Victim Phenomenon: The Way Out. In M. Riga (Ed.), *Impact of Medical Errors and Malpractice on Health Economics, Quality, and Patient Safety* (pp. 197–222). Hershey, PA: IGI Global. doi:10.4018/978-1-5225-2337-6.ch008

Sllame, A. M. (2017). Integrating LAB Work With Classes in Computer Network Courses. In H. Alphin Jr, R. Chan, & J. Lavine (Eds.), *The Future of Accessibility in International Higher Education* (pp. 253–275). Hershey, PA: IGI Global. doi:10.4018/978-1-5225-2560-8.ch015

Smirnov, A., Ponomarev, A., Shilov, N., Kashevnik, A., & Teslya, N. (2018). Ontology-Based Human-Computer Cloud for Decision Support: Architecture and Applications in Tourism. *International Journal of Embedded and Real-Time Communication Systems*, *9*(1), 1–19. doi:10.4018/IJERTCS.2018010101

Smith, C. R. (2018). Medical Students' Quest Towards the Long White Coat: Impact on Mental Health and Well-Being. In C. Smith (Ed.), *Exploring the Pressures of Medical Education From a Mental Health and Wellness Perspective* (pp. 1–42). Hershey, PA: IGI Global. doi:10.4018/978-1-5225-2811-1.ch001

Smith, S. I., & Dandignac, M. (2018). Perfectionism: Addressing Lofty Expectations in Medical School. In C. Smith (Ed.), *Exploring the Pressures of Medical Education From a Mental Health and Wellness Perspective* (pp. 68–91). Hershey, PA: IGI Global. doi:10.4018/978-1-5225-2811-1.ch003

Smith-Ditizio, A. A., & Smith, A. D. (2018). Computer Fraud Challenges and Its Legal Implications. In M. Khosrow-Pour, D.B.A. (Ed.), Encyclopedia of Information Science and Technology, Fourth Edition (pp. 4837-4848). Hershey, PA: IGI Global. doi:10.4018/978-1-5225-2255-3.ch419

Soczywko, J., & Rutkowska, D. (2018). The Patient/Provider Relationship in Emergency Medicine: Organization, Communication, and Understanding. In A. Rosiek-Kryszewska & K. Leksowski (Eds.), *Healthcare Administration for Patient Safety and Engagement* (pp. 74–105). Hershey, PA: IGI Global. doi:10.4018/978-1-5225-3946-9.ch005

Soni, P. (2018). Implications of HIPAA and Subsequent Regulations on Information Technology. In M. Gupta, R. Sharman, J. Walp, & P. Mulgund (Eds.), *Information Technology Risk Management and Compliance in Modern Organizations* (pp. 71–98). Hershey, PA: IGI Global. doi:10.4018/978-1-5225-2604-9.ch004

Sosnin, P. (2018). Figuratively Semantic Support of Human-Computer Interactions. In *Experience-Based Human-Computer Interactions: Emerging Research and Opportunities* (pp. 244–272). Hershey, PA: IGI Global. doi:10.4018/978-1-5225-2987-3.ch008

Souza, T. de V. I. E. (2020). Certifications for Medical Interpreters: A Comparative Analysis. In I. Souza, & E. Fragkou (Eds.), *Handbook of Research on Medical Interpreting* (pp. 26-53). IGI Global. https://doi.org/10.4018/978-1-5225-9308-9.ch002

Srilakshmi, R., & Jaya Bhaskar, M. (2021). An Adaptable Secure Scheme in Mobile Ad hoc Network to Protect the Communication Channel From Malicious Behaviours. *International Journal of Information Technology and Web Engineering*, *16*(3), 54–73. https://doi.org/10.4018/IJITWE.2021070104

Srivastava, A., & Aggarwal, A. K. (2018). Medical Image Fusion in Spatial and Transform Domain: A Comparative Analysis. In M. Anwar, A. Khosla, & R. Kapoor (Eds.), *Handbook of Research on Advanced Concepts in Real-Time Image and Video Processing* (pp. 281–300). Hershey, PA: IGI Global. doi:10.4018/978-1-5225-2848-7.ch011

Srivastava, S. K., & Roy, S. N. (2018). Recommendation System: A Potential Tool for Achieving Pervasive Health Care. In J. Machado, A. Abelha, M. Santos, & F. Portela (Eds.), *Next-Generation Mobile and Pervasive Healthcare Solutions* (pp. 111–127). Hershey, PA: IGI Global. doi:10.4018/978-1-5225-2851-7.ch008

Stanimirovic, D. (2017). Digitalization of Death Certification Model: Transformation Issues and Implementation Concerns. In S. Saeed, Y. Bamarouf, T. Ramayah, & S. Iqbal (Eds.), *Design Solutions for User-Centric Information Systems* (pp. 22–43). Hershey, PA: IGI Global. doi:10.4018/978-1-5225-1944-7.ch002

Subbaraman, K., Singh, M., & Johar, I. P. (2021). Medical Tourism: History, Global Scenario, and Indian Perspectives. In M. Singh & S. Kumaran (Eds.), *Growth of the Medical Tourism Industry and Its Impact on Society: Emerging Research and Opportunities* (pp. 1–18). IGI Global. https://doi.org/10.4018/978-1-7998-3427-4.ch001

Sukhwani, N., Kagita, V. R., Kumar, V., & Panda, S. K. (2021). Efficient Computation of Top-K Skyline Objects in Data Set With Uncertain Preferences. *International Journal of Data Warehousing and Mining*, *17*(3), 68–80. https://doi.org/10.4018/IJDWM.2021070104

Sukkird, V., & Shirahada, K. (2018). E-Health Service Model for Asian Developing Countries: A Case of Emergency Medical Service for Elderly People in Thailand. In M. Khosrow-Pour (Ed.), *Optimizing Current Practices in E-Services and Mobile Applications* (pp. 214–232). Hershey, PA: IGI Global. doi:10.4018/978-1-5225-5026-6.ch011

Susanto, H., Yie, L. F., Setiana, D., Asih, Y., Yoganingrum, A., Riyanto, S., & Saputra, F. A. (2021). Digital Ecosystem Security Issues for Organizations and Governments: Digital Ethics and Privacy. In Z. Mahmood (Ed.), *Web 2.0 and Cloud Technologies for Implementing Connected Government* (pp. 204–228). IGI Global. https://doi.org/10.4018/978-1-7998-4570-6.ch010

Syväjärvi, A., Leinonen, J., Kivivirta, V., & Kesti, M. (2017). The Latitude of Information Management in Local Government: Views of Local Government Managers. *International Journal of Electronic Government Research*, *13*(1), 69–85. doi:10.4018/IJEGR.2017010105

Talbot, T. B. (2017). Making Lifelike Medical Games in the Age of Virtual Reality: An Update on "Playing Games with Biology" from 2013. In B. Dubbels (Ed.), *Transforming Gaming and Computer Simulation Technologies across Industries* (pp. 103–119). Hershey, PA: IGI Global. doi:10.4018/978-1-5225-1817-4.ch006

Tanque, M., & Foxwell, H. J. (2018). Big Data and Cloud Computing: A Review of Supply Chain Capabilities and Challenges. In A. Prasad (Ed.), *Exploring the Convergence of Big Data and the Internet of Things* (pp. 1–28). Hershey, PA: IGI Global. doi:10.4018/978-1-5225-2947-7.ch001

Tarver, E. (2022). Virtual Simulation: A Flipped Classroom Teaching Tool for Healthcare Education. In L. Coelho, R. Queirós, & S. Reis (Eds.), *Emerging Advancements for Virtual and Augmented Reality in Healthcare* (pp. 65–81). IGI Global. https://doi.org/10.4018/978-1-7998-8371-5.ch005

Teixeira, A., Gomes, A., & Orvalho, J. G. (2017). Auditory Feedback in a Computer Game for Blind People. In T. Issa, P. Kommers, T. Issa, P. Isaías, & T. Issa (Eds.), *Smart Technology Applications in Business Environments* (pp. 134–158). Hershey, PA: IGI Global. doi:10.4018/978-1-5225-2492-2.ch007

Tewari, P., Tiwari, P., & Goel, R. (2022). Information Technology in Supply Chain Management. In V. Garg & R. Goel (Eds.), *Handbook of Research on Innovative Management Using AI in Industry 5.0* (pp. 165–178). IGI Global. https://doi.org/10.4018/978-1-7998-8497-2.ch011

Thompson, N., McGill, T., & Murray, D. (2018). Affect-Sensitive Computer Systems. In M. Khosrow-Pour, D.B.A. (Ed.), Encyclopedia of Information Science and Technology, Fourth Edition (pp. 4124-4135). Hershey, PA: IGI Global. doi:10.4018/978-1-5225-2255-3.ch357

Triberti, S., Brivio, E., & Galimberti, C. (2018). On Social Presence: Theories, Methodologies, and Guidelines for the Innovative Contexts of Computer-Mediated Learning. In M. Marmon (Ed.), *Enhancing Social Presence in Online Learning Environments* (pp. 20–41). Hershey, PA: IGI Global. doi:10.4018/978-1-5225-3229-3.ch002

Tripathi, S., & Musiolik, T. H. (2022). Fairness and Ethics in Artificial Intelligence-Based Medical Imaging. In T. Musiolik & A. Dingli (Eds.), *Ethical Implications of Reshaping Healthcare With Emerging Technologies* (pp. 71–85). IGI Global. https://doi.org/10.4018/978-1-7998-7888-9.ch004

Tripathy, B. K. T. R., S., & Mohanty, R. K. (2018). Memetic Algorithms and Their Applications in Computer Science. In S. Dash, B. Tripathy, & A. Rahman (Eds.), Handbook of Research on Modeling, Analysis, and Application of Nature-Inspired Metaheuristic Algorithms (pp. 73-93). Hershey, PA: IGI Global. https://doi.org/doi:10.4018/978-1-5225-2857-9.ch004

Turcu, C. E., & Turcu, C. O. (2017). Social Internet of Things in Healthcare: From Things to Social Things in Internet of Things. In C. Reis & M. Maximiano (Eds.), *Internet of Things and Advanced Application in Healthcare* (pp. 266–295). Hershey, PA: IGI Global. doi:10.4018/978-1-5225-1820-4.ch010

Turulja, L., & Bajgoric, N. (2017). Human Resource Management IT and Global Economy Perspective: Global Human Resource Information Systems. In M. Khosrow-Pour (Ed.), *Handbook of Research on Technology Adoption, Social Policy, and Global Integration* (pp. 377–394). Hershey, PA: IGI Global. doi:10.4018/978-1-5225-2668-1.ch018

Tutgun Ünal, A., Ekinci, Y., & Tarhan, N. (2022). Health Literacy and Cyberchondria. In H. Aker & M. Aiken (Eds.), *Handbook of Research on Cyberchondria, Health Literacy, and the Role of Media in Society's Perception of Medical Information* (pp. 276–297). IGI Global. https://doi.org/10.4018/978-1-7998-8630-3.ch015

Unwin, D. W., Sanzogni, L., & Sandhu, K. (2017). Developing and Measuring the Business Case for Health Information Technology. In K. Moahi, K. Bwalya, & P. Sebina (Eds.), *Health Information Systems and the Advancement of Medical Practice in Developing Countries* (pp. 262–290). Hershey, PA: IGI Global. doi:10.4018/978-1-5225-2262-1.ch015

Unwin, D. W., Sanzogni, L., & Sandhu, K. (2017). Developing and Measuring the Business Case for Health Information Technology. In K. Moahi, K. Bwalya, & P. Sebina (Eds.), *Health Information Systems and the Advancement of Medical Practice in Developing Countries* (pp. 262–290). Hershey, PA: IGI Global. doi:10.4018/978-1-5225-2262-1.ch015

Usharani, B. (2022). House Plant Leaf Disease Detection and Classification Using Machine Learning. In M. Mundada, S. Seema, S. K.G., & M. Shilpa (Eds.), *Deep Learning Applications for Cyber-Physical Systems* (pp. 17-26). IGI Global. https://doi.org/10.4018/978-1-7998-8161-2.ch002

Ustun, A. B., Yilmaz, R., & Yilmaz, F. G. (2020). Virtual Reality in Medical Education. In S. Umair (Ed.), *Mobile Devices and Smart Gadgets in Medical Sciences* (pp. 56–73). IGI Global. https://doi.org/10.4018/978-1-7998-2521-0.ch004

Vadhanam, B. R. S., M., Sugumaran, V., V., V., & Ramalingam, V. V. (2017). Computer Vision Based Classification on Commercial Videos. In M. S., & V. V. (Eds.), Multi-Core Computer Vision and Image Processing for Intelligent Applications (pp. 105-135). Hershey, PA: IGI Global. https://doi.org/ doi:10.4018/978-1-5225-0889-2.ch004

Vairinho, S. (2022). Innovation Dynamics Through the Encouragement of Knowledge Spin-Off From Touristic Destinations. In C. Ramos, S. Quinteiro, & A. Gonçalves (Eds.), *ICT as Innovator Between Tourism and Culture* (pp. 170–190). IGI Global. https://doi.org/10.4018/978-1-7998-8165-0.ch011

Valverde, R., Torres, B., & Motaghi, H. (2018). A Quantum NeuroIS Data Analytics Architecture for the Usability Evaluation of Learning Management Systems. In S. Bhattacharyya (Ed.), *Quantum-Inspired Intelligent Systems for Multimedia Data Analysis* (pp. 277–299). Hershey, PA: IGI Global. doi:10.4018/978-1-5225-5219-2.ch009

Vamsi, D., & Reddy, P. (2020). Electronic Health Record Security in Cloud: Medical Data Protection Using Homomorphic Encryption Schemes. In C. Chakraborty (Ed.), *Smart Medical Data Sensing and IoT Systems Design in Healthcare* (pp. 22–47). IGI Global. https://doi.org/10.4018/978-1-7998-0261-7.ch002

Vartholomaios, P., Ramdani, N., Christophorou, C., Georgiadis, D., Guilcher, T., Blouin, M., Rebiai, M., Panayides, A. S., Pattichis, C. S., Sarafidis, M., Costarides, V., Vellidou, E., & Koutsouris, D. (2019). ENDORSE Concept: An Integrated Indoor Mobile Robotic System for Medical Diagnostic Support. *International Journal of Reliable and Quality E-Healthcare*, *8*(3), 47–59. https://doi.org/10.4018/IJRQEH.2019070104

Vasant, P. (2018). A General Medical Diagnosis System Formed by Artificial Neural Networks and Swarm Intelligence Techniques. In U. Kose, G. Guraksin, & O. Deperlioglu (Eds.), *Nature-Inspired Intelligent Techniques for Solving Biomedical Engineering Problems* (pp. 130–145). Hershey, PA: IGI Global. doi:10.4018/978-1-5225-4769-3.ch006

Vassilis, E. (2018). Learning and Teaching Methodology: "1:1 Educational Computing. In K. Koutsopoulos, K. Doukas, & Y. Kotsanis (Eds.), *Handbook of Research on Educational Design and Cloud Computing in Modern Classroom Settings* (pp. 122–155). Hershey, PA: IGI Global. doi:10.4018/978-1-5225-3053-4.ch007

Vaz de Almeida, C. (2022). ACP Model-Assertiveness, Clarity, and Positivity: A Communication and Health Literacy Model for Health Professionals. In C. Vaz de Almeida & S. Ramos (Eds.), *Handbook of Research on Assertiveness, Clarity, and Positivity in Health Literacy* (pp. 1–22). IGI Global. https://doi.org/10.4018/978-1-7998-8824-6.ch001

Verma, K. (2022). Modeling Digital Healthcare Services Using NLP and IoT in Smart Cities. In J. Thomas, V. Geropanta, A. Karagianni, V. Panchenko, & P. Vasant (Eds.), *Smart Cities and Machine Learning in Urban Health* (pp. 138–155). IGI Global. https://doi.org/10.4018/978-1-7998-7176-7.ch007

Verma, S., & Jain, A. K. (2022). A Survey on Sentiment Analysis Techniques for Twitter. In B. Gupta, D. Peraković, A. Abd El-Latif, & D. Gupta (Eds.), *Data Mining Approaches for Big Data and Sentiment Analysis in Social Media* (pp. 57–90). IGI Global. https://doi.org/10.4018/978-1-7998-8413-2.ch003

Viswanathan, J., Saranya, N., & Inbamani, A. (2021). Deep Learning Applications in Medical Imaging: Introduction to Deep Learning-Based Intelligent Systems for Medical Applications. In S. Saxena & S. Paul (Eds.), *Deep Learning Applications in Medical Imaging* (pp. 156–177). IGI Global. https://doi.org/10.4018/978-1-7998-5071-7.ch007

Wang, H., Huang, P., & Chen, X. (2021). Research and Application of a Multidimensional Association Rules Mining Method Based on OLAP. *International Journal of Information Technology and Web Engineering*, *16*(1), 75–94. https://doi.org/10.4018/IJITWE.2021010104

Wang, X., Su, K., & Su, L. (2019). Research on Improved Apriori Algorithm Based on Data Mining in Electronic Cases. *International Journal of Healthcare Information Systems and Informatics*, *14*(3), 16–28. https://doi.org/10.4018/IJHISI.2019070102

Wexler, B. E. (2017). Computer-Presented and Physical Brain-Training Exercises for School Children: Improving Executive Functions and Learning. In B. Dubbels (Ed.), *Transforming Gaming and Computer Simulation Technologies across Industries* (pp. 206–224). Hershey, PA: IGI Global. doi:10.4018/978-1-5225-1817-4.ch012

Wickramasinghe, N. (2020). Minority Health and Wellness: A Digital Health Opportunity. In N. Wickramasinghe (Ed.), *Handbook of Research on Optimizing Healthcare Management Techniques* (pp. 116–126). IGI Global. https://doi.org/10.4018/978-1-7998-1371-2.ch008

Wickramasinghe, N., Geholt, V., Sloane, E., Smart, P. J., & Schaffer, J. L. (2021). Using Health 4.0 to Enable Post-Operative Wellness Monitoring: The Case of Colorectal Surgery. In N. Wickramasinghe (Ed.), *Optimizing Health Monitoring Systems With Wireless Technology* (pp. 233–247). IGI Global. https://doi.org/10.4018/978-1-5225-6067-8.ch016

Wilcox, S., Huzo, O., Minhas, A., Walters, N., Adada, J. E., Pennington, M., Roseme, L., Mohammed, D., Dusic, A., & Zeine, R. (2022). The Impact of Medical or Health-Related Internet Searches on Patient Compliance: The Dr. Net Study. In H. Aker & M. Aiken (Eds.), *Handbook of Research on Cyberchondria, Health Literacy, and the Role of Media in Society's Perception of Medical Information* (pp. 72–97). IGI Global. https://doi.org/10.4018/978-1-7998-8630-3.ch005

Wimble, M., Singh, H., & Phillips, B. (2018). Understanding Cross-Level Interactions of Firm-Level Information Technology and Industry Environment: A Multilevel Model of Business Value. *Information Resources Management Journal, 31*(1), 1–20. doi:10.4018/IRMJ.2018010101

Wimmer, H., Powell, L., Kilgus, L., & Force, C. (2017). Improving Course Assessment via Web-based Homework. *International Journal of Online Pedagogy and Course Design, 7*(2), 1–19. doi:10.4018/IJOPCD.2017040101

Witzke, K., & Specht, O. (2017). M-Health Telemedicine and Telepresence in Oral and Maxillofacial Surgery: An Innovative Prehospital Healthcare Concept in Structurally Weak Areas. *International Journal of Reliable and Quality E-Healthcare, 6*(4), 37–48. doi:10.4018/IJRQEH.2017100105

Wong, A. K., & Lo, M. F. (2018). Using Pervasive Computing for Sustainable Healthcare in an Aging Population. In B. Fong, A. Ng, & P. Yuen (Eds.), *Sustainable Health and Long-Term Care Solutions for an Aging Population* (pp. 187–202). Hershey, PA: IGI Global. doi:10.4018/978-1-5225-2633-9.ch010

Wong, S. (2021). Gendering Information and Communication Technologies in Climate Change. In M. Khosrow-Pour D.B.A. (Eds.), *Encyclopedia of Information Science and Technology, Fifth Edition* (pp. 1408-1422). IGI Global. https://doi.org/10.4018/978-1-7998-3479-3.ch096

Wong, Y. L., & Siu, K. W. (2018). Assessing Computer-Aided Design Skills. In M. Khosrow-Pour, D.B.A. (Ed.), Encyclopedia of Information Science and Technology, Fourth Edition (pp. 7382-7391). Hershey, PA: IGI Global. doi:10.4018/978-1-5225-2255-3.ch642

Wongsurawat, W., & Shrestha, V. (2018). Information Technology, Globalization, and Local Conditions: Implications for Entrepreneurs in Southeast Asia. In P. Ordóñez de Pablos (Ed.), *Management Strategies and Technology Fluidity in the Asian Business Sector* (pp. 163–176). Hershey, PA: IGI Global. doi:10.4018/978-1-5225-4056-4.ch010

Wu, W., Martin, B. C., & Ni, C. (2017). A Systematic Review of Competency-Based Education Effort in the Health Professions: Seeking Order Out of Chaos. In K. Rasmussen, P. Northrup, & R. Colson (Eds.), *Handbook of Research on Competency-Based Education in University Settings* (pp. 352–378). Hershey, PA: IGI Global. doi:10.4018/978-1-5225-0932-5.ch018

Yadav, S., Ekbal, A., Saha, S., Pathak, P. S., & Bhattacharyya, P. (2017). Patient Data De-Identification: A Conditional Random-Field-Based Supervised Approach. In S. Saha, A. Mandal, A. Narasimhamurthy, S. V, & S. Sangam (Eds.), Handbook of Research on Applied Cybernetics and Systems Science (pp. 234-253). Hershey, PA: IGI Global. doi:10.4018/978-1-5225-2498-4.ch011

Yamada, H. (2021). Homogenization of Japanese Industrial Technology From the Perspective of R&D Expenses. *International Journal of Systems and Service-Oriented Engineering, 11*(2), 24–51. doi:10.4018/IJSSOE.2021070102

Yang, Y., Zhu, X., Jin, C., & Li, J. J. (2018). Reforming Classroom Education Through a QQ Group: A Pilot Experiment at a Primary School in Shanghai. In H. Spires (Ed.), *Digital Transformation and Innovation in Chinese Education* (pp. 211–231). Hershey, PA: IGI Global. doi:10.4018/978-1-5225-2924-8.ch012

Yilmaz, R., Sezgin, A., Kurnaz, S., & Arslan, Y. Z. (2018). Object-Oriented Programming in Computer Science. In M. Khosrow-Pour, D.B.A. (Ed.), Encyclopedia of Information Science and Technology, Fourth Edition (pp. 7470-7480). Hershey, PA: IGI Global. doi:10.4018/978-1-5225-2255-3.ch650

Yu, B., Wijesekera, D., & Costa, P. C. (2017). Informed Consent in Healthcare: A Study Case of Genetic Services. In A. Moumtzoglou (Ed.), *Design, Development, and Integration of Reliable Electronic Healthcare Platforms* (pp. 211–242). Hershey, PA: IGI Global. doi:10.4018/978-1-5225-1724-5.ch013

Yu, B., Wijesekera, D., & Costa, P. C. (2017). Informed Consent in Electronic Medical Record Systems. In I. Management Association (Ed.), Healthcare Ethics and Training: Concepts, Methodologies, Tools, and Applications (pp. 1029-1049). Hershey, PA: IGI Global. doi:10.4018/978-1-5225-2237-9.ch049

Yu, L. (2018). From Teaching Software Engineering Locally and Globally to Devising an Internationalized Computer Science Curriculum. In S. Dikli, B. Etheridge, & R. Rawls (Eds.), *Curriculum Internationalization and the Future of Education* (pp. 293–320). Hershey, PA: IGI Global. doi:10.4018/978-1-5225-2791-6.ch016

Yu, M., Li, J., & Wang, W. (2017). Creative Life Experience among Students in Medical Education. In C. Zhou (Ed.), *Handbook of Research on Creative Problem-Solving Skill Development in Higher Education* (pp. 158–184). Hershey, PA: IGI Global. doi:10.4018/978-1-5225-0643-0.ch008

Yuhua, F. (2018). Computer Information Library Clusters. In M. Khosrow-Pour, D.B.A. (Ed.), Encyclopedia of Information Science and Technology, Fourth Edition (pp. 4399-4403). Hershey, PA: IGI Global. doi:10.4018/978-1-5225-2255-3.ch382

Zakaria, R. B., Zainuddin, M. N., & Mohamad, A. H. (2022). Distilling Blockchain: Complexity, Barriers, and Opportunities. In P. Lai (Ed.), *Handbook of Research on Social Impacts of E-Payment and Blockchain Technology* (pp. 89–114). IGI Global. https://doi.org/10.4018/978-1-7998-9035-5.ch007

Zanetti, C. A., George, A., Stiegmann, R. A., & Phelan, D. (2020). Digital Health. In R. Gotian, Y. Kang, & J. Safdieh (Eds.), *Handbook of Research on the Efficacy of Training Programs and Systems in Medical Education* (pp. 404–426). IGI Global. https://doi.org/10.4018/978-1-7998-1468-9.ch021

Zangão, M. O. (2020). Self-Perceived Health Status. In C. Fonseca, M. Lopes, D. Mendes, F. Mendes, & J. García-Alonso (Eds.), *Handbook of Research on Health Systems and Organizations for an Aging Society* (pp. 1–11). IGI Global. doi:10.4018/978-1-5225-9818-3.ch001

Zarour, K. (2017). Towards a Telehomecare in Algeria: Case of Diabetes Measurement and Remote Monitoring. *International Journal of E-Health and Medical Communications*, *8*(4), 61–80. doi:10.4018/IJEHMC.2017100104

Zavyalova, Y. V., Korzun, D. G., Meigal, A. Y., & Borodin, A. V. (2017). Towards the Development of Smart Spaces-Based Socio-Cyber-Medicine Systems. *International Journal of Embedded and Real-Time Communication Systems*, *8*(1), 45–63. doi:10.4018/IJERTCS.2017010104

Zeinali, A. A. (2018). Word Formation Study in Developing Naming Guidelines in the Translation of English Medical Terms Into Persian. In M. Khosrow-Pour, D.B.A. (Ed.), Encyclopedia of Information Science and Technology, Fourth Edition (pp. 5136-5147). Hershey, PA: IGI Global. doi:10.4018/978-1-5225-2255-3.ch446

Zhang, Z., Ma, J., & Cui, X. (2021). Genetic Algorithm With Three-Dimensional Population Dominance Strategy for University Course Timetabling Problem. *International Journal of Grid and High Performance Computing*, *13*(2), 56–69. https://doi.org/10.4018/IJGHPC.2021040104

Zineldin, M., & Vasicheva, V. (2018). Reducing Medical Errors and Increasing Patient Safety: TRM and 5 Q's Approaches for Better Quality of Life. In *Technological Tools for Value-Based Sustainable Relationships in Health: Emerging Research and Opportunities* (pp. 87–115). Hershey, PA: IGI Global. doi:10.4018/978-1-5225-4091-5.ch005

About the Contributors

* * *

Devipriya A. is currently working as an Assistant Professor in the Department of Computing Technologies, SRM Institute of Science and Technology, Kattankulathur. She has received Ph.D degree in Information and Communication Engineering from Anna University, Chennai. She is having more than 17 years of experience in Teaching. She has completed AI & ML 6 months Course in Xebia Academy, Delhi and Design Thinking Course in Taylor's University. Her areas of interest is Artificial Intelligence, Machine Learning, Deep Learning, Data Analytics, and Internet of Things.She has published more than 20 papers in various reputed Journals that includes 4 SCI Indexed and 12 Scopus Indexed Journals. She has published 2 books and 2 book chapters and 4 Patent including Springer, Taylor & Francis and presented more than 10 papers in both national and International Conferences. She is acting as a Reviewer of SCI Indexed Journals on "Wireless Personal Communications" and "IET Networks". She has been the Incharge of Machine Learning Special Lab. She has given a Guest Lecturer in various subjects such as Machine Learning, Artificial Intelligence and Deep Learning in Premier Institutions. She has also given an Invited Talk in AICTE Sponsored FDP on Deep Learning and its Applications and NITTTR sponsored FDP on An Enterprise perspective on Blockchain Technology. She has acted as a jury in a National level project contest, Symposium and Various International Conferences. She has been awarded as Excellence in Leadership Award in the year 2014-2015 in SriGuru Institute of Technology and also awarded as a best faculty in the year 2018-2019 in Sri Krishna College of Engineering and Technology, Coimbatore, Tamilnadu. She has acted as a mentor in Hackathon conducted by Xebia Academy. She has been recognized as an evaluator for the Toycathon 2021 organized by MHRD. She is also an active member in ISTE, ACM.

Atul Kumar Agnihotri received his B.Tech. and M. Tech. degree in the field of Electronics Instrumentation & Control from U.P.Technical University (UPTU), Lucknow in 2006 and 2014 respectively. His area of interest is Signal Processing & Wireless sensor network.

N. Noor Alleema, Professor, Department of Computer Science and Engineering working at Saveetha School of Engineering, Saveetha Institute of Medical and Technical Science(SIMATS), Chennai, obtained her Bachelor Degree in Computer Science from Madras University, Chennai in 2004, Master degree in the Department of Computer Science and engineering from Anna University, Chennai in 2006 and Ph.D. Degree in the Department of Computer Science from Sathyabama Institute of Science and Technology in 2021. Having more than 15 years of Teaching Experience and specialized in the various Domains like IOT, Mobile Ad Hoc networks (MANETs). She has published more number of conference papers and journal articles on a range of research areas such as Mobile Ad-hoc Networks, IOT and Networking.

C. V. Suresh Babu is a pioneer in content development. A true entrepreneur, he founded Anniyappa Publications, a company that is highly active in publishing books related to Computer Science and Management. Dr. C.V. Suresh Babu has also ventured into SB Institute, a center for knowledge transfer. He holds a Ph.D. in Engineering Education from the National Institute of Technical Teachers Training & Research in Chennai, along with seven master's degrees in various disciplines such as Engineering, Computer Applications, Management, Commerce, Economics, Psychology, Law, and Education. Additionally, he has UGC-NET/SET qualifications in the fields of Computer Science, Management, Commerce, and Education. Currently, Dr. C.V. Suresh Babu is a Professor in the Department of Information Technology at the School of Computing Science, Hindustan Institute of Technology and Science (Hindustan University) in Padur, Chennai, Tamil Nadu, India. For more information, you can visit his personal blog at .

Mhesh Chitraivel completed his B.E (EEE) from Madras University in the year 1998, M.E (CSE) from Anna University in the year 2006, and Ph.D in the field of Artificial Intelligence from Veltech University in the year 2016. He is having 24 years of experience in teaching experience at various levels and his research interest includes Data Science, Data Security and Block chain technology.

Amar Choudhary is a highly accomplished professional with expertise in Analog and Digital Communication, Wireless Communication, Analog & Digital Electronics, and Technicalities of 5G/6G. He earned his Ph.D. from Amity University, Noida, Uttar Pradesh, with his research focusing on "Analysis & Optimization of Solar Radiation Estimation Models." He holds a Master's degree (M. Tech.) and a Bachelor's degree (B. Tech.) in Electronics & Telecommunication Engineering from Biju Patnaik University of Technology, Rourkela, Odisha. With over nine years of experience in Teaching, Industry, and Research, Dr. Choudhary has made significant contributions to his field. He is a bonafide member of the Institute of Electrical and Electronics Engineers (IEEE) and actively participates in its valuable societies such as IEEE Intelligent Transportation Systems Society, IEEE Vehicular Technology Society, and IEEE Council on Electronic Design Automation. Additionally, he serves as an EXECOM Member of IEEE Vehicular Technology Society. Dr. Choudhary's influence extends to the academic publishing world, where he holds the prestigious position of Chief Editor (India) for the INTERNATIONAL JOURNAL OF INVENTIONS IN ELECTRONICS & ELECTRICAL ENGINEERING. He also serves as a reviewer for several other Scopus & WoS Indexed Journals. Furthermore, Dr. Choudhary has vast experience in obtaining Extension of Approval (EOA) from the All India Council for Technical Education, New Delhi, showcasing his commitment to maintaining the highest educational standards.

Vinod D. has around 18 years of experience in teaching and research in various Institutes under the department of Computer Science and Engineering. Completed his Ph.D. in the Domain of Information Security in the year 2018, with highly commendable reviews at Sathyabama Institute of Science and Technology. Completed his Masters of Engineering, in the department of Computer Science and Engineering at GKM Engineering College, Anna University in 2009. Completed the Bachelor of Technology in Information Technology in Adhiyamaan Engineering College, Anna University. He is currently acting as Scientific Advisor in Ja-Assure Singapore. He has published around 3 Science indexed and 30 Scopus Indexed Journals and more than 25 International Conference presentations across prestigious Universities of India and other Countries. Has an h-index of 3, Reviewer for 6 Scopus indexed journals, and 3 Science indexed journal. Presently working as Assistant Professor in Department of Computing Technologies, School of Computing, College of Engineering and Technology, SRM Institute of Science and Technology, SRM Nagar, Kattankulathur, Chennai, TN, India.

Anand Kumar Dohare, Ph. D. (CSE), M. Tech. (CSE), is presently working as an Assistant Professor in the Information Technology Department at Greater Noida Institute of Technology (Engineering Institute), Greater Noida. India. He has Intellectual acumen with 15 years of teaching experience. He published Various Patent and Research Papers in National and International Indexed Journals. He also participated and organized Various seminars/ Workshops/ Conferences. He is an active member of various academic and technical committees.

Sunil Kadyan is working as an Associate Professor in School of Management & Commerce Manav Rachna University Faridabad Haryana. He is a Bachelor of Ayurved, Medicine and Surgery (BAMS) Doctor from MDU Rohtak. He completed his MBA (Insurance) and PhD (Management- Insurance) from Amity University. He is a Fellow from Insurance Institute of India, Mumbai. He has also completed Specialized Diploma in Health Insurance and Diploma in Life Insurance underwriting from III, Mumbai. He has cleared UGC NET in Management. He also did Insurance Professional Certifications from LOMA USA and CII London. His area of specialization is General Management, Marketing and Insurance. He is also a Resource Person for Audio/Video programmes for NIOS learners; LIVE PCP Programmes; Standardization of Marking Scheme; Preparation of learning material, at NIOS for Insurance domain. He has presented various Research Papers in National as well as International Conferences and Seminars in the areas of Insurance and General Management. Author of multiple publications in reputed SCOPUS, ABDC Category B Journals UGC Care journals. He is an Author of a Book "Marketing of Financial Products and Services."

Rakesh Kancharla, M. Tech (CSE), Ph.D., is presently working as an Assistant Professor in the Computer Science and Engineering Department at SASI Institute of Technology & Engineering, Tadepalligudem, Andhra Pradesh, India. He has taught for eleven years and possesses technical acuity. He published Various Research Papers in National and International Indexed Journals. He also participated and organized Various seminars/Workshops/ Conferences. He is an active member of various academic and technical committees.

Rita Komalasari is a lecturer at YARSI University. Her current work is focused on Safeguarding the Future: Cutting-Edge Time-Stamping Services and Blockchain Technologies for Maintaining EHR Data Integrity Over the Long Term.

Rakshit Kothari is a research scholar in the Department of Computer Science and Engineering at College of Technology and Engineering, Maharana Pratap University of Agriculture and Technology, Udaipur, Rajasthan, India. He has done B.Tech in Computer Science and Engineering at Rajasthan Technical University, Kota with first division honours. He secured Master of Technology in Computer Science and Engineering at College of Technology and Engineering, Maharana Pratap University of Agriculture and Technology, Udaipur, Rajasthan, India under the guidance of Dr. Naveen Choudhary, Professor and Head, CTAE, MPUAT. He has teaching experience for more than 2 years and IT industry experience of 1 year. He has presented number of papers in National and International Journals, Conference and Symposiums He is currently a member in Soft Computing Research Society. His main area of interest include the Internet of Things, Cryptography and Blockchain.

Sresh Anand M. is presently working as an Assistant Professor at Department of Computing Technology, in SRM Institute of Science and Technology, Kattankulathur. He has completed his Bachelor of Engineering in Computer Science and Engineering from Arunai Engineering College affiliated to Anna University, Chennai, Tamilnadu in the year 2002. He pursued his Master of Technology in Remote Sensing from College of Engineering Guindy, Anna University, Chennai, Tamilnadu in the year 2007. He achieved the Doctor of Philosophy in Information and Communication Engineering from Anna University, Chennai, Tamilnadu in the year 2018. He had published more than 50 papers in UGC approved, Scopus indexed journals and conferences. He had file 13 Indian patent which under in examination stage, Granted three Indian design patent and one Australian patent. He published four paper books. He is having 18 years of experience in teaching. His areas of interest are Image Processing, Computer Vision, Machine Learning, Human Computer Interaction and Deep Learning. He is a member in ISTE, ACM, IEEE and CSI.

G Padmapriya is currently working as Assistant Professor in Department of Computing Technologies, School of Computing, SRM Institute of Science and Technology, Kattankulathur, Chennai. She pursued Masters in Computer Science and Engineering in K.S. Rangasamy College of Technology affiliated to Anna University – Chennai between 2006 to 2008, With a strong desire in research and development she pursued and completed her Doctor of Philosophy in Information and Communication Engineering from Anna University – Chennai in the year 2016. She has more than 15 years of teaching experience in reputed engineering colleges and specialized in Data Mining, Data Analytics, Machine Learning, Soft Computing, Natural Language Language Processing, Quantum Computing but not limited to. She has produced remarkable academic achievements in all the subjects handled in undergraduate and postgraduate. She has published various research papers in reputed international journals, conferences and book chapters. She has active membership in Indian Society for Technical Education [ISTE], Computer Science Teachers Association [CSTA], International Association of Engineers [IAENG], Universal Association of Computer and Electronics Engineers [UACEE]. She is also serving as the Editorial member and reviewer of ASDF International.

Sddhi Rajan has twenty eight years of work experience in academics, industry & research institutions. The area of research of Ph.D work is in Spatial Data Mining. Undergone two months of specialized training on Spatial Data Analysis & GIS, sponsored by IIRS-NNRMS (Ministry of Space, GOI) at IIRS, Dehradun (2013). Was nominated as an invited researcher to work on algorithm development for data mining on a DST sponsored project at ICMR, New Delhi(2009). Was given a grant from AICTE to present a research paper, related to the ICMR-DST sponsored project on Data Mining, at Dalian University of Technology, Dalian, China. Published book on Object Oriented Concepts & programming using C++ (Global Vision Publication). Life time member of Indian Society of Remote Sensing. (ISRS).

Ygita Sharma is currently Professor with School of Management and Commerce at Manav Rachna University, India. She is also handling Entrepreneurship, Incubation and Start-up. She has 15 years plus of academic experience, 10 years of Industry experience. She had also managed her own start-up in publication Industry. She is associated as mentor with National Institute of Entrepreneurship and Small Business Development (NIESBUD) for the Program Udyam Disha to handhold and Guide aspiring and existing Entrepreneurs from remote locations. She is certified as Entrepreneurship Trained Faculty of Entrepreneurship from DST & NEN (National Entrepreneurship Network) with Honors and also certified by NIESBUD for completing Accreditation Program on Entrepreneurial Motivation Trainers. She has been recipient of grants for Entrepreneurship, Employability from Rajeev Gandhi Institute for Youth Development, Government of India; AICTE and NIESBUD, Ministry of MSME. She has been a resource person for online portal SWAYAM in areas of Marketing and Entrepreneurship. She has been a recipient of various awards for entrepreneurship, mentorship and academics at prestigious platforms.

Vshal Upmanu is having Eighteen years of Academic Experience including 4+ years of administrative post. Currently he is working as an Professor in Data science Department in Meerut institute of technology, Meerut. His Ph.D. is in the field of Data Science. He is IBM certified expert in data visualization tools. He is certified Data Analyst having 02 Patent (1Published, 1 Grant).

U. Vignesh is currently an Assistant Professor Senior Grade 2 in School of Computer Science and Engineering, Vellore Institute of Technology (VIT) - Chennai. Prior to his recent appointment at the VIT, he was a Post-Doctoral Fellow in National Institute of Technology (NIT), Trichy – India. Dr. Vignesh received his undergraduate degree in B.Tech (IT) as well as his M.Tech (IT) degree from Anna University - Chennai, and his PhD in Computer Science and Engineering from VIT University - Chennai. Dr. Vignesh published several papers in preferred Journals, patents and chapters in books, and participated in a range of forums on computer science, social science, etc. He also presented various academic as well as research-based papers at several national and international conferences. His research activities are currently twofold: while the first research activity is set to explore the developmental role that society needs with technology such as, Artificial Intelligence; the second major research theme that he is pursuing is focused on the bioinformatics and data mining.

Index

www.ingramcontent.com/pod-product-compliance
Lightning Source LLC
LaVergne TN
LVHW060002031026
849161LV00025B/1248